Ischemic Stroke

Editor

LOTFI HACEIN-BEY

NEUROIMAGING CLINICS OF NORTH AMERICA

www.neuroimaging.theclinics.com

Consulting Editor
SURESH K. MUKHERJI

November 2018 • Volume 28 • Number 4

ELSEVIER

1600 John F. Kennedy Boulevard • Suite 1800 • Philadelphia, Pennsylvania, 19103-2899

http://www.neuroimaging.theclinics.com

NEUROIMAGING CLINICS OF NORTH AMERICA Volume 28, Number 4
November 2018 ISSN 1052-5149, ISBN 13: 978-0-323-64157-9

Editor: John Vassallo (j.vassallo@elsevier.com)
Developmental Editor: Casey Potter

Neuroimaging Clinics of North America (ISSN 1052-5149) is published quarterly by Elsevier Inc., 360 Park Avenue South, New York, NY 10010-1710. Months of issue are February, May, August, and November. Business and editorial offices: 1600 John F. Kennedy Blvd., Suite 1800, Philadelphia, PA 19103-2899. Business and editorial offices: 6277 Sea Harbor Drive, Orlando, FL 32887-4800. Periodicals postage paid at New York, NY, and additional mailing offices. Subscription prices are USD 387 per year for US individuals, USD 622 per year for US institutions, USD 100 per year for US students and residents, USD 440 per year for Canadian individuals, USD 791 per year for Canadian institutions, USD 525 per year for international individuals, USD 791 per year for international institutions and USD 260 per year for Canadian and foreign students and residents. To receive student/resident rate, orders must be accompanied by name of affiliated institution, date of term, and the *signature* of program/residency coordinator on institution letterhead. Orders will be billed at individual rate until proof of status is received. Foreign air speed delivery is included in all *Clinics* subscription prices. All prices are subject to change without notice. POSTMASTER: Send address changes to *Neuroimaging Clinics of North America*, Elsevier Health Sciences Division, Subscription **Customer Service, 3251 Riverport Lane, Maryland Heights, MO 63043. Telephone: 1-800-654-2452 (U.S. and Canada); 314-447-8871 (outside U.S. and Canada). Fax: 314-447-8029. E-mail: journalscustomer service-usa@elsevier.com (for print support); journalsonlinesupport-usa@elsevier.com (for online support).**

Reprints. For copies of 100 or more of articles in this publication, please contact the Commercial Reprints Department, Elsevier Inc., 360 Park Avenue South, New York, NY 10010-1710. Tel.: 212-633-3874; Fax: 212-633-3820; E-mail: reprints@elsevier.com.

Neuroimaging Clinics of North America is covered by *Excerpta Medical/EMBASE,* the RSNA Index of Imaging Literature, *MEDLINE/PubMed (Index Medicus),* MEDLINE/MEDLARS, SciSearch, Research Alert, and Neuroscience Citation Index.

PROGRAM OBJECTIVE

The goal of *Neuroimaging Clinics of North America* is to keep practicing radiologists and radiology residents up to date with current clinical practice in radiology by providing timely articles reviewing the state of the art in patient care.

TARGET AUDIENCE

Practicing radiologists, radiology residents, and other healthcare professionals who utilize neuroimaging findings to provide patient care.

LEARNING OBJECTIVES

Upon completion of this activity, participants will be able to:

1. Review current role of multimodal computed tomography (CT, CTA, and PCT) in the evaluation of patients with acute ischemic stroke.
2. Discuss recent advances in endovascular stroke therapy.
3. Recognize challenges in diagnosis of acute ischemic stroke and methods for improvement.

ACCREDITATION

The Elsevier Office of Continuing Medical Education (EOCME) is accredited by the Accreditation Council for Continuing Medical Education (ACCME) to provide continuing medical education for physicians.

The EOCME designates this enduring material for a maximum of 15 *AMA PRA Category 1 Credit*(s)™. Physicians should claim only the credit commensurate with the extent of their participation in the activity.

All other healthcare professionals requesting continuing education credit for this enduring material will be issued a certificate of participation.

DISCLOSURE OF CONFLICTS OF INTEREST

The EOCME assesses conflict of interest with its instructors, faculty, planners, and other individuals who are in a position to control the content of CME activities. All relevant conflicts of interest that are identified are thoroughly vetted by EOCME for fair balance, scientific objectivity, and patient care recommendations. EOCME is committed to providing its learners with CME activities that promote improvements or quality in healthcare and not a specific proprietary business or a commercial interest.

The planning committee, staff, authors and editors listed below have identified no financial relationships or relationships to products or devices they or their spouse/life partner have with commercial interest related to the content of this CME activity:

Jerome Berge, MD; José Biller, MD, FAAN, FACP, FAHA; Martin Bretzner, MD; Simon F. De Meyer, PhD; R. Gilberto González, MD, PhD; Lotfi Hacein-Bey, MD; Andreas Hartmann, MD; Jeremy J. Heit, MD, PhD; Shannon Hextrum, MD; Joshua A. Hirsch, MD, FACR, FSIR, FSNIS; Bin Jiang, MD, PhD; Angelos M. Katramados, MD; Alison Kemp; Angelos A. Konstas, MD; Gregory Kuchcinski, MD; Pradeep Kuttysankaran; Xavier Leclerc, MD, PhD; Carlos Leiva-Salinas, MD, PhD; Thabele M. Leslie-Mazwi, MD; Jay P. Mohr, MD; Suresh K. Mukherji, MD, MBA, FACR; Govind Mukundan, MD; Jean-Pierre Pruvo, MD, PhD; Pamela W. Schaefer, MD; David J. Seidenwurm, MD; Nina J. Solenski, MD, FAHA; E. Turgut Tali, MD; John Vassallo; Max Wintermark, MD, MPH, MBA; Lei Wu, MD; Wei Wu, MD; William T. Yuh, MD, MSEE; Greg Zaharchuk, MD, PhD.

The planning committee, staff, authors and editors listed below have identified financial relationships or relationships to products or devices they or their spouse/life partner have with commercial interest related to the content of this CME activity:

Waleed Brinjikji, MD: is a consultant/advisor for Cerenovus and Superior Medical Editing; is an employee of Marblehead Medical LLC

Patrick A. Brouwer, MD, MSc: is a consultant/advisor for Cerenovus, Medtronic, and Stryker

Jae H. Choi, MD, MS: owns stock and holds patents and/or receives royalties from Hybernia Medical, LLC.

Michael H. Lev, MD, FAHA, FACR: has participated in a speaker's bureau and acted as a consultant and/or advisor for the General Electric Company and Takeda Pharmaceutical Company Limited. He has also participated in a speaker's bureau and received research support from Siemens Medical Solutions, USA.

John Pile-Spellman, MD: owns stock and holds patents and/or receives royalties from Hybernia Medical, LLC.

Panayiotis N. Varelas, MD, PhD, FNCS: participates in speakers bureau for UCB SA, Belgium

UNAPPROVED/OFF-LABEL USE DISCLOSURE

The EOCME requires CME faculty to disclose to the participants:

1. When products or procedures being discussed are off-label, unlabelled, experimental, and/or investigational (not US Food and Drug Administration [FDA] approved); and
2. Any limitations on the information presented, such as data that are preliminary or that represent ongoing research, interim analyses, and/or unsupported opinions. Faculty may discuss information about pharmaceutical agents that is outside of FDA-approved labelling. This information is intended solely for CME and is not intended to promote off-label use of these

medications. If you have any questions, contact the medical affairs department of the manufacturer for the most recent prescribing information.

TO ENROLL

To enroll in the *Neuroimaging Clinics of North America* Continuing Medical Education program, call customer service at 1-800-654-2452 or sign up online at http://www.theclinics.com/home/cme. The CME program is available to subscribers for an additional annual fee of USD 244.40.

METHOD OF PARTICIPATION

In order to claim credit, participants must complete the following:
1. Complete enrolment as indicated above.
2. Read the activity.
3. Complete the CME Test and Evaluation. Participants must achieve a score of 70% on the test. All CME Tests and Evaluations must be completed online.

CME INQUIRIES/SPECIAL NEEDS

For all CME inquiries or special needs, please contact elsevierCME@elsevier.com.

NEUROIMAGING CLINICS OF NORTH AMERICA

THE CLINICS ARE AVAILABLE ONLINE!
Access your subscription at:
www.theclinics.com

Contributors

CONSULTING EDITOR

SURESH K. MUKHERJI, MD, MBA, FACR
Professor and Chairman, Walter F. Patenge
Endowed Chair, Department of Radiology,
Michigan State University, Chief Medical
Officer and Director of Health Care Delivery,
Michigan State University Health Team, East
Lansing, Michigan, USA

EDITOR

LOTFI HACEIN-BEY, MD
Interventional Neuroradiology and
Neuroradiology, Department of Medical
Imaging, Sutter Health, Professor, Radiology
Department, University of California, Davis
School of Medicine, Sacramento, California,
USA

AUTHORS

JEROME BERGE, MD
Interventional Neuroradiology, Radiology
Department, Bordeaux University Medical
Center, Bordeaux, France

JOSÉ BILLER, MD, FAAN, FACP, FAHA
Professor, Chairperson, Department
of Neurology, Loyola University Chicago,
Stritch School of Medicine, Loyola University
Medical Center, Maywood, Illinois,
USA

MARTIN BRETZNER, MD
Neuroradiology Department, Lille University
Medical Center, CHU Lille, Lille,
France

WALEED BRINJIKJI, MD
Departments of Radiology and Neurosurgery,
Mayo Clinic, Rochester, Minnesota, USA;
Joint Department of Medical Imaging,
Toronto Western Hospital, Toronto, Ontario,
Canada

PATRICK A. BROUWER, MD, MSc
Neuroradiology Department,
Neurointervention Section, Karolinska
University Hospital, Stockholm, Sweden

JAE H. CHOI, MD, MS
Medical Director, Center for Unruptured Brain
Aneurysms, Neurological Surgery PC, Lake
Success, New York, USA; Adjunct Assistant
Professor, Department of Neurology, SUNY
Downstate Medical Center, Brooklyn, New
York, USA; CEO/Managing Partner, Hybernia
Medical LLC, Uniondale, New York,
USA

SIMON F. DE MEYER, PhD
Laboratory for Thrombosis Research, KU
Leuven, Campus Kulak Kortrijk, Kortrijk,
Belgium

R. GILBERTO GONZÁLEZ, MD, PhD
Neuroradiology, Massachusetts General
Hospital, Harvard Medical School, Boston,
Massachusetts, USA

LOTFI HACEIN-BEY, MD
Interventional Neuroradiology and
Neuroradiology, Department of Medical
Imaging, Sutter Health, Professor, Radiology
Department, University of California, Davis
School of Medicine, Sacramento, California,
USA

ANDREAS HARTMANN, MD
Department of Neurology, Klinikum Frankfurt
(Oder), Frankfurt (Oder), Germany

JEREMY J. HEIT, MD, PhD
Department of Radiology, Division of
Neuroimaging and Neurointervention, Stanford
Health Care, Stanford, California, USA

SHANNON HEXTRUM, MD
Resident Physician, Department of Neurology,
Loyola University Medical Center, Maywood,
Illinois, USA

**JOSHUA A. HIRSCH, MD, FACR, FSIR,
FSNIS**
Neurointerventional Radiology, Interventional
Radiology, Massachusetts General Hospital,
Harvard Medical School, Boston,
Massachusetts, USA

BIN JIANG, MD, PhD
Division of Neuroradiology, Life Science
Research Professional, Department of
Radiology, Stanford University, Stanford,
California, USA

ANGELOS M. KATRAMADOS, MD
Assistant Professor, Department of Neurology,
Wayne State University, Henry Ford Hospital,
Detroit, Michigan, USA

ANGELOS A. KONSTAS, MD
Interventional Neuroradiology and
Neuroradiology, Department of Radiology,
Huntington Memorial Hospital, Pasadena,
California, USA

GREGORY KUCHCINSKI, MD
Neuroradiology Department, Lille University
Medical Center, CHU Lille, Lille, France

XAVIER LECLERC, MD, PhD
Neuroradiology Department, Lille University
Medical Center, Lille University, INSERM
U1171, CHU Lille, Lille, France

CARLOS LEIVA-SALINAS, MD, PhD
Chief, Division of Neuroradiology, Assistant
Professor, Department of Radiology, University
of Missouri, Columbia, Missouri,
USA

THABELE M. LESLIE-MAZWI, MD
Neuroendovascular Program, Neurocritical
Care, Departments of Neurosurgery and
Neurology, Massachusetts General Hospital,
Harvard Medical School, Boston,
Massachusetts, USA

MICHAEL H. LEV, MD, FAHA, FACR
Emergency Radiology, Massachusetts General
Hospital, Harvard Medical School, Boston,
Massachusetts, USA

JAY P. MOHR, MD
Doris & Stanley Tananbaum Stroke Center,
Neurological Institute of New York, Columbia
University Medical Center, New York,
New York, USA

GOVIND MUKUNDAN, MD
Department of Medical Imaging, Sutter
Health, Sacramento, California, USA

JOHN PILE-SPELLMAN, MD
Co-Founder/Managing Partner, Hybernia
Medical LLC, Uniondale, New York,
USA; Co-Director, Center for Unruptured
Brain Aneurysms, Neurological Surgery PC,
Lake Success, New York,
USA

JEAN-PIERRE PRUVO, MD, PhD
Neuroradiology Department, Lille University
Medical Center, Lille University, INSERM
U1171, CHU Lille, Lille, France

PAMELA W. SCHAEFER, MD
Neuroradiology, Radiology, Massachusetts
General Hospital, Harvard Medical School,
Boston, Massachusetts, USA

DAVID J. SEIDENWURM, MD
Department of Medical Imaging, Sutter Health,
Sacramento, California, USA

NINA J. SOLENSKI, MD, FAHA
Associate Professor, Department of
Neurology, University of Virginia School of
Medicine, University of Virginia Health System,
Charlottesville, Virginia, USA

E. TURGUT TALI, MD
Director, Section of Neuroradiology, Professor of Radiology and Neuroradiology, Department of Radiology, Gazi University School of Medicine, Yenimahalle, Ankara, Turkey

PANAYIOTIS N. VARELAS, MD, PhD, FNCS
Division Head, NeuroCritical Care Service, Director, Neurosciences Intensive Care Unit, Senior Staff, Departments of Neurology and Neurosurgery, Henry Ford Hospital, Professor of Neurology, Wayne State University, Detroit, Michigan, USA

MAX WINTERMARK, MD, MPH, MBA
Professor of Radiology and, by courtesy, of Neurology, Neurosurgery, and Psychiatry and Behavioral Sciences, Chief, Division of Neuroradiology, Department of Radiology, Stanford University, Stanford, California, USA

LEI WU, MD
Department of Radiology, University of Washington, Seattle, Washington, USA

WEI WU, MD
Department of Radiology, University of Washington, Seattle, Washington, USA; Department of Radiology, Tongji Hospital, Tongji Medical College Affiliated to Huazhong University of Science and Technology, Wuhan, Hubei, China

WILLIAM T. YUH, MD, MSEE
Department of Radiology, University of Washington, Seattle, Washington, USA

GREG ZAHARCHUK, MD, PhD
Department of Radiology, Division of Neuroimaging and Neurointervention, Stanford Health Care, Stanford, California, USA

Contents

Non–stroke conditions may present in ways suggestive of ischemic stroke (ie, stroke mimic). Alternatively, the clinical presentation of ischemic stroke can vary considerably and may appear similar to another condition (ie, stroke chameleon). Common and uncommon mimics and chameleons are presented with discussion of key considerations to improve diagnostic accuracy.

Teleradiology, transfer of radiology images to a distant diagnostician, has existed for more than 50 years and is a fundamental element in telestroke programs. Teleradiology allows access to expertise for accurate and rapid interpretation of noncontrast CT (NCCT) scans to distinguish ischemic stroke from hemorrhagic stroke. No acute stroke thrombolytic or clot retrieval treatment decision can be made without it. Innovations in CT software and ambulance-based CT scans are significantly improving outcomes by matching patients to effective treatment paradigms. This article reviews telestroke models, NCCT interpretation pearls, and access challenges to the latest neuroradiology technology within rural and underserved regions.

This review outlines the current role of the individual components of multimodal computed tomography (computed tomography, computed tomography angiography, and perfusion computed tomography) in the evaluation of patients with acute ischemic stroke.

Acute stroke caused by large vessel occlusions (LVOs) are common. The time window to treat is up to 24 hours, and the most important factor is the size of the ischemic core. If the core is small (<70–100 mL), the penumbra must be large;

penumbral imaging is unnecessary. MR imaging is precise in measuring the core, and superior to alternatives. The necessary sequences are obtainable rapidly, comparable to computed tomography scans. Available evidence suggests that most patients with LVOs are slow progressors defined as having a small core 6 hours or more after ictus onset.

taking place from rigid time windows for intervention (time is brain) to physiology-driven paradigms that rely heavily on neuroimaging. At this time, one can reasonably anticipate that more patients will be treated, and that outcomes will keep improving. This article discusses in detail recent advances in endovascular stroke therapy.

Given the need for early restoration of blood flow and preservation of partially damaged brain cells after ischemic stroke, the noninterventional treatment of stroke relies heavily on the speedy recognition and classification of the clinical syndrome. Initiation of systemic thrombolysis with careful observation of contraindications within the 3.0 (4.5)-hour time window is the approved therapy of choice. Management of hemorrhagic complications and resumption of oral anticoagulation if indicated are also discussed in this article.

The most feared complication after acute ischemic stroke is symptomatic or asymptomatic hemorrhagic conversion. Neuroimaging and clinical criteria are used to predict development of hemorrhage. Seizures after acute ischemic stroke or stroke-like symptoms from seizures are not common but may lead to confusion in the peristroke period, especially if seizures are repetitive or evolve into status epilepticus, which could affect neuroimaging findings. Malignant infarction develops when cytotoxic edema is large enough to lead to herniation and death. Post-stroke neuroimaging prognosticators have been described and should be assessed early so that appropriate treatment is offered before herniation leads to additional tissue injury.

Reperfusion is the first line of care in a growing number of eligible acute ischemic stroke patients. Early reperfusion with thrombolytic drugs and endovascular mechanical devices is associated with improved outcome and lower mortality rates compared with natural history. Reperfusion is not without risk, however, and may result in reperfusion injury, which manifests in hemorrhagic transformation, brain edema, infarct progression, and neurologic worsening. In this article, the functional and structural changes and underlying molecular mechanisms of ischemia and reperfusion are reviewed. The pathways that lead to reperfusion injury and novel neuroprotective strategies with endogenous properties are discussed.

Stroke is a major health burden worldwide with attendant mortality, morbidity, and cost. In 2010, there were approximately 16.9 million strokes and an estimated 33 million stroke survivors worldwide. Also, in the United States, stroke is the third leading cause of death, with ischemic stroke resulting in 8% 30-day mortality (20% for hemorrhagic stroke). The staggering economic cost of the disease is driven largely by disability and long term care. Efforts in stroke healthcare delivery are focusing on performance, efficiency and value to better serve the consumer.

Stroke, a major burden to society, can now be treated in increasingly larger numbers of patients. Intravenous thrombolysis and mechanical thrombectomy are both now standard of care with class I, level of evidence A. Various local, regional, and national challenges are present, preventing equality in access to care for many patients. France is a developed country with a centralized national health care system accessible for all citizens. This article discusses current challenges in the implementation of the delivery of stroke care and some solutions that are being evaluated by the medical community.

Foreword
Ischemic Stroke

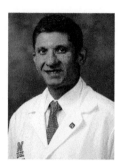

Suresh K. Mukherji, MD, MBA, FACR
Consulting Editor

"Time is Brain," and I would suggest that stroke imaging and treatment have a more direct impact on patient care that any other field in Radiology. There have been major recent advancements in the understanding, evaluation, imaging, and treatment of stroke, especially in rapid intervention and clot retrieval.

I would like to express my sincere gratitude to the article authors for their very impressive contributions. The topics covered in this issue include clinical signs and symptoms, pathophysiology, imaging biomarkers, medical management, interventional techniques, and socioeconomic challenges and opportunities. As Dr Hacein-Bey states in his preface, this is a truly outstanding group, and I am very honored that they participated in this important issue.

Finally, I want to personally thank Dr Lotfi Hacein-Bey for his willingness to guest edit this important issue. I was thrilled when he accepted our invitation as he is someone I have admired throughout my career. This important, timely, and....wonderful issue will benefit all stakeholders involved in stroke care, but most importantly...our patients!

Suresh K. Mukherji, MD, MBA, FACR
Department of Radiology
Michigan State University
Michigan State University Health Team
846 Service Road
East Lansing, MI 48824, USA

E-mail address:
sureshkm@msu.edu

Preface

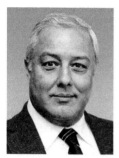

Lotfi Hacein-Bey, MD
Editor

During the decade since the last *Neuroimaging Clinics* issue on this topic, major progress has been made as to the understanding, evaluation, imaging, and treatment of stroke, which remains the leading cause of death and disability worldwide, and continues to be on the rise in developed countries. I wish to express my immense gratitude to the authors and coauthors, all experts in their field, many who are personal friends, for their invaluable contributions.

- Shannon Hextrum and Jose Biller educate us on proper clinical identification of stroke syndromes, and recognition of stroke mimics and chameleons, which remains key, especially with extended therapeutic time windows.
- Nina Solenski, a telestroke expert, explains how Internet-based telecommunications technologies are undergoing standardization in developed countries to triage patients.
- Carlos Leiva-Salinas and Max Wintermark provide a detailed update to their previous work a decade ago on CT-based imaging of stroke, the most widely available and used technique in the United States.
- The Massachusetts General Hospital team, led by R. Gilberto Gonzalez, which includes Pamela Schaefer and Michael Lev (both Editors of past *Neuroimaging Clinics* issues on stroke) share their valuable experience with MR imaging–based stroke protocols.
- Jeremy Heit and colleagues from Stanford introduce the reader to advanced imaging techniques that may find future use in assessing penumbral tissue and collaterals, such as MR imaging–based arterial spin labeling or blood-oxygen-level dependent contrast imaging techniques, and multiphase CT angiography.
- William Yuh and colleagues eloquently remind us of our currently imperfect understanding of cerebrovascular physiology, leading to humbling limitations of neuroimaging in sorting out oligemia, hypoperfusion, ischemia, apoptosis, and viable tissue (penumbra).
- Patrick Brouwer and colleagues provide insight on the effect of thrombus composition on rheology and on mechanical thrombectomy; they also educate us on potential novel pharmacologic approaches targeting neutrophils and blood factors.
- Hacein-Bey and colleagues describe the current status of stroke interventional techniques. The best outcomes are seen when successful thrombectomy is completed within 30 minutes of intervention, as resistant thrombi become increasingly tightly adherent to the arterial wall, while persistent occlusion allows penumbra to progress to infarction.
- Andreas Hartmann and J.P. Mohr provide an excellent update on the medical management of those stroke patients who have not received intervention.
- Angelos Katramados and Panayiotis Varelas provide their useful insight as neurointensive care specialists on how to follow patients in the aftermath of a stroke.
- Jae Choi and John Pile-Spellman deliver extremely important new knowledge on cerebral molecular changes following ischemia, and successful or unsuccessful reperfusion. More importantly, they introduce the reader to adjunctive neuroprotective methods that may soon find important clinical applications.

Neuroimag Clin N Am 28 (2018) xvii–xviii
https://doi.org/10.1016/j.nic.2018.08.001
1052-5149/18/© 2018 Published by Elsevier Inc.

- Govind Mukundan and David Seidenwurm provide useful information on stroke public policy and payment models in the United States.
- Jean-Pierre Pruvo and colleagues describe their valuable experience with successfully addressing some of the challenges of managing stroke in France. Their approach relies heavily on MR imaging for patient triaging (with near-zero rates of inappropriate delivery of thrombolysis), simulation-based training programs, and creative ways of addressing major shortages in the specialized workforce which are already facing all countries.

I also wish to express gratitude to Dr Suresh Mukherji for providing the opportunity for this work, and to the Editorial team at Elsevier, primarily John Vassallo, Casey Potter, Pradeep Kuttysankaran, Nicole Congleton, Reni Thomas, and many others, whose skilled help has contributed to this collective effort, which we hope useful to physicians, and more so to patients.

Lotfi Hacein-Bey, MD
Interventional Neuroradiology and
Neuroradiology
Department of Medical Imaging
Sutter Health
Sacramento, CA 95815, USA

Radiology Department
University of California Davis
School of Medicine
4860 Y Street
Sacramento, CA 95817, USA

E-mail address:
lhaceinbey@yahoo.com

Clinical Distinction of Cerebral Ischemia and Triaging of Patients in the Emergency Department

Mimics, Wake-ups, Late Strokes, and Chameleons

Shannon Hextrum, MD[a],*, José Biller, MD[b]

KEYWORDS

- Stroke mimics • Stroke chameleons • Thrombolysis • Migraines • Seizures • Dizziness • Vertigo
- Facial paralysis

KEY POINTS

- Several clinical entities closely mimic acute ischemic stroke and pose diagnostic challenges for clinicians.
- Stroke chameleons are ischemic strokes that present similar to non–stroke conditions, and these may interfere with prompt recognition and treatment of acute ischemic stroke.
- Consideration of key discriminating features of stroke mimics and chameleons can assist clinicians in proper triaging of suspected acute ischemic strokes.

INTRODUCTION

The heterogeneity in signs and symptoms of arterial ischemic strokes may pose a challenge to clinicians. In the acute setting, diagnostic accuracy is critical for decisions of intravenous (IV) thrombolysis with recombinant tissue plasminogen activator (alteplase) and may be complicated by the abundance of both "stroke mimics" and "stroke chameleons." A stroke mimic represents a non–stroke disorder with a presentation suggestive of acute ischemic stroke, whereas a chameleon is an ischemic stroke presenting similarly to a non–stroke condition.[1] In this review, the authors discuss the challenges in diagnosis of acute ischemic stroke and propose methods for improvement.

STROKE MIMICS

Although the prevalence of stroke mimics is difficult to quantify, estimates range from as low as 1.4% to as high as 38% of admissions for suspected acute ischemic stroke.[2,3] A wide variety of conditions account for stroke mimics, and not all are neurologic in nature (Table 1). Metabolic derangements, central nervous system (CNS) or systemic infection, cardiovascular events, and psychiatric issues may masquerade as acute ischemic strokes.[4] Although MR imaging has become an important tool in the diagnosis of acute stroke, its sensitivity is not 100%.[5] In the acute and subacute setting, a negative diffusion-weighted imaging (DWI) does not exclude the possibility of true ischemic stroke.[6,7] As such, ischemic stroke remains a clinical

Disclosure Statement: The authors report no disclosures.
a Department of Neurology, Loyola University Medical Center, 2160 South First Avenue, Building 105, Room 2700, Maywood, IL 60153, USA; b Department of Neurology, Loyola University Chicago, Stritch School of Medicine, Loyola University Medical Center, 2160 South First Avenue, Building 105, Room 2700, Maywood, IL 60153, USA
* Corresponding author.
E-mail address: Shannon.hextrum@gmail.com

neuroimaging.theclinics.com

Table 1
List of stroke mimics and chameleons

Mimics	Chameleons
Seizures	Purely motor stroke
Headaches	with monoparesis
• Migraines	• Hand-knob area
• HaNDL	infarction
• SMART syndrome	Stroke with
Metabolic disturbances	predominately
• Sepsis	cognitive symptoms
• Hepatic	• Gerstmann
encephalopathy	syndrome
• Hypo/	• Balint syndrome
hyperglycemia	• Hippocampal
• Hypo/	infarctions
hypernatremia	• Top of the basilar
• MELAS	syndrome
Drug and Alcohol	• Artery of
toxicity	Percheron infarct
• SESA	Stroke with
Space-occupying	seizure-like activity
lesions	• Limb-shaking TIAs
Syncope/Presyncope	• Capsular warning
Peripheral vertigo	syndrome
Neurovascular	• Brainstem infarcts
conditions	with convulsions
• CAA	
• PRES	
Autoimmune &	
Inflammatory	
disorders	
• MS	
• CLIPPERS	
• MG	
Channelopathies	
• Primary episodic	
ataxia	
• Hypo/hyperkalemic	
periodic paralysis	

Abbreviations: CAA, cerebral amyloid angiopathy; CLIPPERS, chronic lymphocytic inflammation with pontine perivascular enhancement responsive to steroids; HaNDL, headache and neurological deficits with cerebrospinal fluid (CSF) lymphocytosis; MELAS, Mitochondrial encephalomyopathy with lactic acidosis and stroke-like episodes; MG, myasthenia gravis; MS, Multiple sclerosis; PRES, posterior reversible encephalopathy syndrome; SESA, Subacute encephalopathy with seizures in chronic alcoholism; SMART, stroke-like migraine attacks after radiation therapy; TIAs, transient ischemic attacks.

diagnosis, and recognition of stroke mimics is important for clinical decision making.

Seizures

Among the most common stroke mimics are seizures and postictal phenomena that may present with focal neurologic deficits, including weakness, sensory changes, aphasia, and neglect. Postseizure unilateral weakness, referred to as Todd paralysis, may last for hours or days. Details regarding the onset of symptoms, including adventitious movements and automatisms, may help clarify the diagnosis. However, it is often the case that these events are unwitnessed.[1,8] Furthermore, classic signs of seizure activity, including oral lacerations and urinary incontinence, may not always help with diagnostic accuracy. A systematic review of 5 studies by Brigo and colleagues[9] reported low sensitivity (38%) and specificity (57%) for urinary incontinence as a predictive factor for epileptic seizures versus nonepileptic spells. A separate 2012 review by Brigo and colleagues[10] assessed the value of tongue biting as a predictor of epileptic seizures or syncope. Their findings showed high specificity (96%), although low sensitivity (33%), for tongue biting to correctly identify epileptic seizures, suggesting the absence of tongue biting is one clinical examination finding that may help rule out seizure activity. Although such statistics are compelling, the authors caution against any absolute rules regarding oral lacerations or tongue biting and the likelihood of epileptic seizures.

Seizures may also cause restricted diffusion on DWI sequence of MR imaging, adding to the complexity of this stroke mimic. Nevertheless, there are key qualities in the pattern of distribution that help distinguish seizures from an ischemic infarction. In seizure activity, the DWI changes do not follow a clear vessel distribution.[11] For instance, seizures commonly result in DWI changes of the entire hippocampus. A posterior cerebral artery (PCA) infarction affecting the hippocampus would not generally include the pes hippocampus, a region supplied by the anterior choroidal artery (AChA).[11,12] Cortical DWI changes related to ictal activity will tend to respect the gray-white junction, showing minimal involvement of white matter.[13]

In addition to diagnostic challenges, a treatment approach to the seizure patient with stroke-like features may be difficult. The possibility of coexisting seizure at stroke onset complicates matters. However, this is not an absolute contraindication for IV alteplase administration in ischemic infarction.[1] A further consideration in the triaging and management of stroke patients at presentation is whether IV thrombolysis increases the likelihood of early seizures after ischemic stroke. Xu and colleagues[14,15] analyzed data available on seizure activity from the large-scale ENCHANTED (Enhanced Control of Hypertension and Thrombolysis Stroke) Study, which randomized patients to receive IV alteplase at low dose (0.6 mg/kg) or standard dose (0.9 mg/kg). Seizures data were analyzed on a total of 3139 patients having received either dose of alteplase; only 42 (1.3%) suffered clinical seizures in the first 7 days from thrombolysis. Male gender, greater severity of stroke, and fever were associated with greater likelihood of seizures. However, the overall seizure rate was encouragingly low and should not deter a clinician from using alteplase in the appropriate clinical context.

Migraine and Headache Disorders

The International Classification of Headache Disorders (ICHD) defines migraine as attacks of headache symptoms lasting 4 to 72 hours, characterized as unilateral, pulsatile, worse with activity, and commonly associated with nausea, photophobia, and phonophobia. Migraine with aura includes various CNS phenomena that may be mistaken for vascular insults. These recurrent symptoms often last minutes in duration and typically result in headache with migraine features.[16] Visual auras are present in 90% of those patients with migraine and do not always precede the headache pain component of migraine with aura. Characteristic visual auras, including scintillating scotomas, may be clearly distinct from symptoms of ischemic infarct. However, sensory auras may include numbness. Language deficits such as aphasia are also documented as migraine auras. When diagnosing migraine with aura, the clinician should note that positive phenomena (paresthesias, flashing lights) rather than negative phenomena (numbness, visual loss) present in the beginning of an attack. The gradual spread of symptoms, often from positive to negative, is likely due to the pathophysiologic process termed cortical spreading depression and is quite distinct from the sudden onset of a cerebrovascular event.[17]

The ICHD classifies hemiplegic migraine separately from migraine with aura. Of key clinical significance is the fact that hemiplegic migraine is defined by both reversible motor symptoms (lasting <72 hours) as well as nonmotor aura. Headache, although not a required feature, is often present concurrently or within 60 minutes of aura.[16] In addition to the presence of nonmotor symptoms such as headache, the gradual nature of symptom onset may again aid the clinician in diagnosing hemiplegic migraine instead of ischemic cerebral infarction. Another important clue to migraines in the patient's history is the existence of premonitory symptoms, such as fatigue, impaired concentration, photophobia, and neck stiffness, which may occur hours to days before migraine onset.[16] A careful and detailed account of symptoms, with close attention to symptom onset, is critical for the diagnosis of various migraine disorders that may mimic ischemic infarction.

Migraines as stroke mimics can be particularly difficult to diagnose in older populations at greater risk for stroke and transient ischemic attack (TIA). In 1980, Fisher[18] described "late-life migraine accompaniments" as TIA-appearing attacks (ie, speech deficits, visual disturbances, paresthesias) in those past the third decade of life. Of note, these migrainous attacks were not always accompanied by headache. Although migraines tend to decrease with advanced age, clinicians should recognize their existence in older patient populations.[19,20]

Another consideration in the spectrum of headache disorders is that of headache and neurologic deficits with cerebrospinal fluid (CSF) lymphocytosis, or HaNDL. This rare condition was well described in a case series of 9 patients, with headache and neurologic disturbances resolving within 12 hours from presentation. Other features to consider when establishing a diagnosis are the predominance of women (77% of the patients) and the young age of onset (median age in this sample was 25).[21] An additional headache disorder associated with reversible neurologic deficits is stroke-like migraine attacks after radiation therapy (SMART syndrome).[22] The proposed diagnostic criteria of Bartleson and colleagues[23] include the following features: remote radiation treatment without evidence of recurrent malignancy, attacks consistent with migraine and complicated migraine, temporary gadolinium enhancement on MR imaging, and full recovery from symptoms in the span of weeks. The exact pathophysiology of this syndrome is unclear, and it has been observed in cases of focal and whole brain radiation.[22] At the authors' institution, a 60-year-old man presented with discrete episodes of alexia, gait difficulty, and aphasia, as well as one episode of presumed homonymous hemianopia with preceding headache. He had a history of seizures as well as a remote history of medulloblastoma treated with resection, chemotherapy, radiation, and requiring placement of ventriculoperitoneal shunt. CSF studies were negative for an infectious, autoimmune, or paraneoplastic process, and MR brain imaging showed diffuse gadolinium enhancement of the left parietal, occipital, and temporal lobes (Fig. 1). Although left hemispheric temporal intermittent rhythmic delta activity was captured on electroencephalogram (EEG), the authors found no ictal activity correlating with his symptoms, and the final diagnosis was SMART syndrome. His alexia and aphasia have improved since hospital discharge, and subsequent MR imaging showed resolution of his prior areas of contrast enhancement (see Fig. 1).

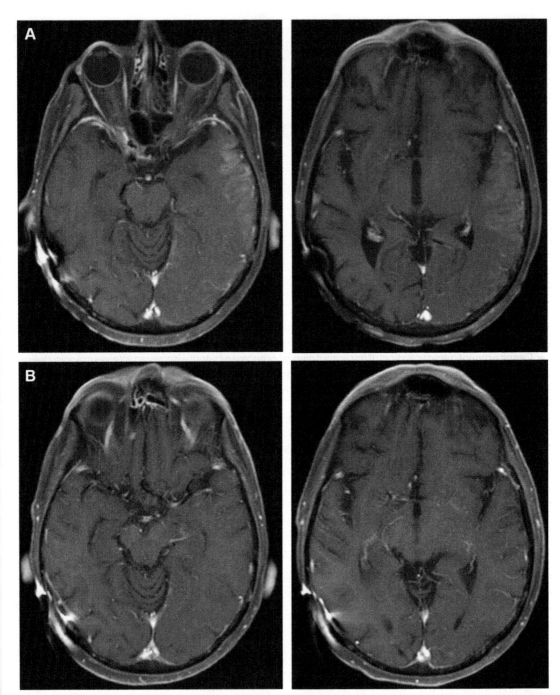

Fig. 1. Postcontrast MR imaging sequence of a patient with SMART syndrome. (*A*) Two axial views during hospital admission, showing left hemispheric contrast enhancement. (*B*) Two axial views 7 weeks later, without enhancement.

Metabolic Disturbances

Sepsis, hepatic encephalopathy, and electrolyte and glucose disturbances are common stroke mimics.[24] Hypoglycemia has long been recognized as a cause of focal neurologic deficits, including hemiplegia.[25,26] As such, routine blood glucose checks are a necessary component of any investigation for acute ischemic infarction; however, symptoms may persist after blood glucose has been normalized. The clinician should be attuned to hallmark indicators of hypoglycemia, chiefly autonomic signs, as well as seizures and decreased level of arousal.[8,27] Hyperglycemia is another important stroke mimic, typically observed when blood glucose levels elevate to the point of causing diabetic ketoacidosis or hyperosmolar hyperglycemic state.[28,29] Shah and colleagues[30] present a case report of severe hyperglycemia (initial blood glucose 825 mg/dL) in a 67-year-old diabetic woman who presented with symptoms suggestive of a classic left middle cerebral artery (MCA) territory large vessel occlusion. The patient's examination demonstrated left gaze deviation, right hemiplegia, and global aphasia, all of which improved with correction of blood glucose.

Hyponatremia is a less common stroke mimic and must be recognized as a potential cause of reversible, focal neurologic deficits. Hemiparesis, ataxia, and tremor have been documented in cases of severe hyponatremia, usually in instances of rapid decline in serum sodium level to less than 120 mmol/L. As with other metabolic disturbances, it is worth noting that confusion is classically present.[31,32] With nonspecific symptoms such as confusion, the possibility of encephalitis should remain high on the differential diagnosis. It is important to consider metabolic derangements as a cause of stroke mimic without neglecting to diagnose and treat other serious neurologic conditions.

Certain inherited disorders, such mitochondrial encephalomyopathy with lactic acidosis and stroke-like episodes (MELAS), may also lead to metabolic issues and stroke-like symptoms. MELAS is a rare condition involving dysfunction in intracellular energy production that may present as transient neurologic deficits concurrent with areas of restricted diffusion on MR imaging.[33] Such MR imaging changes do not respect vascular territories and will disappear and then recur, although chronic structural changes are observed over time, suggestive of the accumulating disease burden. Presentation of symptoms routinely occurs before age 40, and various non-neurologic conditions are apparent, including myopathy, diabetes, exercise intolerance, and growth failure.[34]

Infection and Drug Toxicity

Although CNS infections, such as herpes simplex virus encephalitis, often present with generalized signs and symptoms, including fever, encephalopathy, and headache, it is important to recognize the potential for localizing signs mimicking acute stroke. This clinical presentation is illustrated in the case of a 79-year-old woman with several vascular risk factors and rapid onset of right hemiparesis and aphasia. Computed tomography (CT) perfusion and CT angiography demonstrated no evidence of occlusive disease or perfusion defects. The patient spiked a fever 11 hours after initial symptom onset, with subsequent CSF studies positive for herpes simplex virus type 1.[35] The manifestation of neurologic deficits preceding fever is unusual in this case, although a similar temporal pattern has been described.[36]

Medication toxicity is another key stroke mimic that may be easy to overlook, especially in a patient with several vascular risk favors. Classic signs of phenytoin toxicity (nystagmus, ataxia, dysarthria) may be confused for a posterior circulation stroke. A retrospective case series revealed 14% of cases of phenytoin intoxication were first diagnosed as cerebellar or brainstem infarct.[37,38] In addition, the similarity of phenytoin toxicity to alcohol intoxication may further complicate or delay the diagnosis.[39] Neurotoxicity from other agents, including chemotherapeutic drugs and cefepime, may also be confused for acute stroke. High-dose methotrexate has long been recognized as a cause of acute and transient neurologic deficits. Recognition of this condition is important, because administration of dextromethorphan is an effective treatment.[40] A systematic review of cefepime neurotoxicity by Appa and colleagues[41] pooled 198 cases to better characterize trends in symptoms. Although generalized features including decreased mentation and disorientation were the more commonly reported symptoms, aphasia was reported in 9% of cases. Of cases with recorded data on renal function (171), a full 87% of patients with cefepime toxicity demonstrated renal dysfunction. Furthermore, Appa and colleagues[41] found 110 cases that included renal function documented at that time of cefepime toxicity diagnosis, and 50% of these cases included cefepime dosing above that recommended for their renal function. It is imperative that clinicians quickly recognize iatrogenic contributions to cefepime neurotoxicity or other medication-related stroke mimics.

A great deal can be said about the neurologic deficits associated with acute alcohol intoxication as well as chronic alcohol use. The authors would like to highlight a less commonly discussed syndrome termed subacute encephalopathy with seizures in chronic alcoholism (SESA). In addition to seizure activity (focal or generalized) and periodic lateralized discharges on EEG, SESA presents with focal and transient neurologic deficits. This condition may be hard to delineate in the setting of intoxication or concern for alcohol withdrawal alone. However, this is a distinct clinical entity in chronic alcoholics, and the mainstay of treatment is antiepileptic medication.[42,43]

Space-Occupying Lesions

Intracranial tumors may be associated with episodes of stroke-like symptoms, sometimes called "tumor attacks."[44] Although the exact cause is unclear, symptoms may stem from vascular steal or compression, tumor embolus, changes in intracranial pressure, and postictal paralysis. Small tumors without significant mass effect may not be visualized on routine nonenhanced head CT in the evaluation of suspected acute infarction. High-grade gliomas may be radiographically confused for acute ischemic stroke, given possible hypoattenuation on noncontrast CT and even lack of contrast enhancement and DWI changes on MR imaging.[44] It is worth noting that the use of IV alteplase is contraindicated in patients with intracranial intra-axial neoplasms. However, isolated cases have been reported in the literature without subsequent intracranial hemorrhage.[45]

Cerebral abscesses are other space-occupying cerebral lesions that may mimic acute stroke, and these may not present with typical signs of infection. In fact, a comprehensive systematic review and meta-analysis of intracranial abscesses by Brouwer and colleagues[46] identified fever in 53% of patients and leukocytosis in 60% of patients (for those studies specifying such patient details). Otitis and mastoiditis were the leading conditions cited as underlying causes of cerebral abscesses, and most abscesses identified were seen in immunocompetent individuals. Younger age of onset (33.6 years) as well as predisposing infections may assist the clinician in considering cerebral abscess over ischemic infarction.

Dizziness/Vertigo

Conditions such as vertigo, gait unsteadiness, and presyncope can all be captured under the broader symptom of "dizziness." However, it is important for the clinician to clarify the distinction when assessing the likelihood of stroke. An acute episode of vertigo may be caused by a posterior circulation infarction even in the absence of other neurologic deficits. Advanced age, the presence of vascular risk factors, sudden onset of symptoms, and craniocervical pain (often seen in vertebral artery dissection) should raise concern for a possible CNS cause of vertigo.[47] With regards to the physical examination, subtle features in the patient's ocular movements may point toward a higher likelihood of peripheral vertigo. Kattah and colleagues[48] define a reliable 3-step approach called the "HiNTS" examination (ie, Head-

impulse–Nystagmus–Test-of-Skew). First, a horizontal head impulse test often demonstrates a normal vestibular-ocular reflex in the setting of acute stroke, although it is usually abnormal in peripheral causes. Second, the nystagmus of peripheral vertigo will more likely be horizontal and unidirectional, whereas any vertical or torsional nystagmus should signal higher likelihood of acute stroke. Finally, skew deviation (vertical ocular misalignment) on alternate cover testing is more indicative of central vertigo when present on examination.

Another cause of dizziness may be syncope or presyncope, and in a comprehensive review of stroke mimics, Long and Koyfman[24] cite syncope as comprising up to 20% of all stroke mimics. A wide variety of mechanisms may lead to syncopal events, including hypoglycemia, orthostasis, subclavian steal, and heat-related illness. Such events may be confused for strokes within the posterior circulation that may cause decreased mentation. However, focal neurologic changes and especially cranial nerve abnormalities are more significant clues toward a vertebrobasilar territory infarction.

Neurovascular Conditions

Several primary neurologic conditions of various mechanisms and severity may mimic the time course and symptoms of acute stroke. Cerebral amyloid angiopathy (CAA) is a neurovascular condition caused by deposition of amyloid-β in arterial vessels primarily of the cerebral cortex and leptomeninges. CAA is age related, associated with lobar intracerebral hemorrhage, and has a higher prevalence in patients with dementia. It can also cause transient neurologic deficits, so-called amyloid spells, often involving spreading paresthesias, and commonly occurring for minutes at a time. Cerebral microbleeds or convexity subarachnoid hemorrhage may be observed in a corresponding region of cerebral cortex; however, the exact mechanism of such spells is yet to be determined.[49,50]

Posterior reversible encephalopathy syndrome (PRES) is a neurovascular process defined by cortical and subcortical vasogenic edema with episodic neurologic symptoms, such as headache, seizures, and visual changes. This syndrome has been described in the context of uncontrolled hypertension, eclampsia, sepsis, and chemotherapeutic agents (notably tacrolimus and cyclosporine).[51,52] Commonly, MR imaging findings include hyperintense fluid-attenuated inversion recovery (FLAIR) sequence in the parieto-occipital or posterior frontal lobes.[50] The prevailing theory of the cause of PRES is that severe hypertension triggers dysfunctional autoregulation and subsequent edema, although it is worth noting that PRES is observed in the absence of hypertension.[53] Removing the offending agent or treating the underlying condition is the hallmark of therapy.[51]

Autoimmune and Demyelinating Disorders

Paroxysmal attacks in the setting of demyelinating disease may also present similarly to stroke or TIA. In a retrospective study of 2700 multiple sclerosis (MS) patients, Lacour and colleagues[54] found 22 cases of acute aphasia (.81%), 8 of which (36%) demonstrated the aphasic episode as the first sign of their disease. In a similar vein, Yates and Crawley[55] highlight the case of a 45-year-old man with no significant medical history who presented with recurrent "heaviness" of his left arm and blurred vision, with full resolution of symptoms between episodes. He had been referred to the TIA clinic; however, initial cranial imaging showed lesions consistent with MS. A careful history taking in this case revealed further details to confirm the diagnosis, once again demonstrating the importance of comprehensive history for proper diagnosis and treatment.

Other inflammatory conditions of the CNS should be recognized as potential stroke mimics, including chronic lymphocytic inflammation with pontine perivascular enhancement responsive to steroids (CLIPPERS). This condition was described by Pittock and colleagues[56] in a 2010 case series of 8 patients. Clinically, all patients demonstrated ataxia and diplopia, as well as gadolinium contrast enhancement scattered throughout the pons, medulla, brachium pontis, and midbrain. Four of 8 patients received brain biopsies demonstrating lymphocytic infiltration of the white matter, preferentially in perivascular spaces. Although the progressive nature of symptoms speaks against a diagnosis of acute stroke,[57] the presentation may be confused for subacute infarction.

Myasthenia gravis (MG) and other disorders of the neuromuscular junction may present in a similar fashion to acute stroke. Shaik and colleagues[58] present a case of an 85-year-old man with acute onset isolated speech and swallowing difficulty. He was admitted to a stroke unit for further diagnosis and treatment. However, his MR imaging was negative for acute infarction, and his symptoms persisted. Although there was no evidence of fatigability present on examination, the patient described to family that his symptoms were less severe in the morning, and this broadened the differential to include bulbar MG. Given the widely different treatment approaches between acute stroke and MG, it is important to recognize such features in the patient's history that are critical for diagnostic accuracy.

Channelopathies

Transient neurologic deficits mimicking acute stroke may be observed in various inherited channelopathies, including primary episodic ataxia. This autosomal dominant condition involves mutations of voltage-gated potassium and calcium channels, both of which are prevalent in the cerebellum. Dysfunction of the cerebellum predominates the clinical picture, in the form of episodic ataxia and imbalance. Progressive ataxia is often observed as well. Episodic ataxia type 1 includes brief attacks (minutes or less) and is distinguished by myokymia (fine repetitive muscle movements) persisting between episodes.[59,60] Episodic ataxia type 2 commonly involves attacks persisting for hours, with other symptoms that may be confused for posterior circulation infarction, including vertigo, nystagmus, nausea, and emesis. Both types generally present before age 20, a fact that may be helpful in distinguishing from stroke. Although a family history may aid in the diagnosis, spontaneous mutations may cause either type of episodic ataxia.[59]

Other inherited channelopathies can result in sudden, transient episodes of paralysis that may potentially be mistaken for acute stroke. Hypokalemic periodic paralysis involves variable severity of paralysis following high carbohydrate meals, stress, and rest following exercise. Its cause involves mutations in calcium channels, or less commonly, sodium channels. Hyperkalemic periodic paralysis, a sodium channelopathy, causes similar symptoms, but is triggered by fasting, consumption of potassium, and rest following exercise. It should be noted that both conditions typically cause generalized, flaccid weakness, which is less likely to be confused for an acute ischemic infarction. However, severe cases of hypokalemic periodic paralysis may include bulbar manifestations.[61] This feature combined with the sudden onset of attacks may mislead an examiner to localize a vascular insult to the brainstem.

Thrombolysis in Stroke Mimics and Wake-up Strokes

The American Heart Association and American Stroke Association (AHA/ASA) have established metrics encouraging hospitals to decrease the time to IV alteplase, and concern has been raised that hastened delivery will lead to increased use of thrombolysis in stroke mimics.[62,63] However, a prospective study and meta-analysis in 2015 identified stroke mimics given IV thrombolysis and found significantly lower rates of intracerebral hemorrhage when compared with IV thrombolysis in diagnosed ischemic stroke.[63] A 2017 Swedish study of 48 stroke mimics given IV thrombolysis documented zero cases of symptomatic intracerebral hemorrhage in the stroke mimic group, although given low rates in the stroke cohort, this did not prove to be statistically significant by comparison. Improved functional outcomes were demonstrated in the stroke mimic group at 3 months, although it is worth noting that the patients found to have stroke mimics were significantly younger than those in the ischemic stroke cohort (median age 54 vs 72).[64] The 2018 AHA/ASA guidelines address the relative safety in IV alteplase in stroke mimics, recommending the initiation of IV alteplase in potential stroke mimics as opposed to delaying of treatment in favor of further diagnostic efforts (a class IIa recommendation).[65]

Another important consideration with regards to stroke mimics is the prevalence of unintended stroke mimics in clinic trials of IV thrombolysis. In 2017, a phase 3 trial of the thrombolytic agent tenecteplase showed no benefit in functional outcomes at 3 months when compared with IV alteplase. Although this study was well randomized, it included a high proportion of stroke mimics in the tenecteplase and alteplase trial arms (18% and 17%, respectively). Safety profiles were similar in each trial arm, and the rate of any intracranial hemorrhage was 9% in each group. Perhaps one explanation for the high rate of mimics is the fact that the median National Institutes of Health Stroke Scale (NIHSS) score was 4 in each trial arm, representing mild symptoms. A highly relevant feature of this trial was its inclusion of patients outside of the traditional time window for IV thrombolysis. A subset of patients received tenecteplase with stroke symptoms upon awakening or of unknown time of onset if an MR imaging indicated a mismatch between DWI and FLAIR sequences. This demographic only represented 4% of the patient population in each trial arm, but it may suggest a trend in future studies of IV thrombolysis.[66]

STROKE CHAMELEONS

Less than 10% of ischemic infarcts receive IV alteplase, and fewer still receive endovascular therapy. Stroke chameleons, or ischemic infarctions with signs and symptoms suggestive of another condition, may contribute to delayed recognition or treatment of ischemic infarction (Table 1).[67] It has even been speculated that, given the prevalence of ischemic infarctions, an unusual

presentation of stroke is more likely than a typical presentation of a rare disease.[27] Developing a more detailed understanding of rare stroke syndromes is an important way that neurologists and other clinicians can do their part to improve prompt diagnosis and treatment of ischemic infarcts.

Monoplegia

Isolated monoplegia of an extremity has been documented in both cortical and subcortical infarctions, although it remains a rare presentation of acute stroke.[27,68] Maeder-Ingvar and colleagues[68] published a retrospective study of 4802 patients in a registry of first time strokes, showing that 4.1% suffered a purely motor deficit of the face, arm, or leg. Arm monoplegia was most often due to superficial MCA territory cortical infarction, and face paresis was more likely due to subcortical infarction. The well-described "hand-knob" area located over the precentral gyrus has been recognized as causing isolated hand paresis in the event of stroke to this region.[69,70] Jusufovic and colleagues[71] reported a case of "pseudoperipheral palsy" involving cerebral angiitis with infarction of the hand-knob area resulting in a classic peripheral "claw hand." In addition to a peripheral nervous system disease, monoparesis may commonly be confused for an insult to the spinal cord, or a demyelinating or neuromuscular condition, thus recognition of this chameleon is critical in the acute setting.[72]

With regards to cases of isolated monoparesis, the musculature of the face should be considered as well. Muscles of the upper face receive dual innervation from the cortex of each hemisphere, a fact that commonly aids in differentiating between a peripheral and a central cause of facial weakness.[73] However, it is not always the case that a central lesion spares the upper face. The facial nucleus resides in the pontine tegmentum, and an infarct in the dorsal pons may lead to isolated upper and lower facial weakness, which may be mistaken for Bell's palsy. In contrast, the diagnosis of Bell's palsy may be clarified by several associated symptoms. For example, damage to the facial nerve distal to it branches from the geniculate ganglion interferes with lacrimation, salivation, and sense of taste. Another characteristic feature of Bell's palsy is hyperacusis, resulting from interruption of efferent inputs to the stapedius muscle.[74]

Impaired Cognition

Nonspecific impairments in cognitive function may be difficult to recognize as a manifestation of acute stroke; however, classic syndromes should be unmistakable to the clinician performing a detailed neurologic examination. Josef Gerstmann's[75] hallmark publications described a syndrome of finger agnosia (inability to recognize and differentiate fingers), acalculia (impaired calculation skills), agraphia (impaired writing skills), and right-left disorientation. Now known as Gerstmann syndrome, this constellation of findings localizes to the patient's dominant parieto-occipital lobe. The patient may not volunteer all of these symptoms, and a careful neurologic examination, including tests of writing and calculation skills, is necessary for diagnosis. Balint syndrome is another classically described neurologic disorder that may be confused for a purely psychiatric or ophthalmic condition. It is characterized by impairment of attention to visual phenomena, disability of visual fixation, and "optic ataxia" or discoordination of purposeful eye movements.[76] This presentation is associated with bilateral infarction of the posterior parietal cortices.[77]

Nonspecific memory impairment may also be mistaken for a component of delirium or dementia. However, memory impairment may manifest in strokes involving the PCA territory and including the hippocampus, often associated with other PCA deficits such as visual impairment.[78] An important stroke chameleon is that of isolated amnesia, which may masquerade as an acute delirium. In a case series on amnestic strokes, Ott and Saver[79] included 2 patients where amnesia was the sole neurologic deficit: one with involvement of left anteromesial temporal lobe (AChA territory) and another with accompanying anomia that was due to infarction of the left anterior thalamus (tuberothalamic artery).

An occlusion of the basilar artery demonstrates a highly variable presentation dependent on the location and extent of occlusion, and the symptom profile may mask the diagnosis of this potentially life-threatening condition. Occlusions of a proximal segment of the basilar artery may result in locked-in syndrome from infarction of a large territory of the ventral pons. Alternatively, occlusions of the distal segment of the basilar artery may cause a condition known as top of the basilar syndrome, marked by symptoms such as somnolence, agitation, cortical blindness, and hemianopia. Decreased level of alertness is commonly seen in this syndrome due to involvement of the paramedian tegmental gray matter and may be confused for disorders such as metabolic encephalopathies.[80] A similar impairment in consciousness may be observed with bilateral thalamic infarctions, a rare clinical entity due

to an anatomic variant termed the artery of Percheron. This variant includes a single branch supplying bilateral thalamic regions that stems from one PCA. In addition to mental status changes, this condition may include dysarthria, motor impairment, and cerebellar signs.[81]

Complicating matters further is the fact that posterior circulation infarctions may include a prodrome of symptoms, such as nausea and vertigo, that occur for days or even months before stroke onset.[82] Strokes and TIAs are characteristically sudden in onset, whereas migraines with aura may include gradual and protracted symptoms.[83] Given these clinical challenges, concern has been raised regarding the time to IV thrombolysis in posterior circulation infarctions. In a cross-sectional study of 252 patients treated with IV alteplase, Sarraj and colleagues[84] identified 31 (12%) posterior circulation strokes. The median NIHSS score was 6 for posterior circulation strokes, significantly lower than the median score of 13 for strokes of anterior circulation. The mean door-to-needle time was significantly longer ($P = .003$) for those with posterior circulation strokes (90 minutes) versus anterior circulation (74 minutes). The investigators also showed statistically significant differences regarding delay in neurologic evaluation between these cohorts, which in part may be explained by dissimilar NIHSS scores between groups.[84]

Seizurelike Activity

Nonepileptic hyperkinetic movements, including hemiballism, asterixis, and limb-shaking, have been described in acute stroke and may be mistaken for focal seizures or underlying movement disorders.[85] Limb-shaking TIAs have been documented in the setting of severe steno-occlusive disease of the contralateral internal carotid artery. The resolution of symptoms with carotid endarterectomy has established further evidence for the existence of this condition.[86] One case report identifies a presentation of limb-shaking TIA involving electromyographically confirmed asterixis, and later resolved with carotid stenting.[87]

In 1993, Donnan and colleagues[88] characterized fluctuating episodes of focal deficits in the arm, face, and leg, which they termed "capsular warning syndrome." In their study, 42% of patients developed capsular stroke. When capsular warning syndrome involves pure sensory deficits, it can even mimic the classic Jacksonian march characteristic of focal seizures. Caporale and colleagues[89] reported a case involving transient episodes of numbness and tingling starting on the right foot and progressing to include the right arm. This patient was asymptomatic between episodes and treated with seizure medications for presumed Jacksonian march phenomenon. However, a subsequent episode included right-sided weakness, and the patient was found to have an infarct in the posterior limb of the left internal capsule. A troubling aspect of this case was that the patient had no vascular risk factors to suggest that a cerebrovascular event should be high on the list of differential diagnoses.

Atypical movements mimicking seizures can also be observed in brainstem infarctions. Saposnik and Caplan[90] reported a case of a 72-year-old man with sudden onset of impaired level of alertness and witnessed convulsions. On presentation to the Emergency Department, the patient was noted to have episodic upper limb jerking movements and later found to have a right pontine infarct as well as basilar artery occlusion. An EEG showed no epileptiform discharges. Saposnik and Caplan[90] then compiled several case series of pontine strokes, concluding that, of the reports documenting seizure-like activity, 66 of 287 (23%) pontine strokes showed convulsive-appearing movements.

SUMMARY

An accurate diagnosis of ischemic stroke relies on a detailed history and neurologic examination, which should not be compromised in attempts to reduce time to administration of IV alteplase. Stroke chameleons with nonspecific symptoms, such as nausea, vomiting, and decreased mentation, pose a particular challenge in the triaging of patients in the emergency room. However, such cases often present with additional neurologic findings (nystagmus, ataxia, motor deficits) that localize to a particular vascular territory.[77] Although the timing of symptom onset is often useful in distinguishing strokes (rapid onset) from mimics such as migraines (gradual onset),[83] the authors have demonstrated several exceptions to this general principle. A careful consideration of vascular risk factors may guide a clinician's index of suspicion; however, this too may be misleading in many stroke mimics and chameleons. Attention to subtleties of the neurologic examination and listening closely to patients remain critical for both diagnostic accuracy and development of sound clinical judgment.

REFERENCES

1. Fonseca AC. Transient ischemic attacks and stroke mimics and chameleons. In: Biller J, Ferro JM, editors. Common pitfalls in cerebrovascular disease: case-based learning. Cambridge (England): Cambridge University Press; 2015. p. 1–12.

2. Artto V, Putaala J, Strbian D, et al. Stroke mimics and intravenous thrombolysis. Ann Emerg Med 2012;59: 27–32.

3. Quenardelle V, Lauer-ober V, Zinchenko I, et al. Stroke mimics in a stroke care pathway based on MRI screening. Cerebrovasc Dis 2016;42(3–4): 205–12.

4. Huff JS. Stroke mimics and chameleons. Emerg Med Clin North Am 2002;20(3):583–95.

5. Kim BJ, Kang HG, Kim HJ, et al. Magnetic resonance imaging in acute ischemic stroke treatment. J Stroke 2014;16(3):131–45.

6. Makin SD, Doubal FN, Dennis MS, et al. Clinically confirmed stroke with negative diffusion-weighted imaging magnetic resonance imaging: longitudinal study of clinical outcomes, stroke recurrence, and systematic review. Stroke 2015;46(11): 3142–8.

7. Doubal FN, Dennis MS, Wardlaw JM. Characteristics of patients with minor ischaemic strokes and negative MRI: a cross-sectional study. J Neurol Neurosurg Psychiatry 2011;82(5):540–2.

8. Vilela P. Acute stroke differential diagnosis: stroke mimics. Eur J Radiol 2017;96:133–44.

9. Brigo F, Nardone R, Ausserer H, et al. The diagnostic value of urinary incontinence in the differential diagnosis of seizures. Seizure 2013;22(2):85–90.

10. Brigo F, Nardone R, Bongiovanni LG. Value of tongue biting in the differential diagnosis between epileptic seizures and syncope. Seizure 2012; 21(8):568–72.

11. Boulter DJ, Schaefer PW. Stroke and stroke mimics: a pattern-based approach. Semin Roentgenol 2014; 49(1):22–38.

12. Förster A, Griebe M, Gass A, et al. Diffusion-weighted imaging for the differential diagnosis of disorders affecting the hippocampus. Cerebrovasc Dis 2012;33(2):104–15.

13. Chatzikonstantinou A, Gass A, Förster A, et al. Features of acute DWI abnormalities related to status epilepticus. Epilepsy Res 2011;97(1–2):45–51.

14. Anderson CS, Woodward M, Arima H, et al. Statistical analysis plan for evaluating low- vs. standard-dose alteplase in the ENhanced Control of Hypertension and Thrombolysis strokE stuDy (EN-CHANTED). Int J Stroke 2015;10(8):1313–5.

15. Xu Y, Hackett ML, Chalmers J, et al. Frequency, determinants, and effects of early seizures after thrombolysis for acute ischemic stroke: the ENCHANTED trial. Neurol Clin Pract 2017;7(4):324–32.

16. Headache Classification Committee of the International Headache Society (IHS). The International classification of headache disorders, 3rd edition (beta version). Cephalalgia 2013;33(9):629–808.

17. Lioutas VA, Sonni S, Caplan LR. Diagnosis and misdiagnosis of cerebrovascular disease. Curr Treat Options Cardiovasc Med 2013;15(3):276–87.

18. Fisher CM. Late-life migraine accompaniments as a cause of unexplained transient ischemic attacks. Can J Neurol Sci 1980;7(1):9–17.

19. Prencipe M, Casini AR, Ferretti C, et al. Prevalence of headache in an elderly population: attack frequency, disability, and use of medication. J Neurol Neurosurg Psychiatry 2001;70(3):377–81.

20. Vongvaivanich K, Lertakyamanee P, Silberstein SD, et al. Late-life migraine accompaniments: a narrative review. Cephalalgia 2015;35(10):894–911.

21. Guillan M, Defelipe-Mimbrera A, Alonso-Canovas A, et al. The syndrome of transient headache and neurological deficits with cerebrospinal fluid lymphocytosis mimicking an acute stroke. Eur J Neurol 2016;23(7):1235–40.

22. Goldfinch AI, Kleinig TJ. Stroke-like migraine attacks after radiation therapy syndrome: a case report and literature review. Radiol Case Rep 2017;12(3):610–4.

23. Bartleson JD, Krecke KN, O'neill BP, et al. Reversible, strokelike migraine attacks in patients with previous radiation therapy. Neuro Oncol 2003;5(2):121–7.

24. Long B, Koyfman A. Clinical mimics: an emergency medicine-focused review of stroke mimics. J Emerg Med 2017;52(2):176–83.

25. Malouf R, Brust JC. Hypoglycemia: causes, neurological manifestations, and outcome. Ann Neurol 1985;17(5):421–30.

26. Wallis WE, Donaldson I, Scott RS, et al. Hypoglycemia masquerading as cerebrovascular disease (hypoglycemic hemiplegia). Ann Neurol 1985;18(4):510–2.

27. Fernandes PM, Whiteley WN, Hart SR, et al. Strokes: mimics and chameleons. Pract Neurol 2013;13(1):21–8.

28. Magauran BG, Nitka M. Stroke mimics. Emerg Med Clin North Am 2012;30(3):795–804.

29. Maccario M. Neurological dysfunction associated with nonketotic hyperglycemia. Arch Neurol 1968;19(5):525–34.

30. Shah NH, Velez V, Casanova T, et al. Hyperglycemia presenting as left middle cerebral artery stroke: a case report. J Vasc Interv Neurol 2014;7(4):9–12.

31. Daggett P, Deanfield J, Moss F. Neurological aspects of hyponatraemia. Postgrad Med J 1982;58(686):737–40.

32. Wareing W, Dhotore B, Mahawish K. Hyponatraemic encephalopathy: an unusual stroke mimic. BMJ Case Rep 2015;2015 [pii:bcr2014207397].

33. Henry C, Patel N, Shaffer W, et al. Mitochondrial encephalomyopathy with lactic acidosis and strokelike episodes-MELAS syndrome. Ochsner J 2017;17(3):296–301.

34. Sproule DM, Kaufmann P. Mitochondrial encephalopathy, lactic acidosis, and strokelike episodes: basic concepts, clinical phenotype, and therapeutic management of MELAS syndrome. Ann N Y Acad Sci 2008;1142:133–58.

35. Abdelmalik PA, Ambrose T, Bell R. Herpes simplex viral encephalitis masquerading as a classic left MCA stroke. Case Rep Neurol Med 2015;2015:673724.

36. Abduljabbar M, Ghozi I, Haq A, et al. Sudden 'stroke-like' onset of hemiparesis due to herpetic encephalitis. Can J Neurol Sci 1995;22(4):320–1.

37. Craig S. Phenytoin poisoning. Neurocrit Care 2005;3(2):161–70.

38. Hwang WJ, Tsai JJ. Acute phenytoin intoxication: causes, symptoms, misdiagnoses, and outcomes. Kaohsiung J Med Sci 2004;20(12):580–5.

39. Brostoff JM, Birns J, Mccrea D. Phenytoin toxicity: an easily missed cause of cerebellar syndrome. J Clin Pharm Ther 2008;33(2):211–4.

40. Walker RW, Allen JC, Rosen G, et al. Transient cerebral dysfunction secondary to high-dose methotrexate. J Clin Oncol 1986;4(12):1845–50.

41. Appa AA, Jain R, Rakita RM, et al. Characterizing cefepime neurotoxicity: a systematic review. Open Forum Infect Dis 2017;4(4):ofx170.

42. Fernández-Torre JL, Agirre Z, Martínez-martínez M, et al. Subacute encephalopathy with seizures in alcoholics (SESA syndrome): report of an unusual case. Clin EEG Neurosci 2006;37(3):215–8.

43. Preçi G, Vyshka G. Alcohol abuse and seizures: an overview of clinical notions and pathogenetic theories. International Journal of Clinical and Experimental Neurology 2014;2(1):4–7.

44. Liu X, Almast J, Ekholm S. Lesions masquerading as acute stroke. J Magn Reson Imaging 2013;37(1):15–34.

45. Guillan M, Alonso-canovas A, Garcia-caldentey J, et al. Off-label intravenous thrombolysis in acute stroke. Eur J Neurol 2012;19(3):390–4.

46. Brouwer MC, Coutinho JM, Van de beek D. Clinical characteristics and outcome of brain abscess: systematic review and meta-analysis. Neurology 2014;82(9):806–13.

47. Tarnutzer AA, Berkowitz AL, Robinson KA, et al. Does my dizzy patient have a stroke? A systematic review of bedside diagnosis in acute vestibular syndrome. CMAJ 2011;183(9):E571–92.

48. Kattah JC, Talkad AV, Wang DZ, et al. HINTS to diagnose stroke in the acute vestibular syndrome: three-step bedside oculomotor examination more sensitive than early MRI diffusion-weighted imaging. Stroke 2009;40(11):3504–10.

49. Charidimou A, Gang Q, Werring DJ. Sporadic cerebral amyloid angiopathy revisited: recent insights into pathophysiology and clinical spectrum. J Neurol Neurosurg Psychiatry 2012;83(2):124–37.

50. Finelli PF. Cerebral amyloid angiopathy as cause of convexity SAH in elderly. Neurologist 2010;16(1):37–40.

51. Gao B, Lyu C, Lerner A, et al. Controversy of posterior reversible encephalopathy syndrome: what have we learnt in the last 20 years? J Neurol Neurosurg Psychiatry 2017;0:1–7.

52. Mckinney AM, Short J, Truwit CL, et al. Posterior reversible encephalopathy syndrome: incidence of atypical regions of involvement and imaging findings. AJR Am J Roentgenol 2007;189(4):904–12.

53. Bartynski WS. Posterior reversible encephalopathy syndrome, part 2: controversies surrounding pathophysiology of vasogenic edema. AJNR Am J Neuroradiol 2008;29(6):1043–9.

54. Lacour A, De seze J, Revenco E, et al. Acute aphasia in multiple sclerosis: a multicenter study of 22 patients. Neurology 2004;62(6):974–7.

55. Yates TJ, Crawley F. Paroxysmal symptoms in multiple sclerosis masquerading as transient ischaemic attacks. BMJ Case Rep 2010;2010 [pii: bcr0320102831].

56. Pittock SJ, Debruyne J, Krecke KN, et al. Chronic lymphocytic inflammation with pontine perivascular enhancement responsive to steroids (CLIPPERS). Brain 2010;133(9):2626–34.

57. Tobin WO, Guo Y, Krecke KN, et al. Diagnostic criteria for chronic lymphocytic inflammation with pontine perivascular enhancement responsive to steroids (CLIPPERS). Brain 2017;140(9):2415–25.

58. Shaik S, Ul-haq MA, Emsley HC. Myasthenia gravis as a 'stroke mimic'–it's all in the history. Clin Med (Lond) 2014;14(6):640–2.

59. Jen JC, Graves TD, Hess EJ, et al. Primary episodic ataxias: diagnosis, pathogenesis and treatment. Brain 2007;130(Pt 10):2484–93.

60. Graves TD, Cha YH, Hahn AF, et al. Episodic ataxia type 1: clinical characterization, quality of life and genotype-phenotype correlation. Brain 2014;137(Pt 4):1009–18.

61. Statland J, Phillips L, Trivedi JR. Muscle channelopathies. Neurol Clin 2014;32(3):801–15.

62. Leifer D, Bravata DM, Connors JJ, et al. Metrics for measuring quality of care in comprehensive stroke centers: detailed follow-up to Brain Attack Coalition comprehensive stroke center recommendations: a statement for healthcare professionals from the American Heart Association/American Stroke Association. Stroke 2011;42(3):849–77.

63. Tsivgoulis G, Zand R, Katsanos AH, et al. Safety of intravenous thrombolysis in stroke mimics: prospective 5-year study and comprehensive meta-analysis. Stroke 2015;46(5):1281–7.

64. Kostulas N, Larsson M, Kall TB, et al. Safety of thrombolysis in stroke mimics: an observational cohort study from an urban teaching hospital in Sweden. BMJ Open 2017;7(10):e016311.

65. Powers WJ, Rabinstein AA, Ackerson T, et al. 2018 guidelines for the early management of patients with acute ischemic stroke: a guideline for healthcare professionals from the American Heart Association/American Stroke Association. Stroke 2018;49(3):e46–110.

66. Logallo N, Novotny V, Assmus J, et al. Tenecteplase versus alteplase for management of acute ischaemic stroke (NOR-TEST): a phase 3, randomised, open-label, blinded endpoint trial. Lancet Neurol 2017;16(10):781–8.

67. Chompoopong P, Rostambeigi N, Kassar D, et al. Are we overlooking stroke chameleons? A retrospective study on the delayed recognition of stroke patients. Cerebrovasc Dis 2017;44(1–2):83–7.

68. Maeder-Ingvar M, Van melle G, Bogousslavsky J. Pure monoparesis: a particular stroke subgroup? Arch Neurol 2005;62(8):1221–4.

69. Yousry TA, Schmid UD, Alkadhi H, et al. Localization of the motor hand area to a knob on the precentral gyrus. A new landmark. Brain 1997;120:141–57.

70. Peters N, Müller-Schunk S, Freilinger T, et al. Ischemic stroke of the cortical "hand knob" area: stroke mechanisms and prognosis. J Neurol 2009;256(7):1146–51.

71. Jusufovic M, Lygren A, Aamodt AH, et al. Pseudoperipheral palsy: a case of subcortical infarction imitating peripheral neuropathy. BMC Neurol 2015;15:151.

72. Saguil A. Evaluation of the patient with muscle weakness. Am Fam Physician 2005;71(7):1327–36.

73. Gilden DH. Clinical practice. Bell's Palsy. N Engl J Med 2004;351(13):1323–31.

74. Agarwal R, Manandhar L, Saluja P, et al. Pontine stroke presenting as isolated facial nerve palsy mimicking Bell's palsy: a case report. J Med Case Rep 2011;5:287.

75. Gerstmann J. Syndrome of finger agnosia, disorientation for right and left, agraphia and acalculia local diagnostic value. Arch NeurPsych 1940;44(2):398–408.

76. Hecaen H, De Ajuriaguerra J. Balint's syndrome (psychic paralysis of visual fixation) and its minor forms. Brain 1954;77(3):373–400.

77. Andersen RA, Andersen KN, Hwang EJ, et al. Optic ataxia: from Balint's syndrome to the parietal reach region. Neuron 2014;81(5):967–83.

78. Szabo K, Förster A, Jäger T, et al. Hippocampal lesion patterns in acute posterior cerebral artery stroke: clinical and MRI findings. Stroke 2009;40(6):2042–5.

79. Ott BR, Saver JL. Unilateral amnesic stroke. Six new cases and a review of the literature. Stroke 1993;24(7):1033–42.

80. Mattle HP, Arnold M, Lindsberg PJ, et al. Basilar artery occlusion. Lancet Neurol 2011;10(11):1002–14.

81. Arauz A, Patiño-Rodríguez HM, Vargas-González JC, et al. Clinical spectrum of artery of Percheron infarct: clinical-radiological correlations. J Stroke Cerebrovasc Dis 2014;23(5):1083–8.

82. Demel SL, Broderick JP. Basilar occlusion syndromes: an update. Neurohospitalist 2015;5(3): 142–50.

83. Hawkes CH, Swift TR, Sethi KD. Instant neurological diagnosis, a companion to neurobowl. New York: Oxford University Press; 2016.

84. Sarraj A, Medrek S, Albright K, et al. Posterior circulation stroke is associated with prolonged door-to-needle time. Int J Stroke 2015;10(5):672–8.

85. Ghika-Schmid F, Ghika J, Regli F, et al. Hyperkinetic movement disorders during and after acute stroke: the Lausanne Stroke Registry. J Neurol Sci 1997; 146(2):109–16.

86. Baquis GD, Pessin MS, Scott RM. Limb shaking: a carotid TIA. Stroke 1985;16:444–8.

87. Yoon Y, Kim JS. Limb-shaking TIA: an asterixis. Neurology 2013;81(10):931–2.

88. Donnan GA, O'malley HM, Quang L, et al. The capsular warning syndrome: pathogenesis and clinical features. Neurology 1993;43(5):957–62.

89. Caporale CM, Notturno F, Caulo M, et al. Capsular warning syndrome mimicking a jacksonian sensory march. J Neurol Sci 2009;285(1–2):262–4.

90. Saposnik G, Caplan LR. Convulsive-like movements in brainstem stroke. Arch Neurol 2001; 58(4):654–7.

Telestroke

Nina J. Solenski, MD

KEYWORDS

- Telestroke • Telemedicine • Teleradiology • Acute ischemic stroke
- Prehospital telestroke evalution • PACs • Rural telestroke • Head CT

KEY POINTS

- Teleradiology plays a fundamental role in telestroke programs.
- Models of telestroke care differ significantly in purpose, and design with both current mobile, and fixed videoconferencing options.
- Technology software and hardware applications for prehospital telestroke programs are rapidly evolving and in the initial stages of being broadly implemented nationally.
- Rural and underserved communities need assistance to overcome information technology challenges for unlimited access to computed tomography (CT) and CT angiogram.
- Prehospital telestroke programs are growing in volume and hold promise in the future for reducing stroke burden if the cost/benefit ratio can be reduced.

OVERVIEW OF THE CURRENT STATE OF TELESTROKE

Introduction——US System of Care

Telestroke is the delivery of live 2-way vascular neurology consultations using a telecommunications infrastructure, such as a secure telephone, radio, or videoconferencing platform. As far back as the turn of the century, some form of telemedicine has existed; for example, in the 1860s, telegraphy communicated information about medical supplies and casualty lists concerning US civil war victims. In the 1950s, telemedicine was vital to the early success of the US National Aeronautics and Space Administration program, providing critical remote monitoring of astronaut physiology in space. In contrast, telestroke originated fairly recently, approximately 3 decades ago, with the first reports in the late 1980s and 1990s.[1–4] One of the earliest published programs, TeleBAT, was implemented at the University of Maryland using radio-transmitted information from emergency medical services (EMS) ambulances to the receiving hospital.[1,5]

The concept of using telemedicine for stroke first appeared in the late 1990's as data accumulated demonstrating that telestroke programs could increase access to tissue plasminogen activator (t-PA) thrombolytic treatment in a safe manner.[3,4] Early pioneers in the field, including Lamont, Schwamm, Levine, Hess, Meyer, Wechsler, and others, provided important milestones in the development of telestroke programs.[6–11] Importantly this included clinical research data proving that an in-person National Institutes of Health (NIH) Stroke Scale was equivalent to that done by videoconferencing.[9] They and many other experts in the field over the past 2 decades have further published evidenced-based telestroke guidelines and telestroke quality-care benchmarks to guide current telestroke systems of care.[12,13] At the time of this publication, as a consequence of proven quality care and increased reimbursement for telestroke care, there are an estimated 200 or more telestroke programs implemented throughout the United States. These programs are in addition to the many innovative telestroke programs operating internationally in France,

Disclosures: None.

Department of Neurology, University of Virginia School of Medicine, University of Virginia Health System, PO Box 800394, Hospital Drive, Charlottesville, VA 22908, USA

E-mail address: nsolenski@virginia.edu

Neuroimag Clin N Am 28 (2018) 551–563
https://doi.org/10.1016/j.nic.2018.06.012
1052-5149/18/Published by Elsevier Inc.

Germany, United Kingdom, Ireland, Scandinavia, Australia, New Zealand, and many other countries across the world.

Telestroke Models of Care

The most prevalent care model is the hub and spoke. The hub may be an affiliated or nonaffiliated central major hospital, which provides telestroke consultation to multiple usually smaller hospitals, devoid of neurology or neurosurgical services. Different types of telestroke models have emerged to meet the demands of unique hospital environments (Box 1).

The Digital Imaging and Communications in Medicine (DICOM) server is essential for rapid remote viewing of the vital noncontrast CT (NCCT) of the head obtained during the telestroke consult (Fig. 1). Rapid review is critical to rule out any contraindication for intra-arterial thrombolysis with t-PA, such as hemorrhage or metastatic brain malignancy, and to identify any conditions mimicking focal neurologic deficits (abscess or mass, for example). A growing number of telestroke hospitals are capable of performing head and neck CT angiogram, which provides further vital data on location of any retrievable

clots for potential thrombectomy interventional procedures.

The critical workflow for acute stroke telestroke programs, as seen in Fig. 2, includes

1. Prehospital patient EMS transfer (videoconferencing can begin here)
2. Spoke hospital emergency department (ED) rapid patient evaluation
3. Acute telestroke alert (CT, nursing, pharmacy, remote teleneurologist alerted)
4. Rapid acquisition of a NCCT, and in some cases a head and neck CT angiogram
5. Remote teleneurologist evaluation
6. EMS transfer to hub or other hospital, in cases requiring higher level of care (videoconferencing can continue during transfer)

The phrase, drip and ship, refers to the transfer of an acute stroke patient after intravenous (IV) t-PA to a hospital with neurocritical expertise and the ability to perform additional neuroradiological, neurointerventional or neurosurgical procedures as needed. The phrase, door in to door out, refers to the component of acute stroke continuum of care during the initial telespoke ED evaluation, with the goal of streamlining all processes to minimize time, including transfer times of the patient to any higher level of care (see Fig. 2).

The principal duties of the telestroke consultant typically include obtaining a brief case summary from ED provider (phone or audiovisual [AV] link); reviewing any initial brain imaging, typically the NCCT; and establishing a secure remote live 2-way interactive AV link with the patient. The teleneurologist swiftly obtains a brief medical history, reviewing key elements of time of last known well, determines the NIH Stroke Scale score with the assistance of a bedside nurse, and determines eligibility for IV t-PA or other acute stroke treatments. These tasks must be accomplished within 45 minutes or less from the patient arrival to the telespoke ED. They may be further evaluation for thrombectomy candidacy or preparation for transfer to a higher level of care.

Box 1
Common telestroke models

- Hub and spoke within a single health care system
- Hub and spoke with external sites
  - Hub may be academic center, or a private neurology group practice
- Horizontal hubless network
  - Interconnected multisites usually within 1 hospital setting for on call clinical coverage purposes
- Third-party hub distributed model
  - For-profit business frequently serving multistate sites with teleneurologist consulting from location in the United States
- Supervisory training model
  - Academic-based institution with "multipoint" teleneurology platform, which allows supervising physicians to assist trainees within the hospital setting, such as during acute stroke calls in the ED, in a neurocritical care setting (for placement of lines, or during cardiac or neurology code situations)

Brief Telestroke Technical Overview

Most telestroke systems consist of a remote AV conferencing cart with a secure high-speed broadband connection, a pan-tilt and zoom-capable high-definition camera, and the ability to transmit secure DICOM images via a server. Internet speed with a bandwidth close to 1.2×10^6 bits per second is ideal for high-quality transmission of images and AV conferencing.

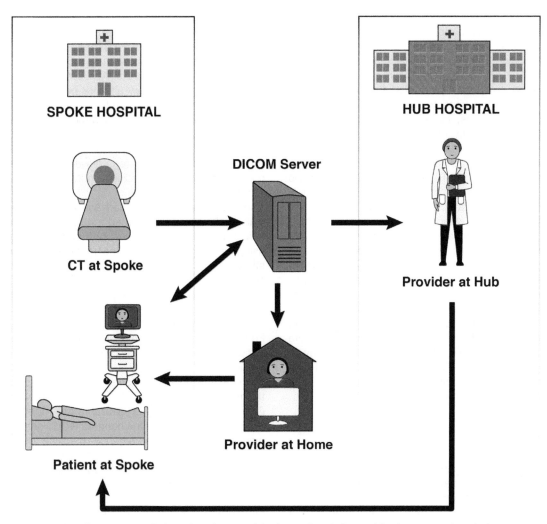

Fig. 1. Graphic illustrating a "hub and spoke" model. The patient is located in the remote hospital emergency department with a videoconferencing system (cart) set up at the bedside. The remote teleprovider may be located at the hub hospital, at home, or with mobile devices in a car or any environment with secure Wi-Fi or Internet web connection. The DICOM server is critical for the rapid transfer of images from the remote PAC system to the hub PAC system to facilitate the critical review by the teleneurologist and by the teleradiologist.

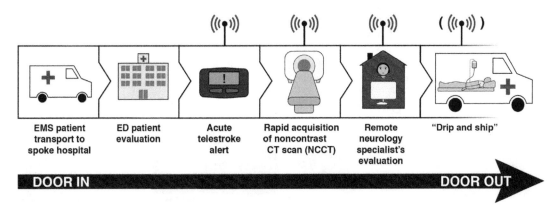

Fig. 2. Summary graphic of the acute stroke continuum of care. The "Door In to Door Out" or "DIDO" refers to minimizing the time from entry of the patient into the remote ED to departure. All processes must be streamlined to ensure a less than 45–60 minutes DIDO time. This entails rapidly evaluating, treating, and transferring to a higher level of care when appropriate.

Commercial vendors offer a wide variety of Food and Drug Administration (FDA)-approved Health Insurance Portability and Accountability Act of 1996 (HIPAA)-compliant clinical videoconferencing equipment platforms. Equipment ranges from desktop units to fixed, mobile, or robotic carts to laptops, tablets, and smartphone endpoints (Fig. 3). In addition, there are various and emerging telemedicine software solutions that offer integration of the video into the electronic medical record (EMR), acute stroke software tools (a timer, NIH Stroke Scale, and calculation of the t-PA dose, for example), and direct viewing of any neuroimaging without accessing the remote EMR. Some software programs offer secure multipoint connections, allowing multiple providers to simultaneously access the videoconference to facilitate live communicate with the teleneurologist, the patient, and/or the ED staff. This application allows the endovascular specialist to discuss the case in real time with the ED physician, patient, and/or neurologist. With the expanding acute stroke therapeutic window for thrombectomy of up to 24 hours, rapid multidisciplinary real-time communication and image sharing are fast becoming the standard.

THE CRITICAL ROLE OF TELERADIOLOGY IN STROKE CARE

Teleradiology systems became commercially available in the 1980s, but their low performance rates and high costs prevented widespread adoption.[14,15] By the early to mid-1990s with the advent of the Internet and of the picture archiving and communications system (PACS), teleradiology advanced to its current state of widespread use.[13,14] For telestroke programs, it became one of the most critical components of remote acute stroke care, and American Heart Association/American Stroke Association acute stroke guidelines strongly support FDA-approved teleradiology services for acute stroke care.[16] With teleradiology, neurologists are able to have rapid outside radiology interpretation of a patient's NCCT or have direct access to the images. Most teleneurologists favor direct interpretation (in addition to an outside interpretation) of a patient's NCCT. Ideally, using shared PAC systems, a teleneurologist can also view all prior neuroimaging studies for direct comparison to the new images.

Data support excellent agreement over the presence or absence of radiological contraindications to t-PA thrombolysis of acute stroke patient CT scan images, regardless if they were read by a telestroke physician, neuroradiologist, or radiologist.[17]

In 2009, the American Heart Association/American Stroke Association issued a statement of their results from an expert review of the evidence for using telestroke services for the treatment of acute stroke patients. In terms of using teleradiology services, they concluded that there was an overwhelmingly high degree of evidence supporting FDA-approved teleradiology services for emergency radiology interpretation (Box 2). Furthermore, the use of mobile devices as a teleradiology platform has also been validated in some studies.[18] One study evaluated the sensitivity and specificity of interpretation of NCCT with subtle hemorrhage using iPad 2 (Apple, Cupertino, California) tablets versus clinical-grade monitors (liquid crystal display). One hundred NCCT studies were evaluated by 5 emergency medicine physicians (50 on the tablet and 50 on the monitor). The data revealed that there was equally high sensitivity and specificity using either device. As artificial intelligence, big data analysis, and faster quantum computers are rapidly developed, it is not difficult to imagine a future of automated algorithmic NCCT interpretations.

Using selected software applications, smartphone and mobile tablet devices can be used to review acute stroke imaging without the image being stored in the device, which enhances protected health information security. One client-server teleradiology system, ResolutionMD (Calgary Scientific Inc, Calgary, Canada), was tested in a retrospective study of NCCT images of patients with acute stroke. Two

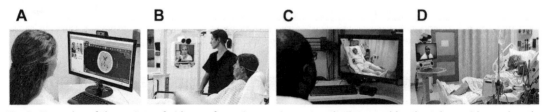

Fig. 3. Examples of the variety of videoconferencing equipment endpoints used by the teleprovider and at the remote site. The provider may use a dedicated HIPAA compliant videoconferencing station, a laptop, desktop, or tablet-based computer (A, C). The remote patient and staff may interact though a mobile cart system placed at the foot of the bed (D) or a fixed endpoint (B).

<table>
<tbody>
<tr><td>

Box 2

Class I recommendations for the use of teleradiology for acute stroke evaluation

1. Teleradiology systems approved by the FDA (or equivalent organization) are recommended for timely review of brain CT scans in patients with suspected acute stroke (class I, level of evidence A).

2. Review of brain CT scans by stroke specialists or radiologists using teleradiology systems approved by the FDA (or equivalent organization) is useful for identifying exclusions for thrombolytic therapy in acute stroke patients (class I, level of evidence A).

3. When implemented within a telestroke network, teleradiology systems approved by the FDA (or equivalent organization) can be effective in supporting rapid imaging interpretation in time for thrombolysis decision making (class I, level of evidence B).

Data from Schwamm LH, Holloway RG, Amarenco P, et al. A review of the evidence for the use of telemedicine within stroke systems of care: a scientific statement from the American Heart Association/American Stroke Association. Stroke 2009;40(7):2616–34.

</td></tr>
</tbody>
</table>

neuroradiologists read the images, one on a medical diagnostic workstation and the other on an iOS device[19,20] (Fig. 4). CT head interpretations of telestroke network patients by vascular neurologists using ResolutionMD on smartphones, were in excellent agreement with interpretations by spoke radiologists using a PAC system station and with those of independent telestroke adjudicators using a desktop viewer. The investigators reported that the sensitivity, specificity, and accuracy of detecting intraparenchymal hemorrhage were each 100% using the iOS device.[20]

Stroke-specific CT and MR imaging analytical image mapping software programs are assisting teleneurologists and endovascular physicians in selecting patients for possible thrombectomy treatment. The automated quantitative RAPID software (iSchemaView, Menlo Park, California) can compute the CT and MR imaging perfusion mismatch, and the Alberta Stroke Program Early CT Score (ASPECTS)[21,22] (Fig. 5). The ASPECTS determines the extent of early ischemic changes on the NCCT on a scale of 1 to 10, with a higher score (≥8) predicting worse outcome.[21,22] This FDA-approved CT and MR imaging analytical tool and the ASPECTS calculation have been shown in multiple trials to successfully select those patients with salvageable brain tissue and, therefore, will have better outcomes from large

vessel thrombectomy.[20–27] The analytical data EW swiftly sent globally to secure text paging mobile devices of the entire acute stroke team expediting treatment decisions for the potential thrombectomy candidate. In the carefully selected subgroup of stroke patients that qualify, thrombectomy after IV t-PA can significantly further improve outcome. Patients enrolled in the DAWN (DWI or CTP Assessment With Clinical Mismatch in the Triage of Wake Up and Late Presenting Strokes Undergoing Neurointervention With Trevo) trial (2016) achieved a 73% chance of significant recovery.[24]

Imaging Network Integration in Rural Communities

Approximately 25% of US hospitals (2018) are known as *critical access hospitals* (CAHs), with a maximum of 25 beds. As of April 2016, there were 1332 critical access hospitals in the United States, of which approximately 25% were accredited by The Joint Commission (see https://www.ruralhealthinfo.org).

They frequently perform as stroke-ready hospitals but may not seek formal stroke care accreditation due to financial costs or lack of resources for rigorous required data processing. Instead by contracting for telestroke services, they are capable of evaluating acute stroke patients, administrating IV t-PA, and rapidly transferring patients within their communities to a higher stroke care facility (drip-and-ship transfers). Telestroke services, however, require active and rigorous quality initiative telespoke programs to ensure clinical benchmarks for timely care are met similar to those in the treating hospital hubs.[28]

Rural regions of the United States have greatly benefited from telestroke services. Telestroke programs for the past 20 years have been increasing access to IV t-PA and improving small hospital cost margins by keeping patients in their communities rather than initiating unnecessary transfers.[29] Radiology resources for evaluation of acute stroke are limited, however, and usually consist of only a head CT scanner, with challenges manning the CT scanner 24 hours a day/365 days a year. Approximately 3 of every 100 ED visits to the rural CAH required transfer for higher level of care, with approximately three-quarters of noncardiac transferred patients having a positive imaging finding related to the reason for transfer.[30]

Multiple US federal programs, such as the Federal Communications Commission, Department of Agriculture, Office for the Advancement of Telehealth, and the Health Resources and Services

Administration are dedicated to funding broadband services to rural and underserved communities. Despite this infrastructure assistance, CAHs still suffer from more Internet outages, high costs for cloud storage or EMR integration applications, and the ability to hire and retain highly qualified IT personnel.

A CAH or small rural community hospital's low-resource state, coupled with a recent demand to evaluate every potential acute stroke patient not only for IV t-PA but also for thrombectomy candidacy, is creating a dilemma for EMS triage decision making in the field. Solutions include development of sophisticated Geographical Information System mapping/Global Position System–guided applications that can assist an EMS driver (or medical helicopter) by calculating the fastest route with real-time data to select to most appropriate hospital ED. Debates are ongoing to determine if telespoke hospitals should or can be equipped to obtain high-quality CT angiogram images image with standard image mapping data software.

Emergency Medical Services and Telestroke

In the 1990s the Maryland Brain Attack Center's Team developed an innovative telestroke

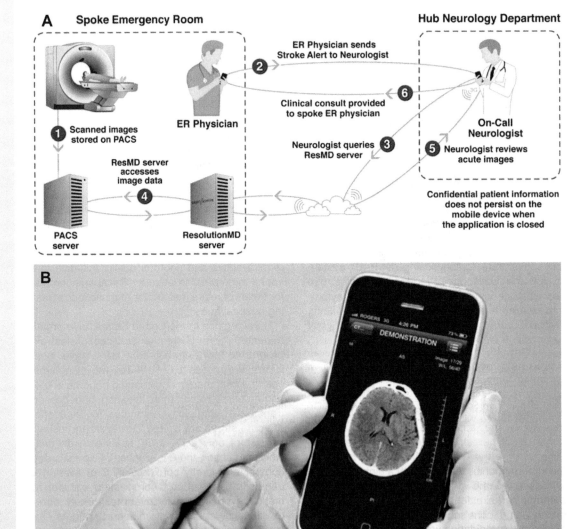

Fig. 4. (A) ResolutionMD software application illustrated on a smartphone. (B) ResolutionMD mobile infrastructure and algorithm. (*From* Demaerschalk BM, Vargas JE, Channer DD, et al. Smartphone teleradiology application is successfully incorporated into a telestroke network environment. Stroke 2012;43:3099; with permission.)

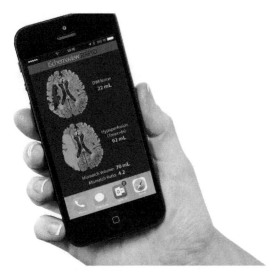

Fig. 5. Quantitative image mapping data (RAPID) is rapidly transmitted to a smart phone assisting the treating physician in deciding which acute stroke patients may benefit from a timely thrombectomy procedure. The ASPECTS is an ordinal scale from 1 to 10, indicating the degree of early ischemic changes; higher scores indicate less edema and better outcome. (*Courtesy of* iSchemaView, Inc, Menlo Park, CA; with permission.)

system.[1,5] The TeleBAT system consisted of an ambulance unit using radio technology to communicate with the hospital base station via a hospital's intranet. Using this system, the NIH Stroke Scale was performed remotely, demonstrating for the first time the feasibility for evaluating prehospital neurologic deficits.

Thirty years later, systems have evolved to incorporate 2-way live streaming patient evaluations during ambulance transport of the acute stroke patient. The rapid evolution to high-fidelity 4G and even 5G cellular connectivity can now support real-time AV streaming en route to conduct remote neurologic screening examinations.[31–35]

By using tablet-based endpoints as a low-cost AV option, there is increasing deployment of prehospital telestroke in both rural and urban EMS networks. Programs, such as the Improving Treatment with Rapid Evaluation of Acute Stroke Via Mobile Telemedicine (iTREAT) study,[36,37] allow rapid prehospital assessment, diminishing the time to obtain a targeted history, review vital sign and medication lists, and perform an NIH Stroke Scale score (Fig. 6). Clinical implementation and additional data collection are ongoing in multiple prehospital telestroke programs, and findings of prospective randomized trials are awaited to determine if stroke outcome is improved and the cost/benefit ratio of any community EMS financial investment incurred versus hospitalization savings.

Prehospital Teleradiology Applications

The faster that t-PA is administered to acute stroke patients (<4.5 hours since last seen normal), the better their outcome. Based on this precept, ambulances in the United States and Europe are being outfitted with modified CT scanners to decrease the time to treatment. Mobile stroke units equipped with a portable CT scanner allow a remote teleneurologist or an on-call neurologist traveling in the ambulance to initiate safe administration of IV t-PA in the field. These units are currently in several US urban centers and in Europe (Fig. 7). Although effective in significantly reducing stroke onset to treatment times, the cost utility remains a barrier to widespread adoption across health systems. Mobile stroke units equipped with fixed or mobile telestroke platforms are also used for prehospital stroke diagnosis and triage for patients with large vessel occlusions to facilities capable of providing endovascular therapy. Whether or not the inevitable scalability can result in significant

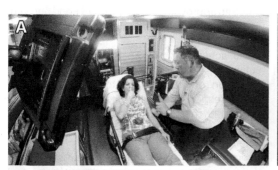 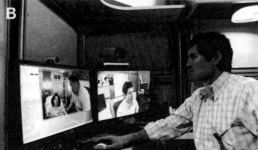

Fig. 6. Prehospital evaluation of the patient in the ambulance by EMS using the iTREAT platform. (*A*) The video-conferencing equipment is mounted on the vehicle wall and the live AV feed is being interpreted by the telestroke neurologist at his office. (*B*) An NIH Stroke Scale is being performed by the EMS provider with verbal guidance and interpretation by the neurologist.

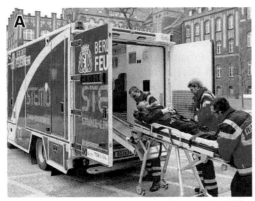
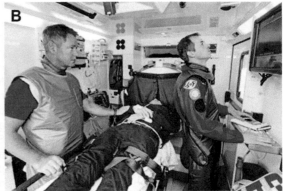

Fig. 7. (*A*) A specialized stroke ambulance (stroke emergency mobile unit) is equipped with AV conferencing capability and with a mobile head CT scanner. (*B*) This allows physicians in Berlin, Germany, to start a prehospital evaluation, including obtaining an NIH Stroke Scale score, and to start specific treatment, such as thrombolysis, at the scene. This is one example of increasing mobile stroke units in the United States and abroad. (*Courtesy of Salynn Boyles; and MEYTEC GmbH Informationssysteme, Seefeld, Germany.*)

cost reduction of CT units per ambulance remains to be seen.

Radiology Challenges in Telestroke

Rapid and accurate reading of the noncontrast CT

The telestroke physician or teleradiologist must quickly assess all noncontrast CT axial images focusing on signs of brain, subdural, or subarachnoid hemorrhage. In addition, surveillance for any hyperdense vessel signs indicating thrombosis or emboli (such as in the middle cerebral arteries or basilar artery or within a branch vessel) (Figs. 8 and 9). A critical evaluation for early or evolving subacute ischemic signs is imperative in decision making for IV t-PA. Approximately 60% of all

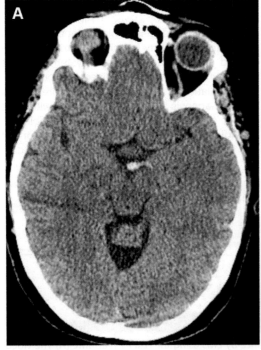
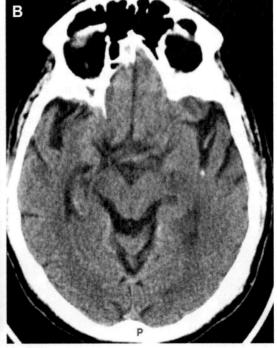

Fig. 8. (*A*) Midline hyperdense basilar artery and proximal left posterior cerebral artery in a patient presenting with vertigo, visual field deficit ataxia, and obtundation. (*B*) Left middle cerebral artery branch occlusion from hyperdense emboli in the temporal insular region.

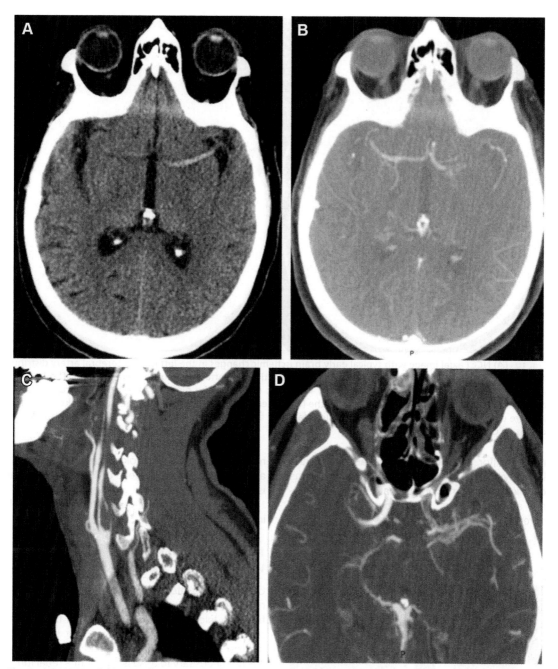

Fig. 9. (*A*) NCCT axial image illustrating a left "dense middle cerebral artery (MCA)" sign with correlation to the intracranial CT-angiogram demonstrating an identical flow void in the left MCA. (*B*) Note the paucity of vessels distant to the left MCA in comparison to the contralateral side. This patient was found to have a dense thrombus at the bifurcation of the cervical internal carotid artery, as seen in the neck magnetic resonance angiogram (*C*). The intracranial magnetic resonance angiogram (*D*) shows the corresponding poor contrast perfusion through the proximal left middle cerebral artery.

cerebral infarctions are seen on an NCCT in the first 3 hours to 6 hours, with overall sensitivity of 64% and specificity of 85%.[38,39] In up to 60%, ischemia in the lentiform nuclei (deep gray-matter nuclei) can be visible in as little as 1 hour

of occlusion. Frank brain tissue hypodensity with edematous changes would be a contraindication for IV t-PA (Fig. 10).

Equally important is to be vigilant to rule out central nervous system stroke mimics, including

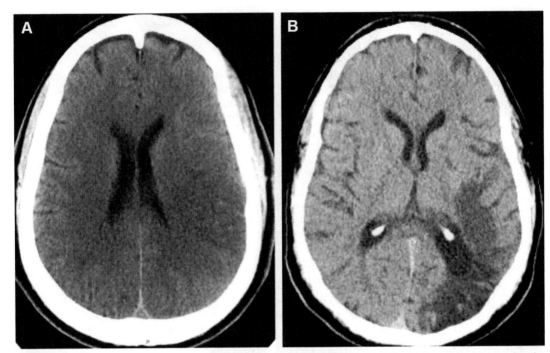

Fig. 10. (A) NCCT axial image with typical early brain ischemic changes in the left middle cerebral artery distribution leading to poor differentiation of the gray-white junction and effacement of the cerebral sulci. The findings are due to initially cellular edema followed by vasogenic edema as the blood-brain barrier is disrupted. Mild developing hypodensity is seen. (B) Over time, the hypoattenuation and swelling become more marked resulting in more distinct regions of evolving irreversible infarction, as seen in the left middle cerebral artery distribution of this NCCT.

masses (for example, tumor, abscess, and large cyst) and vascular abnormalities (such as calcified cavernomas and partially thrombosed giant aneurysm) (Fig. 11). Accurately identifying chronic cerebral infarctions may help diagnosis by suggesting a reactivation syndrome with

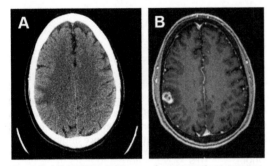

Fig. 11. (A) NCCT axial image from a patient presenting with left hemisensory complaints and mild confusion. The hypoattentuation of the right parietal white matter tracts represent vasogenic edema. (B) The corresponding brain MR imaging with contrast shows a well circumscribed solitary mass in the right parietal cortex with surrounding edema, which could represent an abscess or malignancy.

recrudescence of old stroke signs or symptoms, a frequent masquerader of acute cerebral ischemia.

Table 1 reviews some pearls for reading NCCT images.

The Role of Remote CT Angiogram in Large Vessel Occlusion Triage

Obtaining and interpreting neurovascular intracranial and neck cerebrovascular images obtained from the telespoke, for the purpose of triaging an acute stroke patient for endovascular treatment, can be challenging. Despite good evidence that it is not necessary to assess a patient's renal function prior to administering contrast in the acute stroke setting,[16,40,41] many hospitals still institute this conservative protocol. In too many cases, this can result in up to a 30-minute delay or more waiting for the renal function studies to be processed. Another issue, particularly in hospitals with low stroke volumes, is that rapidly obtaining a CT angiogram may not be feasible due to limited resources or the lack of available trained CT technicians. Lastly, a standard head and neck CT angiogram consists of more than 1000 images, creating a much larger file size, which could take

Table 1
Potential findings on a emergent NCCT for acute stroke

Condition	Pearl
Hemorrhage:	Calcium vs blood—when in doubt, measure Hounsfield units; small cavernomas may be calcified or demonstrate hemosiderin deposits High-density bone creates artifact, particularly in the posterior fossa creating hyperdense streak artifact Calcification of the cerebellar tentorium can appear hyperdense, mimicking subarachnoid hemorrhage
Subarachnoid	Check all ventricular spaces especially posterior horns for possible subacute blood
Intraparenchymal	If atypical hyperdensity pattern, or an unusual location, or bilateral hemorrhages (such as, thalamic), consider cerebral veins or cerebral venous sinuses as the source
Subdural or epidural hematoma	May be subtle—check all axial slices carefully including the uppermost axial cuts
Other—mass	Atypical heterogenous or pattern surrounding edema may represent a hemorrhagic mass, such as tumor, or ischemic hemorrhagic conversion
Cerebral ischemia:	
Early	Sucal effacement (edema), loss of the gray-white junction, obscuration of lentiform nuclei, loss of the insular ribbon Ischemic changes in the cerebellar or brainstem may be difficult to be seen
Subacute	Increasing hypodensity (attenuation) as infarction evolves at ~7–21 d the infarction may appear isodense, known as CT fogging effect
Arteriopathy:	Hyperdense sign of the proximal intracranial vessels may represent clot Look for asymmetry; patients who are dehydrated or have an elevated hematocrit or calcified vessels may have diffuse rather than individual hyperdense appearing proximal vessels Dot sign—on an axial image, a hyperdense middle cerebral artery branch may be clot (rarely can be a calcified embolus)

longer for transmission to external PACs servers or for uploading to a remote physician's viewing device. As discussed previously, the role of cloud-based HIPAA secure server for direct viewing may expand significantly in the future.

The future

The challenges for telestroke and acute teleradiology programs in the future include

- Demonstrating the affordability of using mobile/portable CT scanners through potential scalability, or perhaps developing a new innovative diagnostic modality to distinguish hemorrhagic from ischemic stroke rapidly in the field
- Maximizing broadband Internet speeds and coverage throughout all the United States to allow all EMS units to use prehospital telestroke services
- Guiding the use of artificial intelligence advanced computer programming in teleradiology applications to promote faster, highly accurate interpretations and analysis of the NCCT, head/neck CT angiograph, CT, or brain MR imaging perfusion analysis

Technological solutions will likely develop quickly over the next 5 years to 10 years. Exponential growth in artificial intelligence and machine learning that are automating workflows, health care–centric big data analysis, and the near-future development of the quantum computer are currently being witnessed. Accelerating the development of solutions is the increasing financial pressure from increasing costs for cloud health care data storage, the switch to health care value-based reimbursements, and an insatiable consumer appetite for direct to consumer telemedicine services.

REFERENCES

1. La Monte MP, Cullen J, Gagliano DM, et al. Tele-BAT: mobile telemedicine for the brain attack team. Stroke 1988;29:312.
2. Susman E. Telemedicine to give rural stroke victims fair chance of recovery with new treatment. Telemed Virtual Real 1997;2:1–2.
3. Gagliano D. Wireless ambulance telemedicine may lessen stroke morbidity. Telemed Today 1998;6(1): 22.

4. Shafqat S, Kvedar JC, Guanci MM, et al. Role for telemedicine in acute stroke: feasibility and reliability of remote administration of the NIH stroke scale. Stroke 1999;30(10):2141–5.

5. Lamonte MP, Cullen J, Gagliano DM, et al. TeleBAT: mobile telemedicine for the brain attack team. J Stroke Cerebrovasc Dis 2000;9(3):128–35.

6. Levine SR, Gorman M. Telestroke. Stroke 1999;30: 464–9.

7. Schwamm LH, Rosenthal ES, Hirshberg A, et al. Virtual telestroke support for the emergency department evaluation of acute stroke. Acad Emerg Med 2004;11(11):1193–7.

8. Hess DC, Wang S, Hamilton W, et al. REACH: clinical feasibility of a rural telestroke network. Stroke 2005;36(9):2018–20.

9. Wang S, Lee SB, Pardue C, et al. Remote evaluation of acute ischemic stroke: reliability of national institutes of health stroke scale via telestroke. Stroke 2003;34(10):e188–91.

10. Spokoyny I, Raman R, Ernstrom K, et al. Pooled assessment of computed tomography interpretation by vascular neurologists in the STRokE DOC telestroke network. J Stroke Cerebrovasc Dis 2014; 23(3):511–5.

11. Meyer BC, Raman R, Ernstrom K, et al. Assessment of long-term outcomes for the STRokE DOC telemedicine trial. J Stroke Cerebrovasc Dis 2012;21: 259–64.

12. Schwamm LH, Holloway RG, Amarenco P, et al. A review of the evidence for the use of telemedicine within stroke systems of care: a scientific statement from the American Heart Association/American Stroke Association. Stroke 2009;40(7):2616–34.

13. Wechsler LR, Demaerschalk BM, Schwamm LH, et al. Telemedicine quality and outcomes in stroke: a scientific statement for healthcare professionals from the American Heart Association/American Stroke Association. Stroke 2016;48(1):e3–25.

14. Thrall JH. Teleradiology part I. History and clinical applications1. Radiology 2007;243(3):613–7.

15. Liu Yu, Wang J. PACS and digital medicine: essential principles and modern practice. Boca Raton (FL): CRC Press; 2011. p. 160. Chapter 7-Teleradiology.

16. Powers WJ, Ravinstein AA, Ackderson T, et al. Guidelines for the early management of Patietns with acute ischemic stroke. From the American Heart Association/American Stroke Association. Stroke 2018;49:e1–25.

17. Demaerschalk BM, Bobrow BJ, Raman R, et al. CT interpretation in a telestroke network: agreement among a spoke radiologist, hub vascular neurologist, and hub neuroradiologist. Stroke 2012;43(11):3095–7.

18. Park JB, Choi HJ, Lee JH, et al. An assessment of the iPad 2 as a CT teleradiology tool using brain CT with subtle intracranial hemorrhage under conventional illumination. J Digit Imaging 2013;26: 683–90.

19. Demaerschalk BM, Vargas JE, Channer DD, et al. Smartphone teleradiology application is successfully incorporated into a telestroke network environment. Stroke 2012;43(11):3098–101.

20. Demaerschalk BM, Vegunta S, Vargas BB, et al. Reliability of real-time video smartphone for assessing national institutes of health stroke scale scores in acute stroke patients. Stroke 2012;43(12):3271–7.

21. Barber PA, Demchuk AM, Zhang J, et al. Validity and reliability of a quantitative computed tomography score in predicting outcome of hyperacute stroke before thrombolytic therapy. Lancet 2000; 355(9216):1670–4.

22. Pexman JH, A Barber P. Use of the Alberta Stroke Program Early CT Score (ASPECTS) for assessing CT scans in patients with acute stroke. AJNR Am J Neuroradiol 2001;22:1534–42.

23. Berkhemer O, Fransen PS, Beumer D, et al. A randomized trial of intraarterial treatment for acute ischemic stroke. N Engl J Med 2015;372(4):11–20.

24. Nogueira RG, Jadhav AP, Haussen DC, et al. Thrombectomy 6 to 24 hours after stroke with a mismatch between deficit and infarct. N Engl J Med 2018; 378(1):11–21.

25. Goyal M, Demchuk AM, Menon BK, et al. A randomized assessment of rapid endovascular treatment of ischemic stroke (ESCAPE). N Engl J Med 2015;372:1019–30.

26. Saver J, Goyal M, Bonafe A, et al. "Stent-retriever thrombectomy after intravenous t-PA vs. t-PA alone in stroke. N Engl J Med 2015;372(24):2285–95.

27. Albers GW, Marks MP, Kemp S, et al. "Thrombectomy for stroke at 6 to 16 hours with selection by perfusion imaging. N Engl J Med 2018;378(8):708–18. Available at: http://www.nejm.org/doi/full/10.1056.

28. Solenski NJ, Southerland AS, Shephard T, et al. Improving telestroke performance in rural systems of care - the EQUITe initiative (P6.084). Neurology 2016;86(16 Supplement):P6.084.

29. Hess D. The history and future of telestroke. Nat Rev Neurol 2013;9(6):340–50.

30. Prabhakar AM, Harvey HB, Brinegar KN, et al. Critical access hospital ED to quaternary medical center: successful implementation of an integrated picture archiving and communications system for patient transfers by air and sea. Am J Emerg Med 2016;34(8):1427–30.

31. Audebert HJ, Boy S, Jankovits R, et al. Is mobile teleconsulting equivalent to hospital-based telestroke services? Stroke 2008;39(12):3427–30.

32. Bergrath S, Reich A, Rossaint R, et al. Feasibility of prehospital teleconsultation in acute stroke–a pilot study in clinical routine. PLoS One 2012;7(5): e36796.

33. Liman TG, Winter B, Waldschmidt C, et al. Telestroke ambulances in prehospital stroke management: concept and pilot feasibility study. Stroke 2012; 43(8):2086–90.

34. Van Hooff RJ, Cambron M, Van Dyck R, et al. Prehospital unassisted assessment of stroke severity using telemedicine: a feasibility study. Stroke 2013; 44(10):2907–9.

35. Barrett KM, Pizzi MA, Kesari V, et al. Ambulance-based assessment of NIH stroke scale with telemedicine: a feasibility pilot study. J Telemed Telecare 2016;23(04):476–83.

36. Lippman JM, Smith SN, McMurry TL, et al. Mobile telestroke during ambulance transport is feasible in a rural EMS setting: the iTREAT study. Telemed J E Health 2016;22(6):507–13.

37. Chapman Smith SN, Govindarajan P, Padrick MM, et al. A low-cost, tablet-based option for prehospital neurologic assessment: the iTREAT study. Neurology 2016;87(1):19–26.

38. Wintermark M, Sanelli PC, Albers GW, et al. Imaging recommendations for acute stroke and transient ischemic attack patients: a joint statement by the American Society of Neuroradiology, the American College of Radiology and the Society of NeuroInterventional Surgery. J Am Coll Radiol 2013;10(11): 828–32.

39. Marks MP. Accurate interpretation of outside NCCT images. Neuroimaging Clin N Am 1998;8(3):515–23. in Chapter CT in Ischemic Stroke.

40. Smith WS, Roberts HC, Chuang NA, et al. Safety and feasibility of a CT protocol for acute stroke: combined CT, CT angiograpy, and CT perfusion imaging in 53 consecutive patients. AJNR Am J Neuroradiol 2003;24(4):688–90.

41. Hopyan JJ, Gladstone DJ, Mallia G, et al. Renal safety of CT angiography and perfusion imaging in the emergency evaluation of acute stroke. AJNR Am J Neuroradiol 2003;24: 688–90.

Computed Tomography, Computed Tomography Angiography, and Perfusion Computed Tomography Evaluation of Acute Ischemic Stroke

Carlos Leiva-Salinas, MD, PhD[a], Bin Jiang, MD, PhD[b],
Max Wintermark, MD, MPH, MBA[b],*

KEYWORDS

• CT • CT angiography • Perfusion CT • Stroke • Imaging

KEY POINTS

- Lower ASPECTS score correlates with stroke severity and higher rate of symptomatic hemorrhage after intravenous (IV) recombinant tissue plasminogen activator (rtPA).
- Hypoattenuation on computed tomography angiography (CTA) source images is more sensitive than noncontrast computed tomography to detect early ischemic changes.
- Evaluation of thrombus location and characteristics on CTA predicts recanalization rates after IV rtPA or mechanical thrombectomy.
- Results from latest trials studying the efficacy of mechanical thrombectomy confirm that the association between endovascular reperfusion and improved outcome is not time dependent in patients with a perfusion mismatch; thus, individual patient selection based on perfusion imaging might replace the clock in patients with ischemic stroke far beyond the 6-hour window.
- Because of the interest in expanding the therapeutic window in patients with ischemic stroke, determination of the infarct core volume will become increasingly important. Commercially available fully automated software has proved to provide the best approximation to the final infarct volume.

INTRODUCTION

Stroke is the leading cause of disability and fifth cause of death in the United States.[1] Each year, approximately 800,000 people in the United States and more than 15 million people worldwide experience a stroke. More than 80% of strokes are ischemic in origin.[1]

Neuroimaging is essential for stroke assessment. Given its wider availability, computed tomography (CT) is the most commonly used imaging modality used for acute stroke.[2] The combination of noncontrast computed tomography (NCCT), CT angiography (CTA), and perfusion CT (PCT) can provide the information required to

Disclosure Statement: The authors have no commercial or financial conflict of interest.
[a] Division of Neuroradiology, Department of Radiology, University of Missouri, One Hospital Drive, Columbia, MO 65212, USA; [b] Division of Neuroradiology, Department of Radiology, Stanford University, 300 Pasteur Drive, Stanford, CA 94305, USA
* Corresponding author.
E-mail address: max.wintermark@gmail.com

neuroimaging.theclinics.com

identify candidates for arterial recanalization and decision making in acute stroke.

Since publication of the authors' prior review in *Neuroimaging Clinics* in 2010,[3] results from several multicenter randomized trials[4–8] have changed the management of acute ischemic strokes and provided new information regarding the suitability of neuroimaging for the selection of patients for acute revascularization therapies.

This review provides an update on the current role of the individual components of multimodal CT in the evaluation of patients with acute ischemic stroke, with an emphasis on how they can impact acute treatment decision making.

COMPONENTS OF MULTIMODAL COMPUTED TOMOGRAPHY

Multimodal CT in acute stroke, including non-contrast CT (NCCT) of the brain, CTA of the head and neck, and PCT, provides information regarding the presence of intracranial hemorrhage or other stroke mimics, early ischemic changes, underlying thrombus location and characteristics, collateral circulation, and evaluation of potential ischemic penumbra based on mismatch profile. The ultimate goal of neuroimaging is to help in the triage of patients for acute revascularization therapy, with the underlying idea to select candidates based on individual vascular and physiologic information rather than on rigid time windows.

In the last decade, there has been a significant increase in the utilization of CTA and PCT examinations, and both modalities were associated with increased rates of revascularization treatments.[9,10]

NONCONTRAST COMPUTED TOMOGRAPHY

NCCT of the head remains the first line of imaging for patients with suspected acute ischemia (**Figs. 1 and 2**).[2,9,11]

Brain NCCT is used not only to exclude intracranial hemorrhage but also to assess for early ischemic changes. In the early phases after symptom onset, NCCT relies on the identification of subtle hypoattenuation as a predictor of infarction. In acute ischemia, there is early increased net influx of water into the cells followed by vasogenic edema due to endothelial injury and increased water permeability.[12] Based on animal studies, the increase in water content in the brain parenchyma 3 hours after vessel occlusion is around 1% to 2%, resulting in a decrease of 2 to 4 Hounsfield units on NCCT,[13,14] which is at the limit of what the human eye can identify.[15]

Indeed, only 30% of NCCTs of stroke patients presenting within the 3 hours after symptom onset will show early ischemic changes.[16] In the first 3-hour window, time has no or little effect on the development of identifiable tissue hypoattenuation, when assessed via Alberta Stroke Program Early CT Score (ASPECTS) score; conversely, there is a significant correlation between time and ASPECTS decline beyond the 3-hour timeline.[17] ASPECTS was developed in the year 2000 as an easily applicable, reliable score to evaluate the extent of early ischemic changes on NCCT.[18]

The relationship between the presence of early ischemic changes on NCCT and outcome after reperfusion is complex. Early studies found a relationship between ASPECTS on initial NCCT and functional prognosis.[18,19] However, at that time but also more recently, other publications did not confirm that ASPECTS was associated with the functional outcome after thrombolysis.[16,20–22] More recently, the findings from the MR CLEAN (Multicenter Randomized Clinical Trial of Endovascular Treatment for Acute Ischemic Stroke in the Netherlands) trial were again conflicting to the results from initial trials. In that cohort, patients whose NCCT showed ASPECTS less than 7 did not have a poorer functional outcome, indicating that the extent of early ischemic changes at NCCT within the first 6 hours of stroke might not be correlated with final outcome.[4]

Regarding the prediction of symptomatic intracranial hemorrhage after revascularization, there is also contradicting evidence. In the NINDS recombinant tissue plasminogen activator (rtPA) trial, early ischemic changes scores did not predict increased risk of symptomatic intracranial hemorrhage.[20] The ECASS II trial found opposite results, that is, patients with low ASPECTS have substantially increased risk of thrombolytic-related symptomatic hemorrhage.[21] More recently, the relationship between lower pretherapy ASPECTS scores and parenchymal hemorrhage was also confirmed in patients treated with endovascular thrombectomy. In late 2017, a hemorrhagic transformation index composed of ASPECTS, National Institutes of Health Stroke Scale (NIHSS), atrial fibrillation on admission electrocardiogram, and the presence of a hyperdense middle cerebral artery on NCCT proved successful to predict hemorrhagic transformation, regardless of the administration of IV rtPA.[23]

Finally, ASPECTS has very recently been proposed as a simple tool to identify wake-up stroke patients for mechanical thrombectomy; careful selection using ASPECTS greater than 6 allowed for safe interventions and clinical improvement in this patient population.[24]

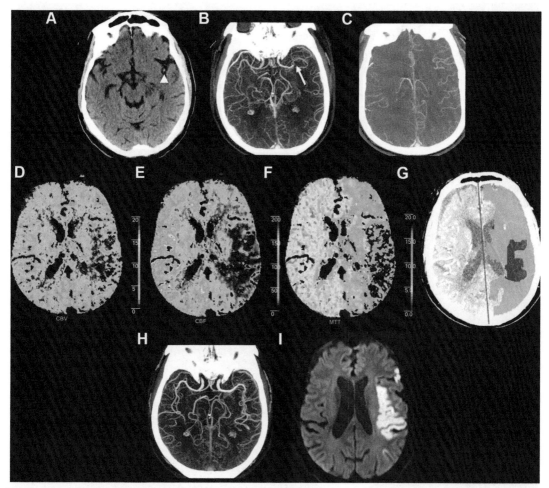

Fig. 1. A 79-year-old male patient with acute stroke. Baseline multimodal CT (*A–G*), posttherapy CTA (*H*), and follow-up axial DWI MR imaging (*I*) performed 1.5 hours, 26.5 hours, and 5 days after symptom onset. Axial NCCT image (*A*) shows a hyperdense M2 left middle cerebral artery (*arrowhead*). ASPECTS score was 7. At baseline CTA (*B, C*), the M1 and M2 segments of the left middle cerebral artery were occluded (*arrow*) with a thrombolysis in myocardial infarction score of 0 and a collateral score of 3. Prognostic map from PCT (*G*) showed an infarct core (*red cluster*, MTT >150%, CBV <2.0 mL) of 37.8 mL and ischemic penumbra (*green cluster*, MTT >150%, CBV >2.0 mL) of 322.1 mL. After a bridging treatment, the vessel was recanalized (*H*), and the final infarct volume was 34.3 mL (*I*).

COMPUTED TOMOGRAPHIC ANGIOGRAPHY

CTA is increasingly used in the evaluation of patients with suspected acute ischemic stroke (**Figs. 1** and **2**).[2,9] Timing of CTA implementation does not affect onset to groin puncture time,[10] but it offers the possibility of promoting a more efficient triage of patients that are candidates for revascularization therapies.

Identification of Thrombus and Evaluation of Thrombus Characteristics

Detection of a filling defect on CTA correlates with higher clinical severity and more pronounced ischemic changes on baseline NCCT.[25,26] Patients with a visible obstruction on CTA are more likely to benefit from IV rtPA or mechanical thrombectomy; the latter should not be attempted in absence of an identifiable target on CTA.[4–8]

The location of the thrombus within the intracranial vasculature influences the recanalization rates after IV rtPA and endovascular therapy. Recanalization of an occluded distal internal carotid artery only occurs in around 5% of patients after IV rtPA,[27,28] as opposed to 30% to 90% for the distal M1 or M2 segments of the middle cerebral arteries.[27,28] Patients with a proximal vessel occlusion are more likely to benefit from additional endovascular intervention.[4–8]

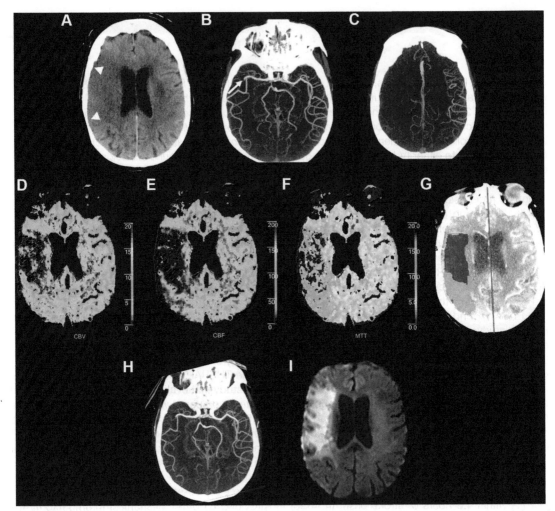

Fig. 2. A 90-year-old female patient with acute stroke. Baseline multimodal CT (*A–G*), posttherapy CTA (*H*), and follow-up axial DWI MR imaging (*I*) performed 1.5 hours, 26 hours, and 9 days after symptom onset. On NCCT (*A*), ASPECTS score was 6 (*arrowheads*). At baseline CTA (*B, C*), the M2 segment of the right middle cerebral artery was occluded with a thrombolysis in myocardial infarction score of 0 and a collateral score of 0. Prognostic map from PCT (*G*) showed an infarct core (*red cluster*, MTT >150%, CBV <2.0 mL) of 41.9 mL and ischemic penumbra (*green cluster*, MTT >150%, CBV >2.0 mL) of 42.1 mL. After IV tPA treatment, the M2 segment was not recanalized, and the final infarct volume was 166.7 mL on follow-up MR imaging (*I*).

Evaluation of the length of the thrombus on vascular imaging also provides information regarding the odds of recanalization after IV thrombolysis.[28,29] The longer the thrombus, the lower the recanalization rate after IV thrombolytics; thrombi longer than 8 mm are unlikely to dissolve after IV rtPA.[29]

The clot burden score provided is a 10-point scale used to determine the extent of the thrombus depending on the location of the clots.[30] A lower score indicates a higher clot burden and predicts lower recanalization rates, larger infarct size, higher risk of hemorrhagic transformation, and poorer functional outcome.[30]

Occasionally, the radiologist can visually identify residual intravascular contrast around or within a thrombus, and such clots are 4 times more likely to recanalize than those that do not show any residual flow.[28] Evaluation of clot permeability can be also evaluated quantitatively by dividing the attenuation of the lumen at the proximal clot interface by the one at the distal interface. A higher ratio indicates a less permeable clot, and thrombi with a ratio greater than 2 are less likely to recanalize than their counterparts.[28]

Proximal vessel occlusion, long thrombus, high clot burden, and absence of thrombus permeability are CTA predictors of low recanalization rates after IV thrombolysis, and thereby, potential markers to take into account to select patients for mechanical thrombectomy.

Evaluation of Collateral Flow

Good collateral circulation on baseline CTA is associated with smaller final infarct volume and better functional outcome. Recent evidence suggests that sustained good collaterals may predict good outcome in patients with cardioembolic stroke, and less so in those with a large artery occlusion.[31] In the first group, collateral flow seems to be associated with time from onset, indicating a benefit of early reperfusion in such subjects. Insufficient collateral flow results in decline of ASPECTS on NCCT,[31,32] likely due to rapid transformation of ischemic penumbra into irreversibly infarcted tissue.

Collateral status on CTA not only is a prognostic biomarker[33,34] but also can be used to select patients for endovascular therapy.[35,36] Recent trials have shown how patients with good collaterals at pretreatment CTA have better functional outcome after endovascular therapy when compared with IV rtPA, whereas patients with poor collaterals did not show a differential effect of successful recanalization.[35,36]

Given the fact that poor collateral flow at admission CTA predicts ASPECTS decay, vascular imaging can add value to the triage of candidates to endovascular treatment and in the decision to transfer them to thrombectomy-capable stroke centers.[32] Delay should be ideally minimized in all patients, but more so in subjects with poor flow,[32] if treatment is indeed indicated. On the other hand, mechanical thrombectomy might still be effective at later stages in patients with strong collaterals.[32,35]

Evaluation of Ischemic Changes

CTA images are usually acquired in the steady-state phase of the contrast bolus injection and are cerebral blood volume (CBV) weighted.[37] Hypoattenuation on source or multiplanar reformations average CTA images correlate with areas of decreased CBV and might thus represent the infarct core. Hypoattenuation on CTA has greater sensitivity to detect ischemia than NCCT.[38]

PERFUSION COMPUTED TOMOGRAPHY

PCT is increasingly used in acute stroke[9] for the evaluation of hemodynamic physiology of the brain parenchyma in an attempt to determine the volume of infarct core and ischemic penumbra (Figs. 1 and 2). The use of PCT does not delay IV rtPA or mechanical thrombectomy when compared with NCCT alone,[10] but is associated with increased use of reperfusion therapies in acute ischemic stroke patients.[9]

The quantitative perfusion data are displayed in color-coded parametric maps, most frequently including cerebral blood flow (CBF), mean transit time (MTT), and CBV. Brain regions with significantly decreased CBV or CBF correspond to the infarct core, and areas with prolonged MTT represent the overall area of low perfusion pressure. Mismatch between both regions can help delineate the ischemic penumbra, ischemic parenchyma at risk of infarction that can be potentially saved from infarction if early successful vessel recanalization and tissue reperfusion.[3]

Selection of acute ischemic stroke patients for revascularization based on physiologic information may potentially shift the treatment paradigm from a rigid time-based paradigm to a more flexible and individualized, tissue-based approach, which may optimize patient selection, and, it is hoped, increase the proportion of patients amenable to treatment.

PCT has been available for years, but there is still no clear consensus regarding the role of perfusion biomarkers for the selection of patients for revascularization treatment. Earlier trials investigating the effect of IV rtPA that used perfusion imaging did not show consistent results.[39–41] One of the factors behind that was the fact that recanalization rates observed with IV thrombolytics were modest, and therefore, did not help clarify if the selection of patients based on physiologic information was meaningful or not.[42] In the past few years, several trials have showed a functional outcome benefit in patients treated with endovascular thrombectomy, based on imaging criteria. Those trials benefited from the use of newer generation mechanical thrombectomy devices that resulted in better recanalization, and this might facilitate clarifying the role of the ischemic penumbra as a biomarker in the triage of patients for acute interventions. Indeed, the penumbra could be seen as a dual-edged sword, in the sense that it can predict good or bad outcome depending on recanalization status.[43] A large ischemic penumbra is associated with a favorable outcome in the setting of successful arterial recanalization, whereas it may predict unfavorable outcome in the absence of recanalization because the large amount of potentially salvageable brain infarction is going to infarct.[42]

Trials involving mechanical devices able to achieve near perfect recanalization rates might facilitate the role of perfusion in the selection of patients.[42] Each of the trials that demonstrated the efficacy of endovascular stroke therapy included at minimum an NCCCT and vascular imaging with CTA.[4–8] Among those, the SWIFT PRIME and EXTEND-IA trials used assessment of ischemic penumbra based on PCT. The magnitude of the clinical benefit in those 2 studies was significantly larger than in the other contemporary trials based solely on NCCT or a combination of NCCT and CTA. In the EXTEND-IA and SWIFT PRIME trials, 71% and 60% of patients respectively who received endovascular therapy achieved functional independence, respectively. One may therefore infer from that information that the use of PCT in the neuroimaging selection criteria may lead to superior patient outcomes.

The results from recent DWI or CTP Assessment with Clinical Mismatch in the Triage of Wake-Up and Late Presenting Strokes Undergoing Neurointervention with Trevo trial (DAWN),[44] and diffusion and perfusion imaging evaluation for understanding stroke evolution 3 (DEFUSE 3)[45] trials confirm that the association between endovascular reperfusion and improved functional and radiologic outcomes is not time dependent[46] in patients with clinical or imaging mismatch, and that individual patient selection based on perfusion imaging can really replace the clock in patients with acute ischemic stroke.

In that respect, DEFUSE 3[45] used perfusion-weighted imaging to randomize patients with a mismatch profile to endovascular treatment or no treatment in the 6- to 16-hour window. Following enrollment of approximately 40% of the maximum predicted sample, an interim analysis showed a high likelihood of benefit in the endovascular group, and the trial was terminated. In the DAWN study, functional outcomes were better after thrombectomy than with standard care alone in patients with acute stroke in the 6- to 24-hour window with a mismatch between the severity of the clinical deficit and infarct volume assessed with PCT or DWI; mean score on the utility-weighted modified rankin scale at 90 days was 5.5 in the thrombectomy group as compared with 3.4 in the control group.[44]

DEFUSE 3 defined target mismatch profile as ischemic core volume less than 70 mL, mismatch ratio ≥1.8, and mismatch volume ≥15 mL.[45] The definition of mismatch on DAWN was more complex: infarct core volume less than 21, 31, or 51 mL depending on patient age and NIHSS.[44] Both studies used automated software (RAPID).[44,45]

Because of DAWN, and because of the interest in expanding the therapeutic window in patients with ischemic stroke, determination of the infarct core volume will become increasingly important. Different commercial PCT software packages predict the infarct core using different approaches.[47] Some rely on absolute values such as CBV less than 2.0 mL/100 g or CBV less than 1.2 mL/100 mL, whereas others rely on relative metrics such as CBF less than 30% of that in normal tissue.[47] The accuracy of the various commercial software packages in predicting the final infarct volume after mechanical thrombectomy differs; fully automated RAPID software has proved to provide the best approximation to the final infarct volume.[47] This software has been used in several major recent revascularization trials,[6,7,44,45] including DAWN.[44]

SUMMARY

CT is the most frequently used imaging modality in the initial workup of acute ischemic stroke patients, and thus, to make treatment decisions regarding the need for vessel recanalization. The addition of CTA and PCT to NCCT does not delay time to groin puncture but offers the possibility of promoting a more efficient triage of patients that are candidates for revascularization therapies. Thrombus location and characteristics on CTA predict recanalization success after IV rtPA and mechanical thrombolysis. Evaluation of collateral score on CTA is useful in the triage of patients for mechanical thrombolysis. Finally, the association between endovascular reperfusion and improved functional and radiologic outcomes is not completely time dependent in patients with a certain target mismatch profiles, and individual selection based on perfusion imaging might replace the clock in patients with ischemic stroke.

REFERENCES

1. Benjamin EJ, Blaha MJ, Chiuve SE, et al. Heart disease and stroke statistics-2017 update: a report from the American Heart Association. Circulation 2017;135:e146–603.
2. Sanossian N, Fu KA, Liebeskind DS, et al. Utilization of emergent neuroimaging for thrombolysis-eligible stroke patients. J Neuroimaging 2017;27:59–64.
3. Leiva-Salinas C, Wintermark M. Imaging of acute ischemic stroke. Neuroimaging Clin N Am 2010;20: 455–68.
4. Berkhemer OA, Fransen PS, Beumer D, et al. A randomized trial of intraarterial treatment for acute ischemic stroke. N Engl J Med 2015;372:11–20.
5. Goyal M, Demchuk AM, Menon BK, et al. Randomized assessment of rapid endovascular treatment of ischemic stroke. N Engl J Med 2015; 372:1019–30.
6. Campbell BC, Mitchell PJ, Kleinig TJ, et al. Endovascular therapy for ischemic stroke with perfusion-imaging selection. N Engl J Med 2015;372:1009–18.

7. Saver JL, Goyal M, Bonafe A, et al. Stent-retriever thrombectomy after intravenous t-PA vs. t-PA alone in stroke. N Engl J Med 2015;372:2285–95.

8. Jovin TG, Chamorro A, Cobo E, et al. Thrombectomy within 8 hours after symptom onset in ischemic stroke. N Engl J Med 2015;372:2296–306.

9. Vagal A, Meganathan K, Kleindorfer DO, et al. Increasing use of computed tomographic perfusion and computed tomographic angiograms in acute ischemic stroke from 2006 to 2010. Stroke 2014; 45:1029–34.

10. Vagal A, Foster LD, Menon B, et al. Multimodal CT imaging: time to treatment and outcomes in the IMS III trial. AJNR Am J Neuroradiol 2016;37: 1393–8.

11. Demaerschalk BM, Kleindorfer DO, Adeoye OM, et al. Scientific rationale for the inclusion and exclusion criteria for intravenous alteplase in acute ischemic stroke: a statement for healthcare professionals from the American Heart Association/American Stroke Association. Stroke 2016;47:581–641.

12. Simard JM, Kent TA, Chen M, et al. Brain oedema in focal ischaemia: molecular pathophysiology and theoretical implications. Lancet Neurol 2007;6: 258–68.

13. Kucinski T, Vaterlein O, Glauche V, et al. Correlation of apparent diffusion coefficient and computed tomography density in acute ischemic stroke. Stroke 2002;33:1786–91.

14. Unger E, Littlefield J, Gado M. Water content and water structure in CT and MR signal changes: possible influence in detection of early stroke. AJNR Am J Neuroradiol 1988;9:687–91.

15. Dzialowski I, Klotz E, Goericke S, et al. Ischemic brain tissue water content: CT monitoring during middle cerebral artery occlusion and reperfusion in rats. Radiology 2007;243:720–6.

16. Patel SC, Levine SR, Tilley BC, et al. Lack of clinical significance of early ischemic changes on computed tomography in acute stroke. JAMA 2001;286:2830–8.

17. Gao J, Parsons MW, Kawano H, et al. Visibility of CT early ischemic change is significantly associated with time from stroke onset to baseline scan beyond the first 3 hours of stroke onset. J Stroke 2017;19: 340–6.

18. Barber PA, Demchuk AM, Zhang J, et al. Validity and reliability of a quantitative computed tomography score in predicting outcome of hyperacute stroke before thrombolytic therapy. ASPECTS Study Group. Alberta stroke programme early CT score. Lancet 2000;355:1670–4.

19. Hill MD, Buchan AM, Canadian Alteplase for Stroke Effectiveness Study (CASES) Investigators. Thrombolysis for acute ischemic stroke: results of the Canadian Alteplase for Stroke Effectiveness Study. CMAJ 2005;172:1307–12.

20. Demchuk AM, Hill MD, Barber PA, et al. Importance of early ischemic computed tomography changes using ASPECTS in NINDS rtPA Stroke Study. Stroke 2005;36:2110–5.

21. Dzialowski I, Hill MD, Coutts SB, et al. Extent of early ischemic changes on computed tomography (CT) before thrombolysis: prognostic value of the Alberta Stroke Program Early CT Score in ECASS II. Stroke 2006;37:973–8.

22. Gonzalez RG, Lev MH, Goldmacher GV, et al. Improved outcome prediction using CT angiography in addition to standard ischemic stroke assessment: results from the STOPStroke study. PLoS One 2012; 7:e30352.

23. Kalinin MN, Khasanova DR, Ibatullin MM. The hemorrhagic transformation index score: a prediction tool in middle cerebral artery ischemic stroke. BMC Neurol 2017;17:177.

24. Konstas AA, Minaeian A, Ross IB. Mechanical thrombectomy in wake-up strokes: a case series using alberta stroke program early CT score (ASPECTS) for patient selection. J Stroke Cerebrovasc Dis 2017;26:1609–14.

25. Qazi E, Al-Ajlan FS, Najm M, et al. The role of vascular imaging in the initial assessment of patients with acute ischemic stroke. Curr Neurol Neurosci Rep 2016;16:32.

26. Sylaja PN, Dzialowski I, Puetz V, et al. Does intravenous rtPA benefit patients in the absence of CT angiographically visible intracranial occlusion? Neurol India 2009;57:739–43.

27. Demchuk AM, Goyal M, Yeatts SD, et al. Recanalization and clinical outcome of occlusion sites at baseline CT angiography in the Interventional Management of Stroke III trial. Radiology 2014;273: 202–10.

28. Mishra SM, Dykeman J, Sajobi TT, et al. Early reperfusion rates with IV tPA are determined by CTA clot characteristics. AJNR Am J Neuroradiol 2014; 35(12):2265–72.

29. Riedel CH, Zimmermann P, Jensen-Kondering U, et al. The importance of size: successful recanalization by intravenous thrombolysis in acute anterior stroke depends on thrombus length. Stroke 2011; 42:1775–7.

30. Tan IY, Demchuk AM, Hopyan J, et al. CT angiography clot burden score and collateral score: correlation with clinical and radiologic outcomes in acute middle cerebral artery infarct. AJNR Am J Neuroradiol 2009;30:525–31.

31. Zhang X, Zhang M, Ding W, et al. Distinct predictive role of collateral status on clinical outcome in variant stroke subtypes of acute large arterial occlusion. Eur J Neurol 2018;25(2):293–300.

32. Boulouis G, Lauer A, Siddiqui AK, et al. Clinical imaging factors associated with infarct progression in patients with ischemic stroke during transfer for

mechanical thrombectomy. JAMA Neurol 2017;74:1361–7.

33. Bang OY, Saver JL, Buck BH, et al. Impact of collateral flow on tissue fate in acute ischaemic stroke. J Neurol Neurosurg Psychiatry 2008;79:625–9.

34. Bang OY, Saver JL, Kim SJ, et al. Collateral flow predicts response to endovascular therapy for acute ischemic stroke. Stroke 2011;42:693–9.

35. Berkhemer OA, Jansen IG, Beumer D, et al. Collateral status on baseline computed tomographic angiography and intra-arterial treatment effect in patients with proximal anterior circulation stroke. Stroke 2016;47:768–76.

36. Menon BK, Qazi E, Nambiar V, et al. Differential effect of baseline computed tomographic angiography collaterals on clinical outcome in patients enrolled in the interventional management of stroke III trial. Stroke 2015;46:1239–44.

37. Bhatia R, Bal SS, Shobha N, et al. CT angiographic source images predict outcome and final infarct volume better than noncontrast CT in proximal vascular occlusions. Stroke 2011;42:1575–80.

38. Coutts SB, Lev MH, Eliasziw M, et al. ASPECTS on CTA source images versus unenhanced CT: added value in predicting final infarct extent and clinical outcome. Stroke 2004;35:2472–6.

39. Albers GW, Thijs VN, Wechsler L, et al. Magnetic resonance imaging profiles predict clinical response to early reperfusion: the diffusion and perfusion imaging evaluation for understanding stroke evolution (DEFUSE) study. Ann Neurol 2006;60:508–17.

40. Davis SM, Donnan GA, Parsons MW, et al. Effects of alteplase beyond 3 h after stroke in the Echoplanar Imaging Thrombolytic Evaluation Trial (EPITHET): a placebo-controlled randomised trial. Lancet Neurol 2008;7:299–309.

41. Furlan AJ, Eyding D, Albers GW, et al. Dose Escalation of Desmoteplase for Acute Ischemic Stroke (DEDAS): evidence of safety and efficacy 3 to 9 hours after stroke onset. Stroke 2006;37:1227–31.

42. Leiva-Salinas C, Patrie JT, Xin W, et al. Prediction of early arterial recanalization and tissue fate in the selection of patients with the greatest potential to benefit from intravenous tissue-type plasminogen activator. Stroke 2016;47:397–403.

43. Zhu G, Michel P, Aghaebrahim A, et al. Prediction of recanalization trumps prediction of tissue fate: the penumbra: a dual-edged sword. Stroke 2013;44:1014–9.

44. Nogueira RG, Jadhav AP, Haussen DC, et al. Thrombectomy 6 to 24 hours after stroke with a mismatch between deficit and infarct. N Engl J Med 2017;378:11–21.

45. Albers GW, Lansberg MG, Kemp S, et al. A multicenter randomized controlled trial of endovascular therapy following imaging evaluation for ischemic stroke (DEFUSE 3). Int J Stroke 2017;12:896–905.

46. Lansberg MG, Cereda CW, Mlynash M, et al. Response to endovascular reperfusion is not time-dependent in patients with salvageable tissue. Neurology 2015;85:708–14.

47. Austein F, Riedel C, Kerby T, et al. Comparison of perfusion CT software to predict the final infarct volume after thrombectomy. Stroke 2016;9:2311–7.

MR Imaging Selection of Acute Stroke Patients with Emergent Large Vessel Occlusions for Thrombectomy

Thabele M. Leslie-Mazwi, MD[a,b,c,d], Michael H. Lev, MD[e],
Pamela W. Schaefer, MD[f,g],
Joshua A. Hirsch, MD, FSIR, FSNIS[h,i],
R. Gilberto González, MD, PhD[j],*

KEYWORDS

• MR Imaging • DWI • Ischemic stroke • Patient selection • Large vessel occlusion

KEY POINTS

• MR imaging offers unparalleled imaging returns for patients with acute stroke.
• Most patients with acute stroke are candidates for an MR imaging scan, and the proportion keeps growing as prior MR imaging contraindications (eg, pacemakers) evolve with better data about risk.
• Necessary sequences can be obtained in very short time intervals, minimizing scan time.
• If the patient has a small core (<70–100 mL), the penumbra must be large, and direct penumbral imaging with perfusion is not needed.
• Future applications include automation and decision support for acute stroke triage.

INTRODUCTION

Imaging of the patient with acute stroke with an anterior circulation large vessel occlusion (LVO) is a cornerstone of management and triage decisions for thrombectomy. With the success of nearly a dozen prospective clinical trials demonstrating the efficacy of mechanical thrombectomy, the focus now is on optimizing the decision to proceed to thrombectomy for the

Financial Disclosure: Dr M.H. Lev reports personal fees from GE, MedyMatch, Takeda, and D-Pharm, and nonfinancial support from Siemens, outside the submitted work; all other authors have no disclosure statements.
[a] Neuroendovascular Program, Massachusetts General Hospital, Harvard Medical School, WAC-7-745, MGH, 15 Parkman Street, Boston, MA 02114-3117, USA; [b] Neurocritical Care, Massachusetts General Hospital, Harvard Medical School, WAC-7-745, MGH, 15 Parkman Street, Boston, MA 02114-3117, USA; [c] Department of Neurosurgery, Massachusetts General Hospital, Harvard Medical School, WAC-7-745, MGH, 15 Parkman Street, Boston, MA 02114-3117, USA; [d] Department of Neurology, Massachusetts General Hospital, Harvard Medical School, WAC-7-745, MGH, 15 Parkman Street, Boston, MA 02114-3117, USA; [e] Emergency Radiology, Massachusetts General Hospital, Harvard Medical School, BLK-SB-0038 MGH, 55 Fruit Street, Boston, MA 02114, USA; [f] Neuroradiology, Massachusetts General Hospital, Harvard Medical School, Founders 228 MGH, 55 Fruit Street, Boston, MA 02114, USA; [g] Radiology, Massachusetts General Hospital, Harvard Medical School, Founders 228 MGH, 55 Fruit Street, Boston, MA 02114, USA; [h] NeuroInterventional Radiology, Massachusetts General Hospital, Harvard Medical School, Gray 241 MGH, 55 Fruit Street, Boston, MA 02114, USA; [i] Interventional Radiology, Massachusetts General Hospital, Harvard Medical School, Gray 241 MGH, 55 Fruit Street, Boston, MA 02114, USA; [j] Neuroradiology, Massachusetts General Hospital, Harvard Medical School, Gray 241 MGH, 55 Fruit Street, Boston, MA 02114, USA
* Corresponding author.
E-mail address: RGGONZALEZ@mgh.harvard.edu

Neuroimag Clin N Am 28 (2018) 573–584
https://doi.org/10.1016/j.nic.2018.06.003
1052-5149/18/© 2018 Elsevier Inc. All rights reserved.

neuroimaging.theclinics.com

benefit of the *individual* patient. Computed tomography (CT) and MR imaging offer options for acute stroke imaging. The major advantage of MR imaging over CT is its capability to detect and *precisely* estimate the volume of the infarct core. This precision leads to better individual patient selection. Precision in measuring the core also makes possible its other advantage: the elimination of the need to attempt to measure the "penumbra" with imaging. In this article, we detail use of MR imaging for acute ischemic stroke due to LVO for optimal triage decisions in individual patients. We recognize that our multidisciplinary stroke program and resources may be uncommon and not easily replicated at every stroke center. Nonetheless, our experience may be a useful guide for others to optimally modify their own stroke imaging protocols for cases of emergent LVO (ELVO).

ANTERIOR CIRCULATION LARGE VESSEL OCCLUSION PHYSIOLOGY

The MR imaging strategy for assessing patients with ELVO derives from the unique physiology produced by the occlusion of a major anterior circulation artery. The occlusion of the proximal middle cerebral artery (MCA) or terminal internal carotid artery (ICA) by an embolus is common, deadly, and potentially treatable. It manifests in alterations in cerebral hemodynamics and physiology, as illustrated in **Fig. 1**. The sudden occlusion reduces blood flow and perfusion, produces ischemia, and results in tissue injury and death. Irreversibly injured tissue is in close proximity to the occluded artery and is termed the ischemic core. The core is surrounded by tissue that may be underperfused but is still viable. This is loosely designated as the "penumbra." The relative size of the core with respect to the penumbra depends on the quality of the pial-pial collateral circulation. A robust collateral circulation results in a small core and simultaneously large penumbra, a circumstance that is ideal for intervention. If the pial-pial collaterals are weak, a large ischemic core rapidly emerges, and the patient is much less likely to benefit from thrombectomy.

A consequence of this special physiology is that if the ischemic core can be measured precisely, the need to directly image the "penumbra" is obviated. All that is necessary is evidence that a penumbra is present, which may be provided by an abnormal neurologic examination. This fact has been validated by the success of the DAWN trial,[1] wherein only core, and no penumbral imaging was performed.

GOALS OF ACUTE STROKE IMAGING

Imaging for the patient with acute stroke aims to accomplish 4 primary goals:

1. Detect presence of hemorrhage
2. Identify a treatable arterial occlusion(s)

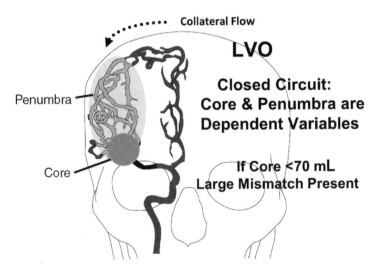

Fig. 1. Physiology of an LVO. Representation of a right MCA occlusion. Reduced blood flow results in irreversible injury to part of the brain (ischemic core) just distal to the site of occlusion. There is a larger area designated as "penumbra," in which the blood flow is abnormal but the tissue is viable because of the pial-pial collateral circulation. This part of the brain may recover if normal flow is reestablished. Because of the collateral circulation, the sizes of the core and penumbra are dependent variables, so if one is small, the other must be large, and vice versa. Because of this dependency, if the core is small, a large mismatch may be assumed and direct measurement of the penumbra is not necessary.

3. Estimate the core infarct volume
4. Establish the presence of a significant amount of penumbral tissue (the viable tissue with altered perfusion)

These goals are listed in order of priority. Excluding hemorrhage is the most important goal. The remaining 3 goals take on increasing importance for patients considered for mechanical thrombectomy. In all cases, a balance exists between obtaining accurate information and the

time taken to obtain such information. An example of a patient who underwent successful thrombectomy after undergoing evaluation with MR imaging is shown in **Fig. 2.**

Detect Presence of Hemorrhage

Accurate detection of hemorrhage is essential for the patient with acute stroke. Hemorrhage may be due to a variety of causes. Sometimes there is hemorrhage in the setting of vascular occlusion.

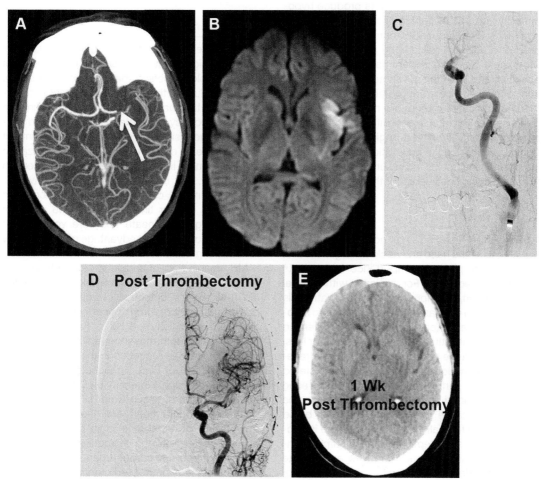

Fig. 2. Case of a woman who experienced sudden right hemiparesis while on a transatlantic flight. The witnessed stroke occurred while flying over the Atlantic Ocean. The patient's condition was radioed to the airport and the hospital was alerted. On arrival, the patient was immediately transported to the hospital emergency department. Noncontrast CT demonstrated a dense left MCA sign (not shown). (*A*) CTA of the head. An image is shown from axial, thick slab, overlapping MIP series. The study demonstrated occlusion of the distal left ICA and proximal left MCA and anterior cerebral artery (ACA) (*arrow*). (*B*) DWI shows the ischemic core involving the insula, left frontal, and left temporal lobes. The volume of the DWI lesion was less than 25 mL. (*C*) Frontal, left internal carotid arteriogram confirms occlusion of the distal left ICA. (*D*) Post-thrombectomy left common carotid arteriogram demonstrates removal of occlusion and anterograde flow within the left ICA, MCA, and ACA arteries and their branches. (*E*) CT scan 1 week after procedure shows small infarct in the left MCA territory. The patient ultimately fully recovered from her neurologic deficits. Full details may be found in case records of the MGH. Case 13 to 2016. (*Data from* Schwamm LH, Jaff MR, Dyer KS, et al. CASE RECORDS of the MASSACHUSETTS GENERAL HOSPITAL. Case 13-2016. A 49-year-old woman with sudden hemiplegia and aphasia during a transatlantic flight. N Engl J Med 2016;374(17):1671–80.)

Delivery of intravenous thrombolytic agents or mechanical reperfusion in the presence of active hemorrhage could be devastating. Cerebral hemorrhage may be visualized by many MR sequences. The most sensitive sequences for detection of blood are those that are sensitive to local disturbances in the magnetic field, typically produced by blood products. In stroke, the primary concern is parenchymal hematoma. Secondary considerations for blood products include thrombus causing vascular occlusion and chronic microhemorrhages. These blood products produce hypointensity on T2*-weighted images. The most commonly used sequences for hemorrhage detection are gradient recalled echo (GRE) sequences. More rapid T2* echo planar images (EPI) are also effective, and have the advantage of freezing motion because slices are obtained very rapidly (<100 ms per slice). There are more sensitive sequences, including susceptibility-weighted imaging and T2 star weighted angiography imaging, but they have longer acquisition times and the increased sensitivity is not essential for the patient with LVO being considered for thrombectomy.

Identify Vascular Occlusion

A variety of MR imaging sequences exist to assess the vessels of the head and neck. Emergent vessel imaging is of particular importance for patients with suspected LVO. For patients with normal renal function, comprehensive information is provided using contrast-enhanced magnetic resonance angiography (ceMRA). This is characterized by fast acquisition times (usually 2 minutes or less) and a large volume of tissue coverage. An intravenous bolus of gadolinium contrast is administered and the scan is performed with short gradient echo sequences. Blood appears hyperintense on the sequence because gadolinium shortens blood T1, and signal from all the remaining tissue is suppressed by the short repetition time. Optimized imaging using this sequence requires appropriate timing, so data are obtained during the peak of arterial enhancement. This may be accomplished by use of a test bolus or more frequently by automatic bolus detection. Ideally ceMRA will be obtained from the aortic arch to the superior temporal lobes, providing visualization of the origins of the great vessels of the neck, the common carotid arteries, the internal carotid and vertebral arteries, the M1 and proximal M2 segments of the MCAs, and the basilar and proximal posterior cerebral arteries.

For patients who have poor renal function (glomerular filtration rate <30 ml/mn) or who have recently undergone CT or MR angiography of the neck, time-of-flight (TOF) MRA of the head may be more appropriate. This can be obtained in 2-dimensional (2D) or 3D acquisitions. Besides avoiding a contrast load, TOF imaging has the advantage of repeatability if imaging is suboptimal (eg, an uncooperative or agitated patient). Two-dimensional TOF imaging has lower spatial resolution but more rapid acquisition than 3D TOF imaging. Two-dimensional MRA is also acquired a single slice at a time, so it may be adequate even if the patient moves.

Estimate of the Core Infarct Volume

Various determinants of patient outcome exist, but the most significant of these are the severity of initial neurologic deficit, the presence and site of arterial occlusion, the success of attempted reperfusion, and the final infarct core volume (a function of both adequacy of collateral circulation and successful reperfusion). The impact of final infarct core volume on outcome[2] has led to the utilization of pretreatment infarct core volumes for selection for therapy. For mechanical thrombectomy pretreatment infarct core volume gains increasing importance in later time windows. The ability of MR imaging to delineate this core volume with high precision is the key advantage of this modality for scanning patients with stroke.

MR imaging is unparalleled for detection of infarct core. MR diffusion-weighted imaging (DWI) allows the detection of acute ischemia as early as 30 minutes from onset, with high sensitivity and specificity (>90%).[3] The reduction of the normal random movement (diffusion) of water molecules causes reduction in the apparent diffusion coefficient of water in ischemic brain tissue and increased signal intensity on DWI. This reduction in diffusion of tissue water is not entirely understood. Contributions are thought to come from failure of membrane ionic pumps with net influx of water from the extracellular to the more osmotic intracellular compartment, reduced extracellular volumes, decreased cytoplasmic mobility, increased intracellular viscosity from the fragmentation of cellular components, and increased cell membrane permeability.

For most patients, the initial DWI lesion volume closely correlates with the final infarct volume if there is successful recanalization. However, in the context of very early reperfusion, partial DWI reversal (tissue that has restricted diffusion but appears normal on follow-up imaging) has been observed. Beyond a certain time threshold, which data suggest is 3.0 to 4.5 hours of cerebral artery occlusion, the DWI abnormality represents tissue that has been irreversibly injured. If diffusion imaging is performed immediately after successful reperfusion, there may be a transient reversal of most or the entire lesion. The apparent temporary reversal of DWI change after reperfusion is therefore described as "pseudonormalization" for these patients. To summarize, between 1 and 3 hours, DWI reversal is variable. Beyond 4.5 hours, the volume of tissue that undergoes reversal is usually no more than 10% of the total DWI lesion, and for most patients is less than 5 mL.[4–6]

Estimate of the Presence of a Significant Volume of Penumbral Tissue

The prospective observational study by Leslie-Mazwi and colleagues[7] and the prospective, randomized DAWN trial by Nogueira and colleagues[1] have demonstrated that direct imaging of the "penumbra" is not necessary for the successful selection of patients for thrombectomy. Indeed, penumbral imaging is beset by the fundamental conundrum that there is no generally accepted definition for such an imaging measurement. The lack of definition has resulted in the adoption of measurements of altered contrast delivery times (Tmax) or contrast transit times (MTT) and the use of a DWI/Tmax or DWI/MTT mismatch for patient selection for thrombectomy. In the presence of an LVO, there may exist oligemic as well as normally perfused tissue beyond the infarct core. For example, a patient with a chronic occlusion of a proximal ICA may have fully compensated, normal arterial blood flow but would meet the criteria of a large "mismatch." As specifically addressed in the DAWN trial, a clinical "penumbra," that is, the presence of a neurologic deficit that is not completely explained by the infarct core visualized on DWI, is adequate to proceed to thrombectomy when there is a small core.

Perfusion imaging with MR imaging may be useful in the assessment of the patient with ischemic stroke that is not caused by an LVO. A patient may present with an acute stroke syndrome due to occlusion of a small branch vessel that is not visualized by MRA or CT angiography (CTA). In this circumstance, dynamic contrast-enhanced perfusion imaging or arterial spin labeling may reveal a small volume of abnormal perfusion caused by the small branch occlusion. These lesions are not amenable to mechanical thrombectomy, but other therapeutic approaches may be attempted.

Application of Additional MR Imaging Sequences

Additional sequences are not necessary for decisions regarding thrombectomy. However, if time permits, T2-weighted fluid-attenuated inversion recovery (FLAIR) provides the most additional information about brain pathology that may be present.

MASSACHUSETTS GENERAL HOSPITAL STROKE IMAGING PROTOCOL 2018

Our approach to imaging patients with acute stroke is based on more than 20 years of experience in imaging and performing endovascular arterial recanalization. Regular, critical reviews of our outcomes, and published data from other stroke centers, provide the evidentiary basis for the Massachusetts General Hospital (MGH) stroke imaging algorithm, which was first published in 2013.[8] The major change implemented in the 2013 protocol was elimination of CT perfusion because our data indicated that it could be unreliable when assessing individual patients.[9] Using this protocol, we performed a prospective observational trial that was published in 2017.[7] The publication of the DAWN[1] and DEFUSE 3[10] trials, as well as recent subgroup analyses of these trials, have added to our understanding, and our protocol has been modified in response to the new data. The current version of our protocol reflecting the new evidence is shown in **Fig. 3**.

Presentation Less Than 6 Hours from Onset

Our imaging protocol for patients who present within 6 hours of ictus is shown in **Fig. 3**A. Imaging typically begins with CT. There are several reasons for this, but the major factors are that CT scans are easily and quickly obtained, and they are reliable for detecting the presence of hemorrhage as well as a treatable LVO. For patients within the window for intravenous thrombolysis (less than 4.5 hours from onset), tissue plasminogen activator (tPA) is transported by pharmacy to the scanner with the patient. If noncontrast head CT demonstrates no hemorrhage, tPA is reconstituted and the bolus is given as a parallel process to preparation for CTA. CTA acquisition occurs from the arch through the vertex with delayed images from the arch through the circle of Willis. CTA data are processed to produce thick slab (30 mm), overlapping (5 mm between the center of each slab) axial, coronal, and sagittal maximum intensity projection (MIP) images. Treatment decisions for thrombectomy are made on the basis of vascular occlusion and the adequacy of collaterals demonstrated on the CTA axial MIPs. The collateral circulation is adequate if they are similar or more prominent on the side of the occlusion when compared with the contralateral side. This is the first of 2 major changes in our new protocol. We have found that

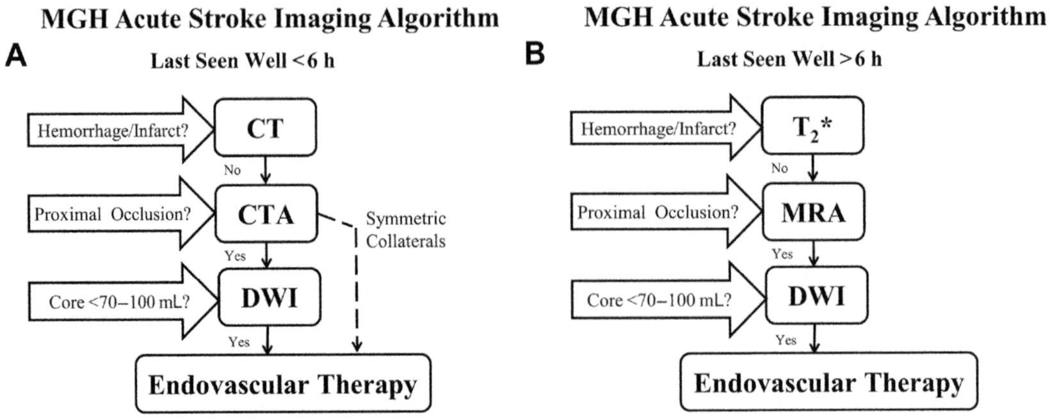

MGH Acute Stroke Imaging Algorithm

A   Last Seen Well <6 h

Hemorrhage/Infarct? → **CT**

No ↓

Proximal Occlusion? → **CTA** --- Symmetric Collaterals

Yes ↓

Core <70–100 mL? → **DWI**

Yes ↓

Endovascular Therapy

MGH Acute Stroke Imaging Algorithm

B   Last Seen Well >6 h

Hemorrhage/Infarct? → **T$_2$***

No ↓

Proximal Occlusion? → **MRA**

Yes ↓

Core <70–100 mL? → **DWI**

Yes ↓

Endovascular Therapy

Fig. 3. MGH stroke imaging protocol 2018. (*A*) Patient last seen well less than 6 hours before possible intervention. Noncontrast CT is performed to assess for hemorrhage or large completed infarct. If neither is present, CTA is performed to identify a large artery occlusion. If present, the collateral circulation is assessed on the axial, thick slab, overlapping MIP images. If the collaterals on the occluded side are similar or hypervascular compared with the contralateral side, the probability of a small ischemic core is high, and patient may proceed to thrombectomy. If the ipsilateral collateral circulation is less robust, the patient proceeds to MR imaging for DWI acquisition. A DWI lesion of less than 70 to 100 mL generally makes the patient eligible for thrombectomy. (*B*) Patient last seen well more than 6 hours before possible intervention. The patient is fully evaluated using MR imaging, if MR imaging is not contraindicated. T2* imaging is used to assess for presence of hemorrhage. LVO is identified with MRA. Ischemic core size is determined with DWI. A DWI lesion of less than 70 to 100 mL generally makes the patient eligible for thrombectomy.

the presence of symmetric collaterals is a reliable marker of a small (<70 mL) core lesion as measured by DWI. If the collateral circulation is clearly decreased compared with the normal side, the diffusion lesion may be small or large. Thus, for any patient for whom therapeutic questions persist after CT scanning, an emergent MR imaging is performed to obtain core measurement using DWI.

Presentation 6 to 24 Hours or Unknown Time from Onset

For all patients presenting in time windows after 6 hours, our protocol uses MR imaging as the sole modality (see **Fig. 3**B). This is the second major change to our stroke imaging protocol and it follows from the DAWN[1] and DEFUSE 3[10] results. T2* imaging is performed using a gradient echo sequence, which takes less than 1 minute; a DWI scan is acquired in less than 2 minutes; and either a 2D TOF MRA of the head or a ceMRA of the head and neck is performed within 2 minutes. We use a core-clinical mismatch, based on information generated by our center and most recently confirmed in the DAWN trial. Patients are considered for thrombectomy if they have a clinical deficit producing an National Institutes of Health Stroke Scale greater than or equal to 6, have an LVO on contrast-enhanced MRA, and have less than 70

to 100 mL of infarct core on DWI. Patients with DWI volumes approaching 100 mL may be excluded based on other factors, such as age and baseline functional status, given that both clinical and imaging parameters must be met to qualify for treatment.

Estimating the Size of the Core Revealed by Diffusion-Weighted Imaging

We use the A*B*C/2 method to estimate the volume of the diffusion abnormality on the DWI scan.[11] The method is simple. At the level at which the DWI lesion appears largest, anteroposterior (A) and transverse lengths (B) are measured. The superoinferior extent (C) is estimated by counting the number of slices in which the diffusion abnormality is present, taking into account the slice thickness and slice gap. The product of A times B times C is divided by 2. This simple method is accurate to approximately 10% and has been validated.[12] An alternative is the use of commercial data processing software that automatically detects and measures the DWI lesion volume. We have used such software, and have found it to be generally reliable, but the software may produce spurious, inaccurate DWI lesion volumes and visual inspection of the measurements is thus extremely important. The software is convenient, but expensive, and so we use the manual method.

Assessing the Core in Patients Who Are Unable to Undergo MR imaging

In our experience, 10% to 15% of patients cannot undergo MR imaging. The most common reason is the presence of a pacemaker. The decision to proceed to thrombectomy relies on the clinical circumstances as well as review of the noncontrast CT, parenchymal images from the CTA (CTA source images), and the CTA. We do not use CT perfusion (CTP). Our studies and those from other groups have confirmed that although CTP may reliably estimate small core lesions, it is unreliable in individual patients with larger core lesions, although it may used for group studies.[9] Because we do not know the size of the core a priori, it is prudent NOT to use this method.

MR IMAGING UTILIZATION IN ISCHEMIC STROKE TRIALS

The scientific foundation for our approach includes our own studies and published work from other centers. In recent years, there has been a plethora of important studies. We review the most pertinent studies here.

PROSPECTIVE OBSERVATIONAL TRIAL USING MR IMAGING FOR PATIENT SELECTION

Major changes in stroke care are occurring following new data available for patients with LVOs. At the time of this writing, the Food and Drug Administration (FDA) has approved at least 1 device for thrombectomy up to 24 hours after stroke onset. The trials evaluating early window therapies were overwhelmingly CT-based trials. Advanced imaging selection was achieved using CTA and CTP imaging in several trials. Fewer than 5% of the total patient population was imaged using MR imaging. Patient selection by MR imaging in the SWIFT Prime trial (in which 19.7% were imaged with MR imaging) had a nearly identical treatment response to the 80.3% selected using CTP.[13]

Trials evaluating patients in later time windows (more than 6 hours after or unknown time of onset) had higher rates of MR imaging utilization. In the DAWN trial, 37.4% of the intervention arm and 35.4% of the control arm were imaged using MR imaging. In the DEFUSE 3 trial, 25% of the thrombectomy patients and 28.9% of the control arm were selected using MR imaging. In these trials, MR imaging parameters were different. The DAWN trial used DWI to quantify core and applied a core-clinical mismatch, whereas the DEFUSE 3 trial used DWI to quantify core and thresholded MR perfusion (Tmax >6) to quantify penumbra

and from those to derive a penumbra/core mismatch ratio.

A very interesting subgroup analysis of the DEFUSE 3 trial was presented by Dr Maarten Lansberg at the 2018 International Stroke Conference.[14] He reported that when considered alone, the 49 patients who were selected using MR imaging inclusion criteria had a significantly higher percentage of good outcomes compared with the 182 patients in the entire DEFUSE 3 cohort that included patients selected by either MR imaging or CTP criteria. Additionally, statistically significant differences between the thrombectomy and medically treated groups were found despite the small size of the MR imaging–selected cohort. Subgroup analysis of the CTP-selected cohort alone was not presented.

These late window trials demonstrated the validity of the "tissue-clock" concept, a refinement of the simplified "time-clock" model of stroke care. Although time is brain, each brain has its own time. The clinical superiority of MR imaging for patient selection, especially in the later time windows, leads to the conclusion that Comprehensive Stroke Center requirements should include immediate MR imaging access for all patients with acute stroke.

SLOW PROGRESSORS AND COMPREHENSIVE/THROMBECTOMY CAPABLE STROKE CENTERS

The DAWN and DEFUSE 3 trials have opened the therapeutic window for endovascular thrombectomy for up to 24 hours after known stroke onset or for up to 24 hours after the patient was last seen well (unknown stroke onset). As "late" treatment of patients with LVO becomes standard of care, comprehensive (or thrombectomy capable) stroke centers must consider how they should modify their LVO patient evaluation programs to accommodate more patients. The individual patient's stroke physiology, especially the size of the infarct core, is of paramount importance in patients who have unknown stroke-onset time, or are evaluated 6 to 24 hours after stroke onset. MR imaging should be the primary imaging modality for these patients because of its superior performance for infarct core measurement.

In light of this new therapeutic window extension, stroke centers need to consider the number of potential patients that may be eligible for treatment. A significant number may be initially evaluated at other institutions that are not equipped to perform thrombectomy. Although data are scarce, there may be a large number of "slow progressors," which we define here as patients who have proximal LVOs with ischemic core lesions smaller than 70 mL at 6 or more hours after stroke onset. Copen and colleagues[15] first reported an unexpectedly large proportion of "slow progressors." A histogram derived from that publication is shown in **Fig. 4**. A total of 109 consecutive patients who underwent MR imaging studies, including diffusion and perfusion imaging, within 24 hours of acute ischemic stroke symptom onset were evaluated. Sixty-eight had LVOs. Unexpectedly, more than 60% of the patients with LVOs imaged at both less than and greater than 9 hours had small infarct cores and diffusion/perfusion mismatches of greater than 160%. What was perhaps even more surprising, there was no relationship between time from stroke symptom onset and the presence of the large mismatch.

The study by Copen and colleagues[15] motivated another study to assess the size of the DWI core lesion in patients with LVO at the time of presentation in the emergency department. Hakimelahi and colleagues[16] reported the ischemic core volumes for a series of 186 consecutive patients with LVO who presented up to 24 hours after stroke onset. A plot of the DWI lesion volume with respect to time after stroke onset is shown in **Fig. 5**.

Statistically and by visual inspection, there was no significant relationship between the ischemic core size and time after ictus. Moreover, most patients had core lesions smaller than 100 mL in every time period (for example 6–9 hours or 15–18 hours). This study confirmed the earlier work by Copen and colleagues.[15]

When considering slow progressors, it is important to consider the rate of growth of the core ischemic lesion. Clearly, there is a large variability in core growth when one considers the data of **Figs. 5** and **6**. In experimental stroke studies that have used DWI to measure infarct volumes, the ischemic core grows in a logarithmic fashion, with rapid early growth, which then tapers to a slower rate. Although it is likely that the ischemic core growth rates in people is similarly logarithmic, data supporting this are rare because it requires that multiple imaging studies be performed over a short period of time. Nevertheless, in a series of 14 patients with acute ischemic stroke with LVOs imaged at a mean baseline of 7.5 hours as well as 4 hours later, 24 hours later, and 1 week later, we observed relatively little growth from the baseline scan to the 1-week scan.[17] Similarly, **Fig. 6** shows the DWI and MTT images of a patient with a left MCA stem occlusion who was imaged with MR imaging 3 times over 24 hours. Close

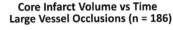

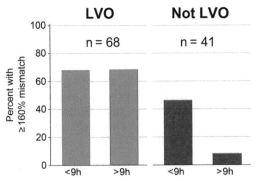

Fig. 4. Presence of a large mismatch in patients with LVO up to 24 hours after onset. The criterion for a large mismatch was a perfusion (MTT)/diffusion (DWI) mismatch of greater than 160%. Patients were grouped into those who had the presence or absence of LVO when they underwent MR imaging. Patients in each group were further subdivided by the time of imaging after stroke onset (less than or >9 hours). More than 60% of all patients with LVO had large mismatches irrespective of the time after ictus. (*Adapted from* Copen WA, Rezai Gharai L, Barak ER, et al. Existence of the diffusion-perfusion mismatch within 24 hours after onset of acute stroke: dependence on proximal arterial occlusion. Radiology 2009;250(3):878–86; with permission.)

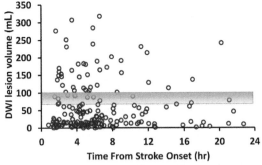

Fig. 5. Ischemic core size versus time in patients with LVO. Scatterplot of consecutive patients who presented to the emergency department with anterior circulation large artery occlusions. The plot shows the size of the DWI lesion abnormality with respect to time last seen well. There is no correlation between ischemic core size and time after stroke onset. Most patient core sizes are below the 70 to 100 mL blue bar when considered as a whole or any time interval from 0 to 24 hours. (*Adapted from* Hakimelahi R, Vachha BA, Copen WA, et al. Time and diffusion lesion size in major anterior circulation ischemic strokes. Stroke 2014;45(10):2936–41.)

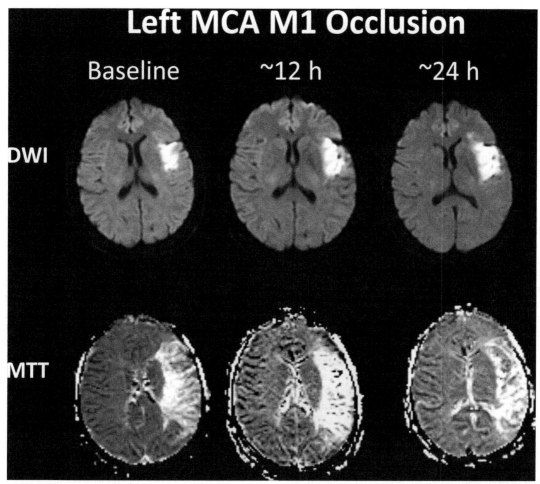

Fig. 6. Serial MR imaging scans in patient with persistent left MCA occlusion. The patient was initially scanned approximately 6 hours after last seen well. The artery occlusion was documented on CTA. Repeat imaging performed approximately 12 and approximately 24 hours after stroke onset showed persistent occlusion and large perfusion deficit (MTT), but very little growth in the size of the ischemic core revealed by DWI.

examination of the DWI images shows that most of the lesion volume is already present at baseline with very slow growth over 24 hours, despite the persistence of an LVO and a large diffusion perfusion mismatch.

In summary, the available data indicate that there is wide variation in the growth of ischemic core in patients with anterior circulation LVOs. The growth rate is likely similar to that observed in experimental animal studies, with rapid early followed by slower later growth that has a logarithmic character. Moreover, the data suggest that most patients with LVOs are "slow progressors," defined as patients with ischemic core volumes of less than 70 to 100 mL when imaged 6 or more hours after stroke onset. If true, this presents an enormous opportunity to benefit many patients with LVOs using mechanical thrombectomy.

Advantages of MR Imaging for Stroke Imaging

MR imaging provides the undisputed advantage of detailed characterization of the ischemic core lesion. Detection of ischemia is much improved with MR imaging compared with CT, with a sensitivity of greater than 90% for DWI compared with approximately 60% for noncontrast CT scans. CTP increases the detection of ischemia compared with CT, but remains inferior to DWI. Furthermore, measurement error between intrarater and interrater lesion volumes is much lower for DWI compared with thresholded CTP. However, true volume thresholds to define excellent versus poor outcomes remain a shifting target. A lesion volume less than 70 mL has been associated with good outcomes when the patient undergoes thrombectomy.[2] For volumes greater than 100 mL, over 90% will have less favorable outcomes (modified Rankin score 3–6) even with thrombectomy. An additional concern has been increased risk of intracranial hemorrhage (possible harm, not just absence of benefits). These notions have come under recent scrutiny based on subgroup analysis from randomized trials and separate reports of patients with larger core volumes achieving either good or improved functional outcomes. Beyond infarct volume alone, the precise anatomic localization that DWI sequences provide aids in determining culprit vascular compromise as well as prognosis.

MR imaging provides the advantage of vascular imaging without the need for contrast media. TOF MRA evaluation of the intracranial circulation allows identification of vascular occlusion for patients with poor renal function for whom gadolinium is contraindicated or CT contrast may be harmful. Use of a 2D as opposed to a 3D TOF sequence allows for rapid image acquisition, and is probably the best choice in less cooperative patients. Because images of each slice are acquired serially and rapidly, individual images are not significantly degraded by motion and an LVO can be readily easily identified. Imaging of cervical vasculature is often challenged by patient motion and image resolution using TOF techniques.

Finally, tailored imaging and the use of accelerated techniques that include parallel imaging and EPI has allowed significant reductions in MR imaging acquisition time; in fact, MR imaging sequences can now be obtained in time frames that are comparable to the speed of CT scanning. For example, Nael and colleagues[18] developed a relatively comprehensive 6-minute MR imaging protocol for evaluation of acute ischemic stroke. This rapid acquisition maintains a high degree of image diagnostic quality and is increasingly used by centers that routinely apply MR imaging for acute stroke evaluation.

The MR imaging protocols adopted at MGH are listed in Tables 1 and 2. The MR imaging

Table 1
MR imaging protocol for patients with preceding CT/CTA

Target	Sequence	Time	Comments
Core	DWI	2 min	—
Other pathology	FLAIR	2 min	Optional

Abbreviations: CT, computed tomography; CTA, computed tomography angiography; DWI, diffusion-weighted imaging; FLAIR, fluid-attenuated inversion recovery.

Table 2
MR imaging protocol for patients without preceding CT/CTA

Target	Sequence	Time	Comments
Hemorrhage	EPI GRE	1 min	—
Occlusion	2D TOF	1 min	—
Core	DWI	2 min	—
Neck vessels	Gd+ 3D TOF	2 min	Optional
Other pathology	FLAIR	2 min	Optional

Abbreviations: CT, computed tomography; CTA, computed tomography angiography; D, dimensional; DWI, diffusion-weighted imaging; EPI, echo planar imaging; FLAIR, fluid-attenuated inversion recovery; Gd, gadolinium; GRE, gradient recalled echo; TOF, time of flight.

examination must be tailored to each individual patient. One of the most common scenarios is a patient with an acute stroke syndrome who was initially evaluated with CT and CTA. If CT imaging reveals an LVO and no hemorrhage, only the DWI sequence is essential (see Table 1). The other common scenario is of the patient with acute stroke syndrome who is imaged first by MR imaging. Patients presenting more than 6 hours post ictus or with an unknown time of onset will be typically imaged with MR imaging first. There are other scenarios. For example, a patient may be transferred from a nearby care health facility where a head CT but not a CTA was performed. Such a patient would go directly to MR imaging, but the sequences obtained would depend on the imaging findings, the patient transfer time, change in signs and symptoms, and other potential confounders. In general, we obtain DWI (to characterize infarct core), EPI GRE (to identify hemorrhage and LVO) and 2D TOF through the circle of Willis (to identify LVO) on all patients who are imaged first by MR imaging, with a total imaging time of less than 5 minutes.

Challenges with MR Imaging for Stroke

Several limitations prevent more common use of MR imaging. Scanner availability is variable in emergency departments worldwide, with access to MR imaging much more limited than the availability of CT scanning. However, all comprehensive stroke centers (including thrombectomy-capable stroke centers) should have MR imaging available, even if it is not physically located in the emergency department.

Only 80% to 85% of patients with acute stroke are candidates for MR imaging. True contraindications include the presence of retained metal (historically this has been mainly because of cardiac pacemakers), and are present in approximately 10% of patients with stroke. The remaining 5% to 10% of patients who are not candidates for MR imaging are excluded because they are too unstable medically (eg, poor airway control, blood pressure instability, repeated vomiting) or have severe agitation. Unlike CT, screening is required to ensure that a patient is appropriate to enter an MR imaging scanner. In many centers, this is accomplished most efficiently by prescreening where possible. However, for patients presenting with unknown medical histories and no family members to provide screening data, either MR imaging is not an imaging option, or scout radiographs are required to exclude the presence of ferromagnetic metals.

The need for prescreening is coupled with the need for patient safety in the MR imaging environment. This may require the removal of electrocardiogram leads placed by ambulance staff or referring hospital emergency departments, changing infusion pumps or priming infusion lines, application of MR imaging safe pulse oximetry, and so forth. These requirements introduce delay. Given the powerful interaction between time and treatment effect for both intravenous and endovascular therapies in patients with stroke presenting within the first few hours, the impact of these delays may be a concern. However, it has been demonstrated that MR imaging can be sufficiently efficient to be the primary imaging method even for tPA administration.[6]

Although MR imaging can reliably detect hyperacute intraparenchymal hemorrhage, it may not be as reliable for detecting hyperacute blood products that contain predominantly oxyhemoglobin within the cerebral spinal fluid. The diamagnetic properties of oxyhemoglobin give it minimal susceptibility effect. For parenchymal hematomas, this is not a concern, but in the subarachnoid space where dilution of blood products by cerebrospinal fluid and high oxygen tension further reduce the sensitivity of susceptibility-weighted imaging, the possibility of missing a hemorrhage is a persistent concern. The use of and additional FLAIR sequence can minimize this concern.

Although MR imaging provides a detailed volumetric analysis of the pretreatment infarct core, the possibility of DWI reversibility discussed previously should be remembered. This is particularly true for patients who are candidates for mechanical thrombectomy in very early time frames (<3 hours). After endovascular therapy, as many as one-third of patient MR imaging scans obtained immediately afterward may demonstrate DWI reversibility; however, most of the brain tissue demonstrating this phenomenon progresses to infarction. The volume of tissue that permanently recovers is typically minimal and not clinically significant. Despite these drawbacks, MR imaging remains far superior to CT methods for core assessment.

FUTURE APPLICATIONS OF MR IMAGING

Although the role of MR imaging in acute stroke imaging continues to be a subject of debate, certain developments should be anticipated in the near future. Automation is likely to increasingly play a role in the interpretation of scans for patients with stroke. At the moment, automation is restricted to programs that process perfusion maps, but the potential for machine-learning algorithms to be able to identify affected tissue volume, hemorrhage, the presence of an LVO, and other salient aspects of MR imaging in acute stroke is large. It is anticipated that automation augmented with artificial intelligence will extend beyond merely descriptive content of the scan to assistance with treatment decisions and prognostication, by incorporating various other patient characteristics and using extensive comparative historical data.

Accelerated scanning is also likely to improve. There continues to be development of faster MR imaging methods, such as parallel imaging. In addition, the expected increases in processing power will shorten image reconstruction time. These incremental improvements will progressively shorten the time difference between MR imaging and CT imaging, and minimize the exclusion of patients from MR imaging due to medical instability or agitation. Furthermore, increasing attention will be paid to streamlining the logistics of safely obtaining MR imaging scans on patients with acute stroke.

Furthermore, MR imaging contraindications will diminish. Concerns related to pacemakers may be overstated. A total of 189 brain MR imaging scans performed in 123 patients with pacemakers or implantable cardioverters/defibrillators resulted in only 1 case of loss of pacing. There were no deaths or system revisions.[19] These findings were confirmed in a second, much larger study in which 1509 patients had 2103 MR imaging studies. One pacemaker had to be replaced.[20] Additionally, recent pacemakers are being designed specifically to be safe in an MR imaging scanner.[21] If pacemakers are considered acceptably safe for emergent MR imaging in the future, the proportion of patients eligible for MR imaging scanning will increase.

Finally, the precision of the information available by MR imaging is anticipated to provide opportunities for truly individualized stroke therapy.

Current decisions in acute stroke are based on population-level data. The nuances and intricacies of the individual patient and their response to therapy will be best understood with detailed information about their imaging profiles. This information is available from MR imaging more consistently than from CT.

SUMMARY

MR imaging in acute ischemic stroke provides specific insights into the pathophysiology of the disease in the individual patient. It is widely available and the time needed to perform MR imaging is similar to that of CT imaging. Clinical application of this imaging modality should bear in mind the known limitations, and further insights from future randomized controlled trials will be helpful in this regard. However, MR imaging parameters for stroke treatment selection will be an important component of future tissue-based decision making and truly personalized acute stroke therapeutics.

REFERENCES

1. Nogueira RG, Jadhav AP, Haussen DC, et al. Thrombectomy 6 to 24 hours after stroke with a mismatch between deficit and infarct. N Engl J Med 2018; 378(1):11–21.
2. Yoo AJ, Chaudhry ZA, Nogueira RG, et al. Infarct volume is a pivotal biomarker after intra-arterial stroke therapy. Stroke 2012;43(5):1323–30.
3. Schaefer PW, Grant PE, Gonzalez RG. Diffusion-weighted MR imaging of the brain. Radiology 2000;217(2):331–45.
4. Schaefer PW, Hassankhani A, Putman C, et al. Characterization and evolution of diffusion MR imaging abnormalities in stroke patients undergoing intra-arterial thrombolysis. AJNR Am J Neuroradiol 2004;25(6):951–7.
5. Campbell BC, Purushotham A, Christensen S, et al. The infarct core is well represented by the acute diffusion lesion: sustained reversal is infrequent. J Cereb Blood Flow Metab 2012;32(1):50–6.
6. Labeyrie MA, Turc G, Hess A, et al. Diffusion lesion reversal after thrombolysis: a MR correlate of early neurological improvement. Stroke 2012;43(11): 2986–91.
7. Leslie-Mazwi TM, Hirsch JA, Falcone GJ, et al. Endovascular stroke treatment outcomes after patient selection based on magnetic resonance imaging and clinical criteria. JAMA Neurol 2016;73(1):43–9.
8. Gonzalez RG, Copen WA, Schaefer PW, et al. The Massachusetts General Hospital acute stroke imaging algorithm: an experience and evidence based approach. J Neurointerv Surg 2013; 5(Suppl 1). i7–12.
9. Schaefer PW, Souza L, Kamalian S, et al. Limited reliability of computed tomographic perfusion acute infarct volume measurements compared with diffusion-weighted imaging in anterior circulation stroke. Stroke 2015;46(2):419–24.
10. Albers GW, Marks MP, Kemp S, et al. Thrombectomy for stroke at 6 to 16 hours with selection by perfusion imaging. N Engl J Med 2018. https://doi.org/10.1056/NEJMoa1713973.
11. Sims JR, Gharai LR, Schaefer PW, et al. ABC/2 for rapid clinical estimate of infarct, perfusion, and mismatch volumes. Neurology 2009;72(24): 2104–10.
12. Luby M, Hong J, Merino JG, et al. Stroke mismatch volume with the use of ABC/2 is equivalent to planimetric stroke mismatch volume. AJNR Am J Neuroradiol 2013;34(10):1901–7.
13. Menjot de Champfleur N, Saver JL, Goyal M, et al. Efficacy of stent-retriever thrombectomy in magnetic resonance imaging versus computed tomographic perfusion-selected patients in SWIFT PRIME trial (Solitaire FR with the intention for thrombectomy as primary endovascular treatment for acute ischemic stroke). Stroke 2017;48(6):1560–6.
14. Lansberg MG, Investigators D. Subgroup analyses of the DEFUSE 3 study International Stroke Conference. Los Angeles, CA, January 24–26, 2018.
15. Copen WA, Rezai Gharai L, Barak ER, et al. Existence of the diffusion-perfusion mismatch within 24 hours after onset of acute stroke: dependence on proximal arterial occlusion. Radiology 2009;250(3): 878–86.
16. Hakimelahi R, Vachha BA, Copen WA, et al. Time and diffusion lesion size in major anterior circulation ischemic strokes. Stroke 2014;45(10):2936–41.
17. Gonzalez RG, Hakimelahi R, Schaefer PW, et al. Stability of large diffusion/perfusion mismatch in anterior circulation strokes for 4 or more hours. BMC Neurol 2010;10:13.
18. Nael K, Khan R, Choudhary G, et al. Six-minute magnetic resonance imaging protocol for evaluation of acute ischemic stroke: pushing the boundaries. Stroke 2014;45(7):1985–91.
19. Strom JB, Whelan JB, Shen C, et al. Safety and utility of magnetic resonance imaging in patients with cardiac implantable electronic devices. Heart Rhythm 2017;14(8):1138–44.
20. Nazarian S, Hansford R, Rahsepar AA, et al. Safety of magnetic resonance imaging in patients with cardiac devices. N Engl J Med 2017;377(26): 2555–64.
21. Mitka M. First MRI-safe pacemaker receives conditional approval from FDA. JAMA 2011;305(10):985–6.

Advanced Neuroimaging of Acute Ischemic Stroke
Penumbra and Collateral Assessment

Jeremy J. Heit, MD, PhD*, Greg Zaharchuk, MD, PhD, Max Wintermark, MD

KEYWORDS

- Stroke • Perfusion • Collaterals • Penumbra • Infarction • MR imaging • CT • MRA

KEY POINTS

- Advanced neuroimaging of acute ischemic stroke is essential for correct patient treatment triage.
- The ischemic penumbra is characterized on imaging as regions of reduced blood flow and increased transit time on computed tomography (CT) perfusion, magnetic resonance (MR) perfusion, or arterial spin labeling (ASL).
- Pial collaterals may be imaged noninvasively with CT angiography, MR angiography, perfusion imaging, or ASL techniques.
- Robust pial collaterals may play a significant protective role in brain preservation in acute ischemic stroke.
- Robust pial collaterals may contribute to superior outcomes after the endovascular treatment of acute ischemic stroke.

INTRODUCTION

Acute ischemic stroke (AIS) is the leading cause of disability in the United States and the second-leading cause of death worldwide.[1] AIS is caused by embolic or thromboembolic occlusion of an artery that supplies the brain, which may result in irreversible infarction of brain tissue (core infarction). However, there is often a larger component of brain tissue that is hypoperfused, but viable, surrounding the core infarction; this tissue is termed the penumbra.[2,3] If timely revascularization of the occluded artery is not performed, the penumbra is at risk of progressing to irreversible infarction. Therefore, preservation of the penumbra is the goal of all stroke treatment.

All AIS treatments seek to open the occluded artery and restore blood flow to the brain. Revascularization of the occluded vessel restores blood flow to the brain (reperfusion), and successful revascularization and reperfusion results in improved clinical outcomes and a greater likelihood of living independently following a stroke.[4–10] Intravenous thrombolysis[4] and endovascular mechanical thrombectomy (EMT)[5–10] are effective treatments for AIS.

Five randomized trials comparing medical management with EMT were reported in 2015 for the treatment of AIS due to large vessel occlusion (LVO) of the internal carotid artery or proximal middle cerebral artery, which included (1) Multicenter Randomized Clinical Trial of Endovascular Treatment for Acute Ischemic Stroke (MR CLEAN), (2)

Disclosures: The authors have no financial or other relevant conflicts of interest.
Department of Radiology, Division of Neuroimaging and Neurointervention, Stanford Healthcare, 300 Pasteur Drive, Stanford, CA 94305, USA
* Corresponding author. Department of Radiology, Division of Neuroimaging and Neurointervention, Stanford University Hospital, 300 Pasteur Drive, S0047, Stanford, CA 94305.
E-mail address: jheit@stanford.edu

Neuroimag Clin N Am 28 (2018) 585–597
https://doi.org/10.1016/j.nic.2018.06.004
1052-5149/18/© 2018 Elsevier Inc. All rights reserved.

Endovascular Treatment for Small Core and Anterior Circulation Proximal Occlusion with Emphasis on Minimizing CT to Recanalization Times (ESCAPE), (3) Randomized Trial of Revascularization with Solitaire FR Device versus Best Medical Therapy in the Treatment of Acute Stroke Due to Anterior Circulation Large Vessel Occlusion Presenting within Eight Hours of Symptom Onset (REVASCAT), (4) Solitaire with the Intention for Thrombectomy as Primary Endovascular Treatment (SWIFT-PRIME), and (5) Extending the Time for Thrombolysis in Emergency Neurologic Deficits–Intra-Arterial (EXTEND IA). These studies found an overwhelming benefit for EMT compared with medical therapy (including intravenous thrombolysis) when treatment was performed within 6 hours of symptom onset.[5–9]

More recently, the Diffusion-Weighted Imaging or Computerized Tomography Perfusion Assessment With Clinical Mismatch in the Triage of Wake Up and Late Presenting Strokes Undergoing Neurointervention With Trevo (DAWN) and Endovascular Therapy Following Imaging Evaluation For Ischemic Stroke 3 (DEFUSE 3) trials have been reported.[10,11] These two randomized trials compared EMT with medical therapy in patients with AIS with an LVO who present 6 to 16 hours or 24 hours since symptom onset.[10,11] Both of these late-window trials similarly found an overwhelming benefit of EMT, which has resulted in new guidelines that recommend the treatment of AIS due to LVO up to 24 hours since patients were last known to be normal.[12]

Neuroimaging remains critical in the diagnosis, triage, and treatment of patients with AIS, particularly those with AIS due to an LVO.[2] Advances in AIS treatment with EMT have been coupled with advances in computed tomography (CT) and MR imaging neuroimaging. Here the authors review advanced noninvasive brain imaging by CT and MR imaging for the evaluation of AIS. Given the wide breadth of topics in AIS imaging, the authors focus their discussion to the evaluation of patients with AIS undergoing triage for EMT and the utility of penumbral and collateral imaging in this context.

PENUMBRAL IMAGING

The role of penumbral imaging in AIS has been hotly debated.[2,13–15] Despite this controversy, there is widespread agreement on the importance of the penumbra as a concept and the importance of identifying the presence of a mismatch between the core infarction and the penumbra in selecting patients for EMT treatment of AIS.[2]

Patients who are most likely to benefit from EMT demonstrate imaging and/or clinical evidence of a salvageable penumbra that is larger than the core infarction at the time of triage.[2] The authors now briefly review the neuroimaging techniques for assessment of the ischemic, but viable, penumbra. Of note, some of these techniques also provide information regarding pial collateral vessels, which is discussed in the subsequent section.

Computed Tomography Perfusion and Magnetic Resonance Perfusion Techniques

Perfusion imaging is the most commonly used method to image the penumbra, and both CT perfusion (CTP) and magnetic resonance perfusion (MRP) techniques are used in the evaluation of patients with AIS. CTP and MRP provide a rapid, quantitative, and easily interpretable visual assessment of the penumbra. Furthermore, the ability to automate the processing of CTP and MRP also allows for the rapid transmission of images that quantitatively and qualitatively summarize the size of the penumbra and ischemic core (Fig. 1). These summary maps facilitate the transfer of patients with AIS and treatment triage to comprehensive stroke centers, such as the authors', even when patients cannot be evaluated by specialized stroke neurology and neurointervention physicians.

CTP is the most commonly performed perfusion imaging technique for the evaluation of patients with AIS given the widespread availability of CT. CTP is performed by injection of iodinated contrast into an antecubital vein followed by serial brain imaging, as the contrast is carried by the blood flow through brain tissue.[3] The change in brain tissue density due to the passage of iodinated contrast over time is used to generate brain perfusion maps that commonly include cerebral blood volume (CBV), cerebral blood flow (CBF), mean transit time, and time-to-maximum of the residue function (Tmax) images.[3,14] The core infarction on CTP is represented by severely reduced CBV or CBF, and the penumbra is represented by regions of prolonged mean transit time or Tmax (Fig. 2).[14]

MRP, also referred to as dynamic susceptibility contrast imaging, is also a well-established perfusion imaging technique; but the more limited availability of MR imaging has limited widespread adoption of this technique relative to CTP. MRP is performed by injection of a contrast agent (gadolinium-based rather than iodinated) into an antecubital vein followed by serial brain imaging.[3] Gadolinium creates low

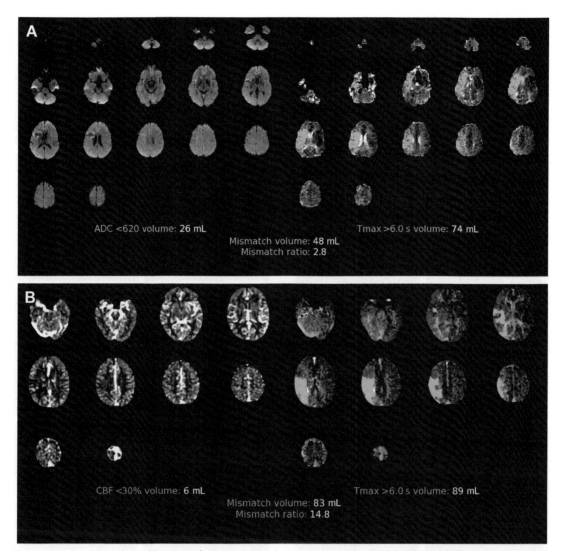

Fig. 1. Target mismatch profile on perfusion imaging in 2 patients with AIS. (*A*) MRP study from a patient with AIS presenting with a right middle cerebral artery syndrome. Diffusion-weighted imaging and MRP images demonstrate a mismatch ratio (difference in volume) between a core infarction of 26 mL (*pink*) and the penumbra of 74 mL (*green*). (*B*) CTP study from a different patient with AIS also presenting with a right middle cerebral artery syndrome. CTP images demonstrate a mismatch ratio between the core infarction of 6 mL (*pink*) and the penumbra of 89 mL (*green*). The core infarction was estimated on CTP as a 70% reduction in CBF relative to the left cerebral hemisphere. Perfusion summary maps (*A, B*) are presented.

susceptibility signal in the brain tissue, and serial brain imaging allows for the processing of brain perfusion images in a manner similar to CTP (**Fig. 3**).[2,16] MRP has several advantages relative to CTP, including the lack of ionizing radiation and greater anatomic definition.[16]

Perfusion imaging has been used in AIS to identify regions of hypoperfused brain tissue, which correspond to the penumbra. In patients with AIS due to LVO, a mismatch between the volume of the core infarction and the penumbra represents brain tissue that may be salvaged

by successful EMT; this target mismatch concept was first validated in the prospective DEFUSE 2 study.[17] More recently, the randomized SWIFT-PRIME and EXTEND-IA trials randomized patients with AIS with a target mismatch to medical therapy or EMT; both studies showed superior clinical outcomes in patients treated by EMT.[8,9] Interestingly, SWIFT-PRIME and EXTEND-IA showed a greater EMT treatment effect relative to the MR CLEAN, REVASCAT, and ESCAPE randomized trials, which did not use perfusion imaging for patient

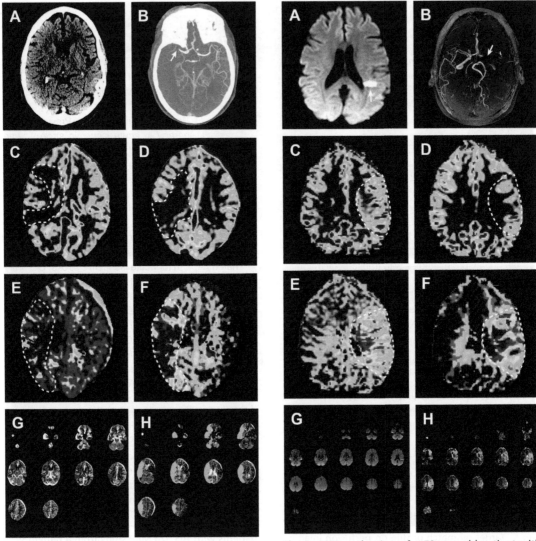

Fig. 2. CTP evaluation of a 76-year-old patient with AIS with occlusion of the right middle cerebral artery. (*A*) Noncontrast head CT demonstrates no evidence of acute infarction. (*B*) Axial maximum-intensity-projection images from a CTA demonstrate occlusion in the distal M1 segment of the right middle cerebral artery (*arrow*). CTP-derived perfusion maps (*C–F*) demonstrate the core infarction (*C, D, dashed outline*) and penumbra (*E, F, dashed outline*) on CBV (*C*), CBF (*D*), mean transit time (*E*), and Tmax (*F*) maps. Perfusion summary maps demonstrate estimates of the core from a 70% reduction of CBF relative to the left cerebral hemisphere (*G, pink*) and the penumbra from the Tmax (*H, green*).

Fig. 3. MRP evaluation of a 50-year-old patient with AIS with occlusion of the left internal carotid artery. (*A*) Diffusion-weighted imaging (DWI) demonstrates a small region of acute infarction in the left periventricular white matter (*arrow*). (*B*) Axial maximum-intensity-projection images from an MRA demonstrate occlusion of the left internal carotid artery (*arrow*). MRP-derived perfusion maps (*C–F*) demonstrate mildly increased CBV (*C, dashed outline*), reduced CBF (*D, dashed outline*), prolonged transit time on MTT (*E, dashed outline*), and Tmax (*F, dashed outline*). Perfusion summary maps demonstrate volumes of the core infarction from DWI (*G, pink*) and the penumbra from Tmax (*H, green*).

selection.[5–9] This difference suggests that perfusion imaging that demonstrates a target mismatch relative to the core infarction may be superior in selecting patients who are most likely to benefit from EMT. However, further studies comparing the imaging selection of patients for AIS treatment are required to test this idea.

Perfusion imaging has also been used to triage patients with AIS presenting in late time windows to EMT. The recently reported DAWN and DEFUSE

3 trials compared medical therapy with EMT for AIS treatment in patients last known to be normal 6 to 24 hours (DAWN) and 6 to 16 hours (DEFUSE 3) before medical evaluation.[10,11] CTP in the DAWN trial was used to estimate the core infarction, and patients with a small core infarction that was mismatched to the severity of their clinical deficits were enrolled in the trial.[10] By contrast, the DEFUSE 3 trial enrolled patients who demonstrated a target mismatch between the core infarction and the penumbra on CTP or MRP.[11] Both trials showed an overwhelming benefit of EMT compared with medical therapy in the treatment of patients with AIS in these late time windows, and it is expected that perfusion imaging will become an essential component of EMT triage in late time windows.

The utility of perfusion imaging extends beyond the initial triage of patients with AIS, and perfusion imaging performed after EMT may provide prognostic information about patient outcomes. Patients who undergo successful EMT and have normal reperfusion on post-EMT CTP or MRP are more likely to achieve a good clinical outcome relative to patients without reperfusion on perfusion imaging.[18] Similarly, reperfusion on CTP after EMT better predicts final infarct volume and patient outcomes irrespective of successful revascularization by EMT.[18,19]

Thus, perfusion imaging is an important tool in the evaluation and prognostication of patients with AIS, particularly in those who undergo EMT. However, patients with impaired renal function or contrast allergies may be ineligible for CTP or MRP evaluation. Other MR imaging techniques, such as arterial spin labeling (ASL) and resting-state functional MR imaging (rs-fMR imaging), may be used to characterize the penumbra in these patients; these techniques are now briefly discussed.

Arterial Spin Labeling

ASL is an MR imaging technique that provides a quantitative measurement of CBF, which may be used to identify the penumbra in patients with AIS. ASL is performed by magnetically labeling blood in the upper neck to create an endogenous blood tracer.[20,21] Next, brain imaging is performed after a short delay to demonstrate the deposition of the labeled blood in the cerebral capillary bed; these images provide a quantitative CBF map (Fig. 4).[21,22] Therefore, ASL does not require the injection of an exogenous contrast agent and it may be serially repeated if necessary, which are distinct advantages relative to MRP.

Regions of hypointense signal on ASL represent regions of decreased CBF, which represent the penumbra in the setting of AIS.[23,24] ASL and MRP demonstrate a high agreement in the detection of a penumbra, but ASL tends to overestimate the size of the penumbra relative to MRP.[24,25] Despite these slight differences, ASL remains a valuable tool in penumbral imaging.

Resting-State Functional MR Imaging

rs-fMR imaging is an advanced MR imaging technique that measures blood oxygen level–dependent (BOLD) changes in brain oxygen utilization when patients are at rest.[26] Several studies have investigated whether BOLD imaging may be used to measure cerebral perfusion.[27–31] Minor changes in blood oxygenation are due to physiologic changes, such as variations in cardiac output or respiration; these subtle variations of the BOLD signal may be measured in the resting state to provide an indication of cerebral perfusion.[29] This rs-fMR imaging is performed by obtaining multiple BOLD imaging time points and plotting the amplitude variation of the BOLD signal as a perfusion map that is sensitive to CBV and oxygenation.[29–31]

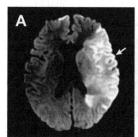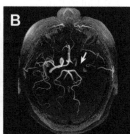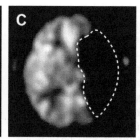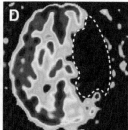

Fig. 4. MRP evaluation of a 57-year-old patient on hemodialysis for renal failure with an AIS due to occlusion of the left internal carotid artery. (*A*) Diffusion-weighted imaging demonstrates a large acute infarction involving nearly all of the left middle cerebral artery territory (*arrow*). (*B*) Axial maximum-intensity-projection images from an MRA demonstrate occlusion of the left internal carotid artery (*arrow*). Axial ASL image in grayscale (*C*) and postprocessed CBF map (*D*) demonstrate severely reduced blood flow in the region of acute infarction (*C, D, dashed outlines*).

Temporal changes in the BOLD signal may then be plotted in a delayed-mapping technique to provide a measure of tissue level cerebral perfusion.[29,30,32]

Tmax images derived from MRP have been compared with rs-fMR imaging delay maps in patients with AIS.[30,31] These studies found a good correlation between rs-fMR imaging delay and Tmax maps, which suggests that rs-fMR imaging may be used to measure penumbra in ischemic stroke. However, no patients in either study were imaged within 3 hours of symptom onset, and the diagnostic accuracy of rs-fMR imaging in the evaluation of AIS has not been established.

PIAL COLLATERALS

The arterial supply to the brain is a complex interconnected network of arterial anastomoses that provides redundant routes for blood flow to the brain. Collateral flow may be provided through large artery-to-artery connections in the circle of Willis, external-to-internal carotid artery connections, and smaller cerebral artery-to-artery (pial) connections.[33] These collateral pathways of blood flow are particularly important in preserved brain viability in the setting of AIS.

The angioarchitecture of the pial anastomotic network is highly variable in patients[33] and in animal models,[34,35] and the genetics governing the biological development and adaptation of collaterals remain poorly understood. Additionally, collateral network robustness has been shown to be influenced by patient age, hypertension, diabetes, chronic reductions in cerebral perfusion, and statin use.[33,36–38] The wide variation in collateral circulation anatomy and robustness in patients with AIS leads to a high variability in resistance to cerebral infarction. The authors now briefly review the importance of collaterals in AIS due to LVO and the advanced neuroimaging techniques that have been developed for collateral vessel imaging.

Collateral Influence on Acute Ischemic Stroke Outcome

Robust collaterals in patients with AIS due to LVO have been shown to be an important predictor of good outcomes.[33,39–49] Patients with good collaterals are thought to be better able to maintain brain viability in the setting of AIS. In support of this hypothesis, patients with good collaterals are more likely to present with a smaller core infarction and a larger target mismatch at the time of imaging triage.[48,50] By contrast, poor collaterals have been associated with larger core infarctions and more rapid infarct growth.[8]

Good collaterals also correlate with improved outcomes after EMT treatment of AIS. Hwang and colleagues[51] found that patients with good collaterals were more likely to have less core infarction growth and superior clinical outcomes after EMT relative to patients with poor collaterals. Similarly, other studies found that clinical outcomes after AIS are superior in patients with good collaterals and successful revascularization by EMT,[52] whereas poor collaterals are associated with poorer reperfusion after EMT.[53] These data indicate that robust collaterals are associated with a favorable prognosis and a favorable response to EMT. However, the mechanism by which robust collaterals result in improved clinical outcomes after successful EMT remains to be determined.

Collateral Imaging Techniques

Several neuroimaging techniques have been developed to image collaterals in the setting of AIS. Vessel imaging by digital subtraction angiography (DSA), CTA, or MRA are the most commonly performed measures; these techniques aim to assess the number, size, and rate of filling of pial collaterals. However, cerebral perfusion techniques also provide collateral status information by indirectly measuring the robustness of blood flow to ischemic brain in the setting of AIS. Of note, multiple scoring systems have been described for the assessment of collaterals, and a thorough discussion of these scales is beyond the scope of this review. Readers are referred elsewhere for an excellent discussion of collateral scoring systems.[54] The authors now briefly review different imaging methods for the assessment of pial collaterals in the setting of AIS.

Digital subtraction angiography

DSA is a minimally invasive procedure in which endovascular access to an artery is obtained by arterial puncture of the common femoral artery or radial artery.[55,56] Once arterial access has been obtained, a catheter is navigated into the cervical internal carotid artery or other artery of interest; a contrast injection through the catheter allows for arterial flow distal to the catheter to be studied in real time. The high spatial and temporal resolution of DSA makes it the gold standard test for the evaluation of pial collateral arteries and collateral blood flow.

Despite its superior spatial and temporal resolution, DSA is infrequently performed to assess collateral robustness for clinical decision-making in AIS because of its invasiveness and decreased availability relative to noninvasive CT or MR imaging techniques.[57] However, collateral robustness

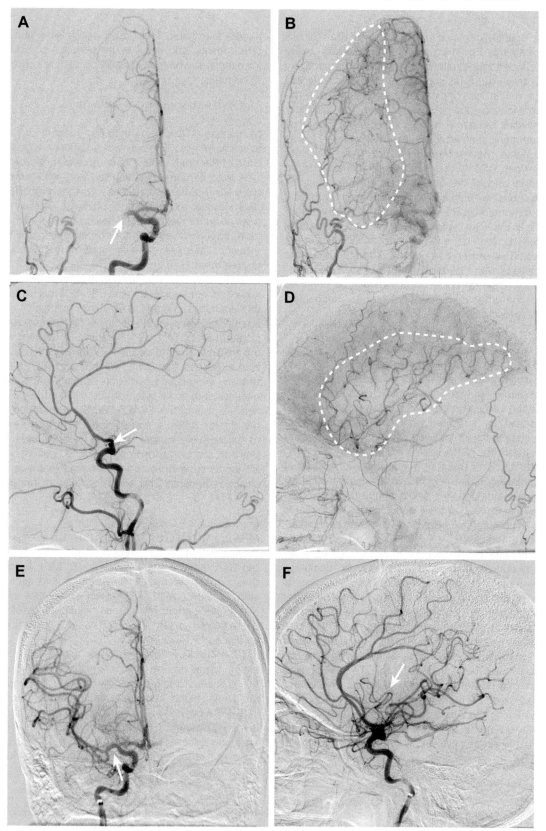

Fig. 5. Robust pial collaterals identified by DSA during EMT treatment of a patient with AIS with a right middle cerebral artery occlusion. Anteroposterior (*A, B, E*) and lateral (*C, D, F*) DSA images after injection of the right

is routinely identified in the context of EMT for AIS treatment. For example, internal carotid artery DSA performed before mechanical thrombectomy of an ipsilateral M1 segment occlusion can identify the robustness of pial collaterals arising from the anterior cerebral artery and even the posterior cerebral artery if a sufficiently large posterior communicating artery is present.

Some neurointerventionalists may elect to perform DSA of the contralateral internal carotid artery and of the posterior circulation to assess the collateral status before performing mechanical thrombectomy. However, most neurointerventionalists think that angiography of these additional vessels does not change endovascular treatment workflow or decision-making. Therefore, in most patients with AIS undergoing endovascular treatment, DSA for collateral assessment is confined to the affected circulation before mechanical thrombectomy (Fig. 5).

Computed tomography angiography

CTA is the most commonly performed study to assess cerebral collaterals given the widespread availability of this technique and excellent identification of cerebral arterial anatomy. CTA is performed by iodinated contrast injection into an antecubital vein followed by CT of the head after a fixed time delay, test bolus, or bolus triggered method.[2,3,58] This CTA acquisition is optimized to capture contrast opacification of the cerebral arteries, although this single acquisition may lead to incomplete arterial opacification in patients with poor cardiac output or a proximal cervical artery stenosis.[58,59]

In patients with AIS due to an LVO, cerebral artery opacification distal to the vascular occlusion represents filling via collaterals (Fig. 6). Collateral filling distal to a vascular occlusion may be better visualized on postprocessed maximum intensity projection (MIP) images (see Fig. 6), which provides treating physicians with a rapid visual assessment of the degree of collateral flow. Patients with poor collaterals on CTA MIP images are more likely to present with a large core infarction and to have a poor clinical outcome.[50] Emerging machine learning techniques to assess pial collaterals on CTA show promise in being able to predict clinical outcomes in patients with AIS.[60] It will be of interest to determine if these newer, automated techniques can reliably separate patients who are likely to benefit from EMT from those in whom an invasive procedure is likely to be futile.

Multiphase computed tomography angiography

Multiphase CTA is performed in a manner similar to single-phase CTA but with additional acquisitions of the brain tissue.[61] The goal of multiphase CTA is to capture time-resolved and more complete filling of the pial arteries in the peak arterial, peak venous, and late venous phases.[61] These images allow for pial collateral flow to be scored in a more time resolved manner so that patients with robust collaterals can be selected for endovascular treatment.

Multiphase CTA was used in the imaging selection of patients enrolled in the ESCAPE trial, which demonstrated a benefit of EMT over medical management.[7] However, the benefit of multiphase over single-phase CTA may be minimal.[62] Moreover, the treatment effect of EMT in the ESCAPE trial was inferior to the SWIFT-PRIME and EXTEND-IA trials, which used perfusion imaging to identify patients with a target mismatch.[8,9,62,63] A post hoc analysis of the SWIFT-PRIME study found a benefit for patients undergoing EMT regardless of collateral status, which further supports the hypothesis that perfusion imaging–based patient selection as superior to collateral-based methods in selecting patients who are most likely to benefit from EMT.[64]

Magnetic resonance angiography

MRA provides a similar spatial resolution to CTA in the evaluation of the cerebral arterial anatomy,[65] but CTA remains slightly superior to MRA in the detection of cerebral artery stenosis and occlusion.[66] There are 2 MRA techniques that are commonly performed in the evaluation of AIS: time-of-flight MRA (TOF-MRA) and contrast-enhanced MRA (CE-MRA).

TOF-MRA is a flow-related technique in which tissue signal in the slab of imaging is nulled by repeated radiofrequency pulses, whereas in-flowing blood remains unsaturated.[67] Thus, TOF-MRA provides high signal in the arteries that is readily distinguished from background brain tissue with excellent spatial resolution. TOF-MRA does not require the injection of an exogenous

---

internal carotid artery demonstrate occlusion of the M1 segment of the right middle cerebral artery (*A, C, arrows*) in the early arterial phase. Robust pial collaterals arising from the right anterior cerebral artery are noted in the late arterial phase (*B, D, dashed outline*). After successful EMT, there is complete recanalization of the right middle cerebral artery (*E, F, arrows*).

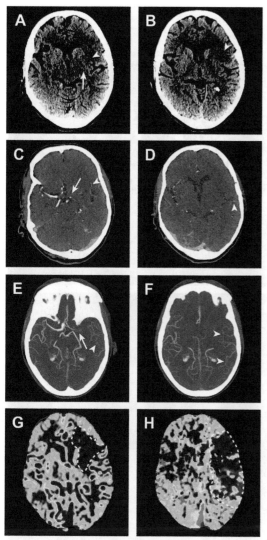

disadvantage in the setting of AIS. Moreover, the flow-related signal of TOF-MRA is only visualized in an antegrade manner, so this technique provides little information regarding collaterals.

By contrast, CE-MRA is performed following the intravenous injection of a gadolinium contrast agent. The use of an exogenous contrast agent, more rapid T1-based imaging, and the ability to rapidly acquire multiple phases of imaging make CE-MRA more similar to CTA than TOF-MRA.[68] CE-MRA better demonstrates arterial collaterals distal to an arterial occlusion because the signal in this technique is related to the T1-shortening effects on the gadolinium contrast agent rather than the flow-related signal of TOF-MRA.[69,70] This superior delineation of collaterals by CE-MRA better predicts the final infarct volume compared with TOF-MRA.[70]

Penumbral imaging by computed tomography perfusion and magnetic resonance perfusion

Although perfusion imaging does not directly assess the size and number of pial collaterals, it provides blood flow and perfusion information, which is directly related to the robustness of collaterals. For example, first-pass CTP was found to be an accurate biomarker for collateral robustness.[71] Nael and colleagues[72] studied patients with AIS who underwent MRP before DSA during EMT and derived a perfusion collateral index from the pretreatment MRP. This perfusion collateral index was reported to be highly accurate in predicting collateral status on the subsequent DSA.[72] Similarly, MRP source images were found to provide accurate collateral grading that was superior to the diffusion-perfusion target mismatch in determining patient outcomes after endovascular treatment of AIS.[73] The segmentation of Tmax maps from MRP into anatomic (pial, cortical, and parenchymal) compartments may be used to derive a pial collateral score that correlates well with DSA.[74] Thus, perfusion imaging by CTP or MRP should be considered as an indirect, but reliable, measure of collaterals.[71–77]

Arterial spin labeling

As noted earlier, ASL is a quantitative measure of CBF and is an alternative technique that may be used to characterize cerebral perfusion in AIS. However, the utility of ASL extends beyond the measurement of the ischemic penumbra, as it has been found to be a more direct measure of pial collaterals as well. Collaterals may be visualized on ASL images as linear hyperintense regions of increased CBF in the periphery of the ischemic penumbra (Fig. 7). Interestingly, ASL performed

Fig. 6. Robust pial collaterals on CTA in a patient with AIS due to a left internal carotid artery occlusion. Noncontrast head CT images (A, B) demonstrate acute infarction with hypodensity of the left lentiform nucleus (A, arrow), left insula (A, arrowhead), left frontal lobe subcortical white matter (B, arrowhead). Source images from a CTA (C, D) demonstrate occlusion of the left internal carotid artery (C, arrow) as the cause of the stroke. However, left middle cerebral artery vessels distal to the occlusion fill via pial collaterals (C, D, arrowheads). The left internal carotid artery occlusion is better demonstrated on axial maximum-intensity projection images (E, arrow) as is the robust filling of the left middle cerebral artery branches (E, F, arrowheads) by pial collaterals. CTP images demonstrate reduced CBF in the left corona radiata (G, dashed outline) and the penumbra on Tmax (H, dashed outline).

contrast agent and is easily reformatted into 3-dimensional images because of its volumetric acquisition. However, the acquisition time of this technique takes several minutes, which may a

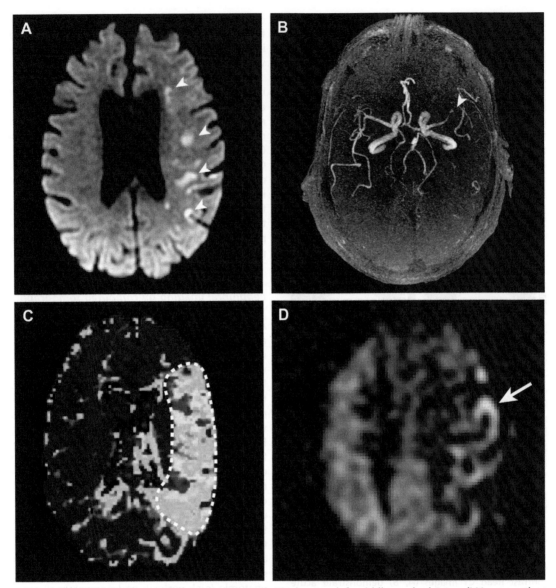

Fig. 7. Robust pial collaterals on ASL in a patient with AIS due to a left middle cerebral artery (M1 segment) occlusion. (*A*) Diffusion-weighted imaging demonstrates small areas of acute infarction involving within the left middle cerebral artery territory (*arrowheads*). (*B*) Axial maximum-intensity-projection images from an MRA demonstrate occlusion of the M1 segment of the left middle cerebral artery (*arrowhead*). (*C*) Axial Tmax image demonstrates a large area of delayed CBF that is consistent with the penumbra (*dashed outline*). (*D*) Axial ASL image demonstrates hyperintense robust collaterals along the lateral edge of the penumbra (*arrow*).

with 2 different postlabel imaging delays may be used to distinguish retrograde from antegrade blood flow in patients with stenosis in the M1 segment of the middle cerebral artery[78]; but this technique has not been evaluated in patients with AIS to the authors' knowledge.

The presence of collaterals detected by ASL are strongly correlated with a good clinical outcome in patients with AIS in retrospective series.[79,80] The ongoing Imaging Collaterals in Acute Stroke (iCAS) study is a prospective cohort study of patients with AIS undergoing MR imaging with ASL before EMT. The iCAS study will determine whether patients with good collaterals on pretreatment ASL are more likely to have a favorable response to EMT and a good clinical outcome after EMT. The results of this study will be of interest and would be a strong validation of the ASL technique in the triage of patients with AIS to EMT.

SUMMARY

The randomized studies that demonstrated the efficacy of EMT treatment of AIS in the past several years[5–9] are the greatest advancements in stroke care since the approval of tissue plasminogen activator for intravenous thrombolysis in 1995.[4] The efficacy of EMT has been closely linked to advancements in neuroimaging by CT and MR imaging to assess the ischemic penumbra and collaterals. The authors expect the coming years to witness even larger changes in the use of advanced neuroimaging in the triage and treatment of AIS as the use of EMT continues to expand.

REFERENCES

1. Writing Group M, Mozaffarian D, Benjamin EJ, et al. Heart disease and stroke statistics-2016 update: a report from the American heart association. Circulation 2016;133(4):e38–360.
2. Heit JJ, Wintermark M. Imaging selection for reperfusion therapy in acute ischemic stroke. Curr Treat Options Neurol 2015;17(2):332.
3. Heit JJ, Wintermark M. Perfusion computed tomography for the evaluation of acute ischemic stroke: strengths and pitfalls. Stroke 2016;47(4):1153–8.
4. National Institute of Neurological Disorders and Stroke rt-PA Stroke Study Group. Tissue plasminogen activator for acute ischemic stroke. N Engl J Med 1995;333(24):1581–7.
5. Berkhemer OA, Fransen PS, Beumer D, et al. A randomized trial of intraarterial treatment for acute ischemic stroke. N Engl J Med 2015;372(1):11–20.
6. Jovin TG, Chamorro A, Cobo E, et al. Thrombectomy within 8 hours after symptom onset in ischemic stroke. N Engl J Med 2015;372(24):2296–306.
7. Goyal M, Demchuk AM, Menon BK, et al. Randomized assessment of rapid endovascular treatment of ischemic stroke. N Engl J Med 2015;372(11): 1019–30.
8. Campbell BC, Mitchell PJ, Kleinig TJ, et al. Endovascular therapy for ischemic stroke with perfusion-imaging selection. N Engl J Med 2015;372(11): 1009–18.
9. Saver JL, Goyal M, Bonafe A, et al. Stent-retriever thrombectomy after intravenous t-PA vs. t-PA alone in stroke. N Engl J Med 2015;372(24):2285–95.
10. Nogueira RG, Jadhav AP, Haussen DC, et al. Thrombectomy 6 to 24 hours after stroke with a mismatch between deficit and infarct. N Engl J Med 2018; 378(1):11–21.
11. Albers GW, Marks MP, Kemp S, et al. Thrombectomy for stroke at 6 to 16 hours with selection by perfusion imaging. N Engl J Med 2018. https://doi.org/10. 1056/NEJMoa1713973.
12. Powers WJ, Rabinstein AA, Ackerson T, et al. 2018 guidelines for the early management of patients with acute ischemic stroke: a guideline for healthcare professionals from the American Heart Association/American Stroke Association. Stroke 2018. https://doi.org/10.1161/STR.0000000000000158.
13. Gonzalez RG. Low signal, high noise and large uncertainty make CT perfusion unsuitable for acute ischemic stroke patient selection for endovascular therapy. J Neurointerv Surg 2012;4(4):242–5.
14. Wintermark M, Sincic R, Sridhar D, et al. Cerebral perfusion CT: technique and clinical applications. J Neuroradiol 2008;35(5):253–60.
15. Liebeskind DS, Parsons MW, Wintermark M, et al. Computed tomography perfusion in acute ischemic stroke: is it ready for prime time? Stroke 2015; 46(8):2364–7.
16. Tong E, Sugrue L, Wintermark M. Understanding the neurophysiology and quantification of brain perfusion. Top Magn Reson Imaging 2017;26(2):57–65.
17. Lansberg MG, Straka M, Kemp S, et al. MRI profile and response to endovascular reperfusion after stroke (DEFUSE 2): a prospective cohort study. Lancet Neurol 2012;11(10):860–7.
18. Cho TH, Nighoghossian N, Mikkelsen IK, et al. Reperfusion within 6 hours outperforms recanalization in predicting penumbra salvage, lesion growth, final infarct, and clinical outcome. Stroke 2015;46(6): 1582–9.
19. Soares BP, Tong E, Hom J, et al. Reperfusion is a more accurate predictor of follow-up infarct volume than recanalization: a proof of concept using CT in acute ischemic stroke patients. Stroke 2010;41(1): e34–40.
20. Zaharchuk G. Better late than never: the long journey for noncontrast arterial spin labeling perfusion imaging in acute stroke. Stroke 2012;43(4): 931–2.
21. Haller S, Zaharchuk G, Thomas DL, et al. Arterial spin labeling perfusion of the brain: emerging clinical applications. Radiology 2016;281(2): 337–56.
22. Telischak NA, Detre JA, Zaharchuk G. Arterial spin labeling MRI: clinical applications in the brain. J Magn Reson Imaging 2015;41(5):1165–80.
23. Wang DJ, Alger JR, Qiao JX, et al. The value of arterial spin-labeled perfusion imaging in acute ischemic stroke: comparison with dynamic susceptibility contrast-enhanced MRI. Stroke 2012;43(4): 1018–24.
24. Zaharchuk G, El Mogy IS, Fischbein NJ, et al. Comparison of arterial spin labeling and bolus perfusion-weighted imaging for detecting mismatch in acute stroke. Stroke 2012;43(7):1843–8.
25. Bivard A, Krishnamurthy V, Stanwell P, et al. Arterial spin labeling versus bolus-tracking perfusion in hyperacute stroke. Stroke 2014;45(1):127–33.

26. Kroll H, Zaharchuk G, Christen T, et al. Resting-State BOLD MRI for Perfusion and Ischemia. Top Magn Reson Imaging 2017;26(2):91–6.

27. Tong Y, Frederick BD. Time lag dependent multimodal processing of concurrent fMRI and near-infrared spectroscopy (NIRS) data suggests a global circulatory origin for low-frequency oscillation signals in human brain. Neuroimage 2010;53(2):553–64.

28. Li Z, Zhu Y, Childress AR, et al. Relations between BOLD fMRI-derived resting brain activity and cerebral blood flow. PLoS One 2012;7(9):e44556.

29. Christen T, Jahanian H, Ni WW, et al. Noncontrast mapping of arterial delay and functional connectivity using resting-state functional MRI: a study in Moyamoya patients. J Magn Reson Imaging 2015;41(2):424–30.

30. Lv Y, Margulies DS, Cameron Craddock R, et al. Identifying the perfusion deficit in acute stroke with resting-state functional magnetic resonance imaging. Ann Neurol 2013;73(1):136–40.

31. Tsai YH, Yuan R, Huang YC, et al. Altered resting-state FMRI signals in acute stroke patients with ischemic penumbra. PLoS One 2014;9(8):e105117.

32. Amemiya S, Kunimatsu A, Saito N, et al. Cerebral hemodynamic impairment: assessment with resting-state functional MR imaging. Radiology 2014;270(2):548–55.

33. Liebeskind DS. Collateral circulation. Stroke 2003;34(9):2279–84.

34. Wang S, Zhang H, Wiltshire T, et al. Genetic dissection of the Canq1 locus governing variation in extent of the collateral circulation. PLoS One 2012;7(3):e31910.

35. Lucitti JL, Mackey JK, Morrison JC, et al. Formation of the collateral circulation is regulated by vascular endothelial growth factor-A and a disintegrin and metalloprotease family members 10 and 17. Circ Res 2012;111(12):1539–50.

36. Menon BK, Smith EE, Coutts SB, et al. Leptomeningeal collaterals are associated with modifiable metabolic risk factors. Ann Neurol 2013;74(2):241–8.

37. Liebeskind DS. Collateral perfusion: time for novel paradigms in cerebral ischemia. Int J stroke 2012;7(4):309–10.

38. Ovbiagele B, Saver JL, Starkman S, et al. Statin enhancement of collateralization in acute stroke. Neurology 2007;68(24):2129–31.

39. Ringelstein EB, Biniek R, Weiller C, et al. Type and extent of hemispheric brain infarctions and clinical outcome in early and delayed middle cerebral artery recanalization. Neurology 1992;42(2):289–98.

40. Kucinski T, Koch C, Eckert B, et al. Collateral circulation is an independent radiological predictor of outcome after thrombolysis in acute ischaemic stroke. Neuroradiology 2003;45(1):11–8.

41. Christoforidis GA, Mohammad Y, Kehagias D, et al. Angiographic assessment of pial collaterals as a prognostic indicator following intra-arterial thrombolysis for acute ischemic stroke. AJNR Am J Neuroradiol 2005;26(7):1789–97.

42. Menon BK, Smith EE, Modi J, et al. Regional leptomeningeal score on CT angiography predicts clinical and imaging outcomes in patients with acute anterior circulation occlusions. AJNR Am J Neuroradiol 2011;32(9):1640–5.

43. Fanou EM, Knight J, Aviv RI, et al. Effect of collaterals on clinical presentation, baseline imaging, complications, and outcome in acute stroke. AJNR Am J Neuroradiol 2015;36(12):2285–91.

44. van den Wijngaard IR, Boiten J, Holswilder G, et al. Impact of collateral status evaluated by dynamic computed tomographic angiography on clinical outcome in patients with ischemic stroke. Stroke 2015;46(12):3398–404.

45. van Seeters T, Biessels GJ, Kappelle LJ, et al. The prognostic value of CT angiography and CT perfusion in acute ischemic stroke. Cerebrovasc Dis 2015;40(5–6):258–69.

46. Sheth SA, Sanossian N, Hao Q, et al. Collateral flow as causative of good outcomes in endovascular stroke therapy. J Neurointerv Surg 2016;8(1):2–7.

47. Hacke W, Kaste M, Fieschi C, et al. Intravenous thrombolysis with recombinant tissue plasminogen activator for acute hemispheric stroke. The European Cooperative Acute Stroke Study (ECASS). JAMA 1995;274(13):1017–25.

48. Miteff F, Levi CR, Bateman GA, et al. The independent predictive utility of computed tomography angiographic collateral status in acute ischaemic stroke. Brain 2009;132(Pt 8):2231–8.

49. Maas MB, Lev MH, Ay H, et al. Collateral vessels on CT angiography predict outcome in acute ischemic stroke. Stroke 2009;40(9):3001–5.

50. Souza LC, Yoo AJ, Chaudhry ZA, et al. Malignant CTA collateral profile is highly specific for large admission DWI infarct core and poor outcome in acute stroke. AJNR Am J Neuroradiol 2012;33(7):1331–6.

51. Hwang YH, Kang DH, Kim YW, et al. Impact of time-to-reperfusion on outcome in patients with poor collaterals. AJNR Am J Neuroradiol 2015;36(3):495–500.

52. Gerber JC, Petrova M, Krukowski P, et al. Collateral state and the effect of endovascular reperfusion therapy on clinical outcome in ischemic stroke patients. Brain Behav 2016;6(9):e00513.

53. Bang OY, Saver JL, Kim SJ, et al. Collateral flow predicts response to endovascular therapy for acute ischemic stroke. Stroke 2011;42(3):693–9.

54. McVerry F, Liebeskind DS, Muir KW. Systematic review of methods for assessing leptomeningeal

collateral flow. AJNR Am J Neuroradiol 2012;33(3): 576–82.

55. Willinsky RA, Taylor SM, TerBrugge K, et al. Neurologic complications of cerebral angiography: prospective analysis of 2,899 procedures and review of the literature. Radiology 2003;227(2):522–8.

56. Yoon W, Kwon WK, Choudhri O, et al. Complications following transradial cerebral angiography: an ultrasound follow-up study. J Korean Neurosurg Soc 2017. https://doi.org/10.3340/jkns.2017.0209.

57. Raymond SB, Schaefer PW. Imaging brain collaterals: quantification, scoring, and potential significance. Top Magn Reson Imaging 2017;26(2):67–75.

58. Mohan S, Agarwal M, Pukenas B. Computed tomography angiography of the neurovascular circulation. Radiol Clin North Am 2016;54(1):147–62.

59. Pulli B, Schaefer PW, Hakimelahi R, et al. Acute ischemic stroke: infarct core estimation on CT angiography source images depends on CT angiography protocol. Radiology 2012;262(2):593–604.

60. Tong E, Patrie J, Tong S, et al. Time-resolved CT assessment of collaterals as imaging biomarkers to predict clinical outcomes in acute ischemic stroke. Neuroradiology 2017;59(11):1101–9.

61. Menon BK, d'Esterre CD, Qazi EM, et al. Multiphase CT angiography: a new tool for the imaging triage of patients with acute ischemic stroke. Radiology 2015; 275(2):510–20.

62. Aviv RI, Parsons M, Bivard A, et al. Multiphase CT angiography: a poor man's perfusion CT? Radiology 2015;277(3):922–4.

63. Patel VP, Heit JJ. Ischemic stroke treatment trials: neuroimaging advancements and implications. Top Magn Reson Imaging 2017;26(3):133–9.

64. Jadhav AP, Diener HC, Bonafe A, et al. Correlation between clinical outcomes and baseline CT and CT angiographic findings in the SWIFT PRIME trial. AJNR Am J Neuroradiol 2017;38(12):2270–6.

65. Hiratsuka Y, Miki H, Kiriyama I, et al. Diagnosis of unruptured intracranial aneurysms: 3T MR angiography versus 64-channel multi-detector row CT angiography. Magn Reson Med Sci 2008;7(4):169–78.

66. Bash S, Villablanca JP, Jahan R, et al. Intracranial vascular stenosis and occlusive disease: evaluation with CT angiography, MR angiography, and digital subtraction angiography. AJNR Am J Neuroradiol 2005;26(5):1012–21.

67. Lim RP, Koktzoglou I. Noncontrast magnetic resonance angiography: concepts and clinical applications. Radiol Clin North Am 2015;53(3):457–76.

68. Wu Y, Johnson K, Kecskemeti SR, et al. Time resolved contrast enhanced intracranial MRA using a single dose delivered as sequential injections and highly constrained projection reconstruction (HYPR CE). Magn Reson Med 2011;65(4):956–63.

69. Yang JJ, Hill MD, Morrish WF, et al. Comparison of pre- and postcontrast 3D time-of-flight MR angiography for the evaluation of distal intracranial branch occlusions in acute ischemic stroke. AJNR Am J Neuroradiol 2002;23(4):557–67.

70. Ernst M, Forkert ND, Brehmer L, et al. Prediction of infarction and reperfusion in stroke by flow- and volume-weighted collateral signal in MR angiography. AJNR Am J Neuroradiol 2015;36(2):275–82.

71. Chen H, Wu B, Liu N, et al. Using standard first-pass perfusion computed tomographic data to evaluate collateral flow in acute ischemic stroke. Stroke 2015;46(4):961–7.

72. Nael K, Doshi A, De Leacy R, et al. MR perfusion to determine the status of collaterals in patients with acute ischemic stroke: a look beyond time maps. AJNR Am J Neuroradiol 2017. https://doi.org/10. 3174/ajnr.A5454.

73. Villringer K, Serrano-Sandoval R, Grittner U, et al. Subtracted dynamic MR perfusion source images (sMRP-SI) provide collateral blood flow assessment in MCA occlusions and predict tissue fate. Eur Radiol 2016;26(5):1396–403.

74. Potreck A, Seker F, Hoffmann A, et al. A novel method to assess pial collateralization from stroke perfusion MRI: subdividing Tmax into anatomical compartments. Eur Radiol 2017;27(2):618–26.

75. Donahue J, Sumer S, Wintermark M. Assessment of collateral flow in patients with cerebrovascular disorders. J Neuroradiol 2014;41(4):234–42.

76. Donahue J, Wintermark M. Perfusion CT and acute stroke imaging: foundations, applications, and literature review. J Neuroradiol 2015;42(1):21–9.

77. Bang OY, Goyal M, Liebeskind DS. Collateral circulation in ischemic stroke: assessment tools and therapeutic strategies. Stroke 2015;46(11):3302–9.

78. Lyu J, Ma N, Liebeskind DS, et al. Arterial spin labeling magnetic resonance imaging estimation of antegrade and collateral flow in unilateral middle cerebral artery stenosis. Stroke 2016;47(2):428–33.

79. de Havenon A, Haynor DR, Tirschwell DL, et al. Association of collateral blood vessels detected by arterial spin labeling magnetic resonance imaging with neurological outcome after ischemic stroke. JAMA Neurol 2017;74(4):453–8.

80. Lou X, Yu S, Scalzo F, et al. Multi-delay ASL can identify leptomeningeal collateral perfusion in endovascular therapy of ischemic stroke. Oncotarget 2017;8(2):2437–43.

Oligemia, Penumbra, Infarction
Understanding Hypoperfusion with Neuroimaging

Lei Wu, MD[a], Wei Wu, MD[a,b], E. Turgut Tali, MD[c],
William T. Yuh, MD, MSEE[a,*]

KEYWORDS

- Acute ischemic stroke • Oligemia • Penumbra • Infarction • Hypoperfusion • Thrombolysis
- Reperfusion

KEY POINTS

- Despite recent demonstration of improved clinical outcomes in acute ischemic stroke with mechanical thrombectomy, considerable inconsistency remains regarding optimal patient selection and ideal treatment algorithms, for a large part because of current insufficiencies with neuroimaging of stroke.
- From a basic physiologic perspective, oligemia, ischemia, infarct core, and penumbra are quantitatively defined by their respective regional cerebral blood flow (rCBF) values, which role is to reflect the severity of the ischemic injury, and therefore to directly and appropriately influence treatment decisions among various possibilities, that is, clear indication, absence of indication, or clear contraindication to reperfusion therapy.
- Imaging-based determination of hypoperfusion using DWI-MR imaging, perfusion CT, or perfusion MR imaging has not yet received consistent validation with rCBF values, and therefore may not allow to reliably differentiate between oligemia, infarct core, and penumbra. As a result, absolute determination of the best therapy may not be possible with imaging alone in the face of oligemia.
- One-size-fits-all treatment algorithms based on a time window or on imaging alone may not fully account for the severity of ischemic injury in the individual patient. Rather, a physiology-based treatment decision tree can best take into account individual variations and guide optimal choice of treatment.
- The "time is brain" paradigm incompletely reflects decision making in stroke treatment. The ability to quickly and reliably identify infarct core and penumbra volumes are key in reducing rates of treatment failure and hemorrhagic transformation, and improving clinical outcomes, even in patients who present late after stroke onset but maintain a favorable infarct to penumbra ratio.
- Inconsistencies in the design and methods of imaging protocols used across various institutions and clinical trials have so far contributed to limiting the reliability of neuroimaging.

Disclosure Statement: None.
[a] Department of Radiology, University of Washington, 1959 Northeast Pacific Street, Room NW011, Seattle, WA 98195, USA; [b] Department of Radiology, Tongji Hospital, Tongji Medical College Affiliated to Huazhong University of Science and Technology, 1095 Jiefang Avenue, Wuhan, Hubei 430074, China; [c] Department of Radiology, Gazi University School of Medicine, Mevlana Blv. No: 89, Yenimahalle, Ankara 06560, Turkey
* Corresponding author.
E-mail address: wyuh@uw.edu

Neuroimag Clin N Am 28 (2018) 599–609
https://doi.org/10.1016/j.nic.2018.06.013
1052-5149/18/© 2018 Elsevier Inc. All rights reserved.

BACKGROUND

Acute ischemic stroke (AIS) remains one of the leading causes of death and significant morbidity in the United States despite a slow decline in its incidence in past decades.[1,2] Each year, approximately 692,000 patients are diagnosed with new or recurrent AIS.[3] Until 2015, intravenous tissue plasminogen activator (tPA) was the mainstay of treatment.[4–6] Recently, the treatment of AIS has been further advanced with positive results from multiple large clinical trials that showed endovascular thrombectomy improved treatment outcome and extended the therapeutic window beyond the traditional 3 to 8 hours.[7–12] Despite the therapeutic window for endovascular thrombectomy now being extended up to 12 to 24 hours for some patients, there is still realistic concern for the risk of hemorrhage after reperfusion in addition to the difficulty of identifying which patients will ultimately benefit from reperfusion intervention.[9,12,13] Hemorrhagic complications have been reported in patients treated during the extended therapeutic windows (8–24 hours) and during the traditional window, and even within 3 hours from symptom onset (Fig. 1).[13–15] Therefore, it remains a major clinical predicament to assess each individual patient's therapeutic window, optimal reperfusion options, and predict outcome before treatment. Currently, there is no well-established means to predict which individual patients with AIS presenting within the therapeutic window will benefit from prompt reperfusion, and which individuals will be harmed (hemorrhagic complication) after prompt successful reperfusion within the conventional and extended therapeutic window. Therefore, the one-size-fits-all time-based ("time is brain") approach remains the common practice for systemic tPA and endovascular recanalization for patients with AIS.[7–12,16,17]

Until recently, the concept that the therapeutic window varies among different individuals has finally gained general acceptance by the stroke community.[12,18,19] To effectively incorporate the concept of individualized therapeutic window for each patient, we should examine the possible factors in the current treatment paradigm, which

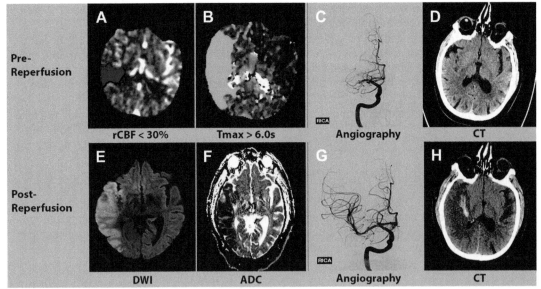

Fig. 1. Hemorrhagic complication from a successfully reperfused patient 1 hour after onset of AIS. A 61-year-old inpatient who developed left hemiparesis while being treated for atrial fibrillation. Code stroke was activated within 1 hour of symptom onset. Prethrombectomy CT perfusion using Rapid (iSchema, Redwood City, CA) demonstrated a small infarction core (31 mL) defined by CBF <30% compared with the contralateral side (A), and a large penumbra (177 mL) defined by Tmax >6.0 seconds at our institution (B). Pretreatment angiogram (C) demonstrated right M1 occlusion with normal noncontrast CT (D). Post-thrombectomy DWI (E) and ADC map (F) demonstrated a large right MCA territory ischemic changes complicated by hemorrhagic conversion (H) despite successful recanalization within 1 hour of symptom onset. (G) This case demonstrates the challenge in treatment selection using time-based therapeutic window without consideration of severity of ischemic injury (rCBF) or physiology-based window. ADC, apparent diffusion coefficient; CT, computed tomography; DWI, diffusion-weighted imaging; MCA, middle cerebral artery; rCBF, regional cerebral blood flow.

limits the ability to triage those who will benefit from treatment and to avoid treating those who will be harmed from reperfusion. One such possibility is the limitation of stroke imaging to differentiate among oligemia, penumbra, and infarction core (their definitions are discussed later) within the hypoperfused tissue. There is a need to better understand how these parameters are defined for parenchymal hypoperfusion and the respective implications of these definitions in guiding optimal treatment selection. To truly optimize stroke treatment decision and outcome while minimizing risks, the one-size-fits-all time-based approach likely has its limitations. Specifically, the time-based approach may exclude patients who may benefit from treatment beyond an arbitrary fixed time window if there is still ischemic tissue with lesser severe ischemic injury (penumbra). Rather than a physiology-based approach, the current fixed time-based approach does not always reflect the severity of the ischemic injury nor the underlying reduction of regional cerebral blood flow (rCBF). Such generalized approach for all patients with AIS is less than ideal because individual patients with the same time of symptom onset may have different degree of ischemic injury and therefore different timelines for conversion from salvageable ischemia (penumbra) to infarction. Similarly, the one-size-fits-all approach may include those patients with hemorrhage risk even for those presenting within the generally accepted therapeutic window if there is severe reduction of rCBF, which quickly converts ischemic tissue into infarction core (see Fig. 1).

Although imaging has been increasingly used in the management of AIS, the current clinical paradigm and inconsistent imaging protocols and interpretation of imaging-based hypoperfusion among different institutions have also limited its potential to optimize patient selection, selection of reperfusion options, and ultimately treatment outcome. Most stroke imaging gold standards, rationales, and approaches are inconsistent and frequently influenced by a few major institutions without reaching consensus and even disproving their own prior conclusions at times. The true potential of advance stroke imaging lies in its ability to detect, delineate, and most importantly to differentiate oligemia, penumbra, and infarction within the hypoperfused brain so that an optimal treatment option is selected before treatment, which includes no reperfusion ("do-no-harm") for those presenting within the traditional or recently extended therapeutic window. To correctly differentiate the various degrees of parenchymal hypoperfusion or ischemic injury is therefore critical, and perhaps just as important

if not more important than the urgent identification of vascular occlusive lesions (Fig. 2). Furthermore, the severity of vascular occlusion may not always reflect the true underlying severity of ischemic injury particularly in patients with chronic occlusive vascular disease because these patients tend to have more opportunity to develop additional collateral circulation (CC) (Fig. 3). Therefore, it is essential to understand the fundamental definitions of parenchymal hypoperfusion and underlying pathophysiology of ischemic injury during AIS, and their implications for optimal treatment selections for individual patients.

STROKE PATHOPHYSIOLOGY: CONTINUUM OF ISCHEMIC INJURY AND DEFINITIONS

Based on clinical data and imaging findings, there are variable definitions of oligemia, penumbra, and infarction core of the hypoperfused brain parenchyma, which critically influence the optimal treatment selection. Fundamentally, these terminologies are quantitatively defined by their respective quantitative rCBF values (Fig. 4) from the primate study, importantly not by imaging.[20] These terminologies are designed for the purpose of reflecting the severity of ischemic injury and therefore facilitate the optimal treatment selection of the hypoperfused tissue.

Hypoperfusion, oligemia, ischemia, penumbra, and infarction core are quantitatively defined by rCBF as the following:

1. Normal rCBF ranges from approximately 60 to 100 mL/100 g/min.[20,21] Hypoperfusion is defined as parenchyma with rCBF lower than 60 mL/100 g/min, which includes oligemia, ischemia, penumbra, and infarction core. Ischemic tissue includes penumbra and infarction core.

2. Oligemia is defined as hypoperfusion that is asymptomatic and recovers without the need for reperfusion treatment (not indicated). It correlates with rCBF values less than 60 mL/100 g/min but greater than the ischemic threshold, usually 22 mL/100 g/min.

3. Ischemia is symptomatic hypoperfusion that occurs at rCBF values less than 22 mL/100 g/min (ischemic threshold). Ischemic tissues include the penumbra and infarction core, which are quantitatively defined by their respective low rCBF values. Reperfusion treatment of ischemic tissue is either indicated or contraindicated depending on the degree of ischemic injury.

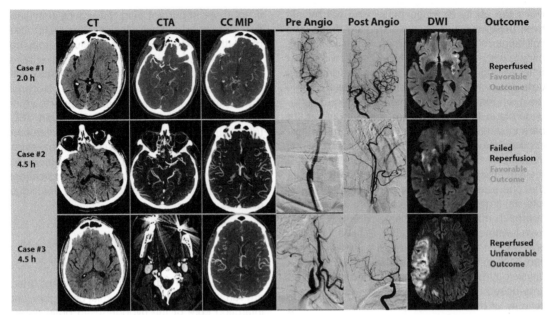

Fig. 2. Different outcomes in three patients with imaging evidence of CC and treatment within therapeutic windows: regardless of the respective success/failure of reperfusion intervention, their different outcomes suggested that vascular lesions and duration of ischemia may not be the only critical factors that influence reperfusion outcome. To increase the impact of imaging on AIS outcome, imaging-based patient selection requires more accurate reflection of rCBF to further improve the differentiation among oligemia, penumbra, and infarction. Case #1: patient with left M1 MCA occlusion who was successfully reperfused within 2 hours of symptom onset had good outcome with a small final infarction. Case #2: patient with proximal right cervical ICA occlusion who was not successfully reperfused but had good outcome with a small final infarction. Case #3: patient with proximal right ICA occlusion who was successfully reperfused with 4.5 hours of symptom onset but had a large infarction volume. CTA, computed tomography angiography; ICA, internal carotid artery; MIP, maximum intensity projection.

4. Infarction core is the irreversible process of near instantaneous conversion from hypoperfused brain with rCBF values less than the infarction threshold (10 mL/100 g/min) to unsalvageable infarcted tissue. It is the most severe form of ischemic injury and associated with high risk of hemorrhage if reperfused; thus, reperfusion is contraindicated.

5. Penumbra is defined as tissues with less severe ischemic injury than the infarction core, and it is reversible. Prompt reperfusion is indicated. It generally correlates with rCBF values of 10 to 22 mL/100 g/min.[16,20,22,23] As time progresses, the penumbra converts into infarction core at a variable rate depending on many anatomic and physiologic factors, particularly the rCBF, and it is the target of reperfusion strategies to salvage tissues with reversible ischemia.

CHALLENGES

The key to improve clinical outcome in AIS is to correctly identify reversible ischemia so that

rapid reperfusion intervention can be undertaken to salvage the penumbra while minimizing the risk of hemorrhage by avoidance of reperfusion of the infarction core. Until recently, the main therapy strategy has been a time-based approach for patients presenting within the respective standard fixed time windows to promptly search for occlusive vascular lesions so that intravenous tPA and/or endovascular thrombectomy can be initiated as soon as possible (time is brain) after hemorrhage and alternative diagnosis have been excluded. The inconsistency in stroke terminologies (oligemia, ischemia, penumbra, infarction core, or tissue-at-risk, which are often used interchangeably in clinical practice and even in scientific presentations/literature) limits optimal treatment selection for which these terminologies have been defined and intended. For instance, imaging-based hypoperfusion is not always indicative of ischemia or tissue at risk, and ischemic tissue is not equal to penumbra. Ischemic tissue is symptomatic hypoperfused tissues that include

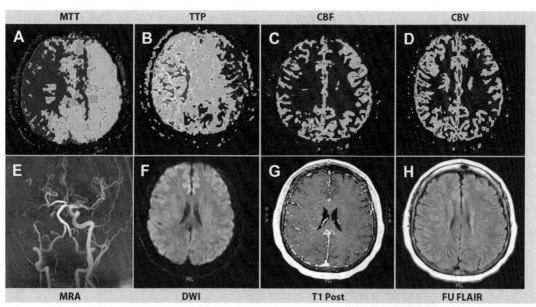

Fig. 3. Potential limitation of perfusion imaging in differentiating oligemia, penumbra, and infarction core. MR imaging perfusion demonstrated hypoperfused right cerebral hemisphere by MTT (*A*), TTP (*B*), CBF (*C*), and CBV (*D*) in an 84-year-old outpatient presented with possible seizure. MRA (*E*) showed complete occlusion of the right ICA without associated ischemia on DWI (*F*). The ICA occlusion was likely chronic in nature as evidenced by extensive CC on the postcontrast MR image (*G*). This patient did not have stroke symptoms and did not receive reperfusion treatment. Follow-up FLAIR (*H*) did not show large territorial infarction of right MCA. Therefore, the MR imaging perfusion abnormalities (*A–D*) likely represent oligemia, which is asymptomatic and has no indication for prompt reperfusion. CBV, cerebral blood volume; MRA, magnetic resonance angiography; MTT, mean transit time; TTP, time to peak.

both penumbra and infarction core depending on severity of ischemic injury (rCBF), which is indicated and contraindicated for reperfusion therapy, respectively. Similarly, neurologic assessments, such as National Institutes of Health Stroke Score measure symptomatic ischemia or severity of clinical presentation but may not readily differentiate the cause of the clinical symptoms by either penumbra or infarction core.

The current patient selection methods are primarily based on the "time is brain" model. This model assumes that all patients with AIS with the same ischemic duration have similar ischemic pathophysiology (same degree of low rCBF or severity of ischemic injury) and assumes that all hypoperfusions consist of only penumbra without the concern of coexisting infarction core. Furthermore, the amount of penumbra may vary for different patients because patients with AIS may have different abilities to maintain rCBF of ischemic tissue higher than the infarction threshold through mechanisms, such as pre-existing CC and compensatory hypertension by autoregulation.[24,25] In addition, maintenance of rCBF by clinical means, such as pharmaceutically induced hypertension and head

positioning, have also been shown to improve outcome, likely by preventing or prolonging penumbral tissue from converting into infarction core (preventing rCBF from dropping lower than the infarction threshold, and therefore increase the size of penumbra and therapeutic window).[26–30] This was also previously demonstrated by Ueda and colleagues[12] that patients had different relative rCBF at given time points from symptom onset, and their outcome (ranging from full recovery to hemorrhage) correlated significantly with the relative rCBF values but not the duration of ischemia. Most notably, patients had neurologic recovery even when successful reperfusion was achieved after almost 12 hours from symptom onset (**Fig. 5**). Their results are concordant with our own experience at our institution that treatment outcome may vary in patients treated within the traditional therapeutic window independent of imaging evidence of collateral circulation and success/failure of the reperfusion therapy (see **Fig. 2**). This suggests that a vascular lesion is not the only key factor that influences rCBF and reperfusion treatment outcome. Patient selection is further limited by the current treatment inclusion

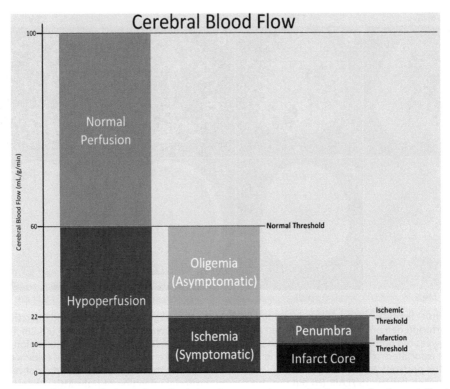

Fig. 4. Parenchymal hypoperfusion, oligemia, ischemia, penumbra, and infarction fundamentally defined by parenchymal rCBF. Continuum of hypoperfusion based on parenchymal rCBF values with three thresholds (normal threshold = 60 mL/100 g/min, ischemic threshold = 22 mL/100 g/min, and infarction threshold = 10 mL/100 g/min). Quantitatively, there are four physiologic states defined by rCBF values: normal (60–100 mL/100 g/min) and hypoperfused parenchyma (<60 mL/100 g/min), which includes oligemia (22–60 mL/100 g/min), penumbra (10–22 mL/100 g/min), and infarction core (<10 mL/100 g/min). Ischemic tissue includes penumbra and infarction core. Reperfusion intervention is indicated for penumbra but contraindicated for infarction core. It is also not indicated for oligemia. (*From* Yuh WT, Alexander MD, Ueda T, et al. Revisiting current golden rules in managing acute ischemic stroke: evaluation of new strategies to further improve treatment selection and outcome. AJR Am J Roentgenol 2017;208(1):37; with permission.)

criteria, which include estimate of infarction size by imaging (usually noncontrast computed tomography [CT] and MR imaging) and National Institutes of Health Stroke Scale, which may not reliably differentiate among oligemia, penumbra, and infarction core.

Therefore, more accurate differentiation between penumbra and infarction core would profoundly impact each individual's therapeutic window, reperfusion option, and ultimately patient outcome.[16,21,31] In our experience, even patients presenting within 1 hour of symptom onset (see **Fig. 1**) may be contraindicated for reperfusion therapy, particularly in patients with AIS with atrial fibrillation in whom there is insufficient time to develop CC, and the penumbra quickly converts into infarction core with sudden severe drop in rCBF. Reperfusion is contraindicated in this group of patients who tend to

have higher risk of hemorrhage.[32,33] In contrast, patients with chronic steno-occlusive disease have been shown to have greater CC, which is a positive predictor of favorable outcome (see **Fig. 3**).[33]

Finally, inconsistent imaging protocols and imperfect imaging-based definitions of different severity of hypoperfusion limit the full potential of imaging and optimal treatment selection. Although quantitative measurement of CBF is possible using O-15 PET, it is impractical in the AIS treatment setting.[34–36] CT- and MR imaging–based perfusion studies provide pseudoquantitative data that approximate physiologic states, but they are imperfect. Specifically, imaging-based hypoperfusion abnormality may become positive during oligemia, and lead to overestimation of the size of penumbra.[18,37–39] Mean transit time maps are particularly prone to this in our experience

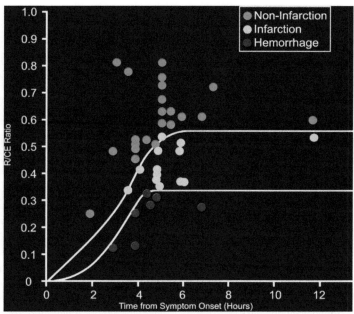

Fig. 5. Severity (y-axis), duration of ischemia (x-axis), and reperfusion outcomes (*colored dots*). Reperfusion outcomes (*red*, hemorrhage; *yellow*, infarction; *blue*, reversible hypoperfusion) of 42 hypoperfusion lesions after successful recanalization within 12 hours after symptom onset are summarized. It is the severity of ischemia compared with the contralateral parenchyma (y-axis), but not the duration of ischemia (x-axis) or National Institutes of Health score, significantly correlated with outcome. By extrapolation from the x-axis, these three different outcomes (reversible hypoperfusion, infarction, and hemorrhage) cannot be readily separated by a given time point within 12 hours. The results showed that patients with relative rCBF between 35% and 55% resulted in infarcts without hemorrhage, and patients suffered hemorrhage if the relative rCBF was less than 35%. Patients with relative rCBF greater than 55% experienced recovery without infarct or hemorrhage after successful recanalization up to 12 hours. These figures demonstrated two important concepts: patients with the same duration of AIS may have suffered different severity of ischemic injury or had different degree of low rCBF; and relative rCBF or physiologic-based therapeutic window is better than time-based therapeutic window for selection of optimal treatment. (*From* Yuh WT, Alexander MD, Ueda T, et al. Revisiting current golden rules in managing acute ischemic stroke: evaluation of new strategies to further improve treatment selection and outcome. AJR Am J Roentgenol 2017;208(1):41; with permission.)

(see **Fig. 3**). This pitfall in perfusion imaging maybe related to the fact that current techniques are sensitive to delay in antegrade flow through large vessels, but they may not adequately account for retrograde flow from CC, particularly through micro-CC when contrast arrival is delayed, or the contrast dose delivery is diminished. Increased macro-CC has been demonstrated to be a positive predictor of good outcome and serve as an indirect measurement of rCBF. However, presence of CC may not be as precise to predict the reperfusion outcome (see **Fig. 2**). Furthermore, determination of penumbra and infarction core by imaging may also be challenging. Relative rCBF by CT perfusion compared with the normal contralateral side can be imprecise in estimating the size of the infarction core and penumbra (see **Fig. 1**, iSchema Rapid, Redwood City, CA), and may mischaracterize chronic encephalomalacia as "infarction core and penumbra" (**Fig. 6**). CT perfusion and MR perfusion are known to overestimate ischemic tissue and tend to include large areas of hypoperfused oligemic tissue, particularly on mean transit time or Tmax maps (see **Fig. 3**). Although diffusion-weighted imaging (DWI) abnormality is commonly accepted as the imaging definition of infarction core, DWI can be positive in patients with oligemia (**Fig. 7**), and can also overestimate the size of infarction core (**Fig. 8**).[38,39] Because DWI and perfusion-weighted imaging can be positive in oligemia, and do not always match the true ischemic injury and differentiate penumbra from infarction core, determination of penumbra or infarction core purely based on diffusion-perfusion mismatch may not always be adequate (**Fig. 9**). Therefore, there is an unmet need to validate the quantitative parameters of imaging hypoperfusion with true underlying rCBF to reflect the

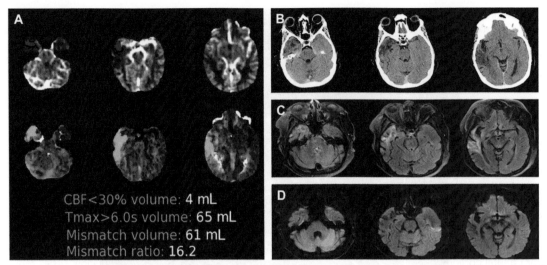

Fig. 6. CT perfusion may mischaracterize chronic encephalomalacia as infarction core and penumbra. 68-year-old patient with a history of prior right middle cerebral artery territory infarct presenting with neglect and possible new or worsening left sided weakness and sensory loss. CT perfusion using Rapid (*A*) showed a "infarction core" and "penumbra" corresponding to the region of chronic encephalomalacia seen on the same day CT head and follow up MRI 1 day later (*B, C*). DWI (*D*) from the same follow up MRI demonstrated no diffusion restriction to suggest acute infarction.

ischemic injury, such as in the original primate stroke model or with the use of O-15 PET.[34,36,37] Meanwhile, more advanced quantitative analysis of imaging parameters from the existing imaging protocols may help to improve the efficacy. Possible avenues include using relative intensity of DWI lesions to increase specificity for infarction core and using arterial spin labeling for

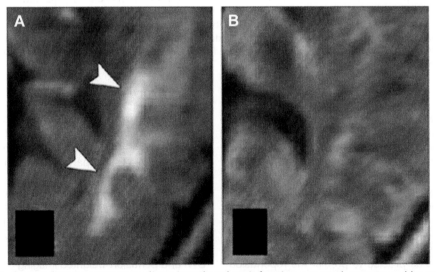

Fig. 7. DWI abnormality may represent oligemia rather than infarction core as demonstrated by spontaneous recovery in a 72-year-old man without reperfusion treatment. Initial DWI (*A*) shows abnormality near trigone of left lateral ventricle (*arrowheads*). Follow-up DWI 25 hours later (*B*) showed full resolution of the DWI abnormality shown in A. This case illustrates that DWI abnormality may not indicate infarction, as generally perceived, and may represent hypoperfused oligemic tissue, which can recover without reperfusion treatment. (*Courtesy of* Moseley ME, MD, Stanford University, Stanford, CA; and *From* Yuh WT, Alexander MD, Ueda T, et al. Revisiting current golden rules in managing acute ischemic stroke: evaluation of new strategies to further improve treatment selection and outcome. AJR Am J Roentgenol 2017;208(1):38; with permission.)

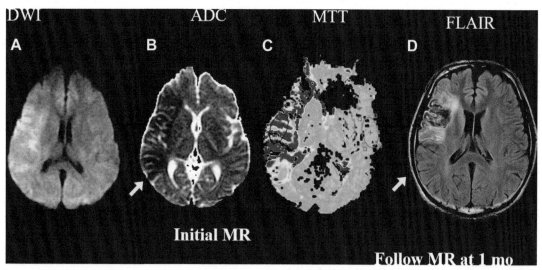

Fig. 8. DWI abnormality and MTT-DWI match may not indicate infarction. This patient had DWI (A) and ADC abnormality (B) in the right MCA territory with corresponding MTT abnormality (C). This is an MTT-DWI match, which is considered as infarction core by the current standards. On his 1-month follow-up MR image (D), the final infarction core was smaller than the original DWI abnormality (A, B). Thus, DWI overestimated the infarction core size. The area of the hypoperfused parenchyma with DWI abnormality (B, arrow), recovered without treatment, and likely represented oligemia (D, arrow).

characterizing CC or rCBF, which was associated with better patient outcome.[40,41] In addition to these challenges, other considerations, such as access to advance imaging especially for remote areas, patient safety (eg, contrast allergy, pacemakers), or rapid image processing time are also areas of further improvement in stroke imaging.

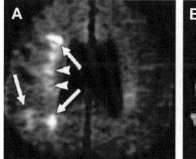 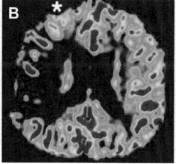 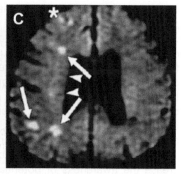

Fig. 9. DWI/perfusion-weighted imaging (PWI) mismatch or match may not represent penumbra or infarct core, respectively. This 76-year-old woman had AIS followed by spontaneous neurologic recovery from spontaneous resolution of right M1 thrombosis confirmed on follow-up MR angiography. Initial DWI (A) showed multiple foci of diffusion restriction (arrows and arrowheads) within right MCA territory. Initial PWI (B) showed that the abnormality in the right MCA territory was more extensive than the DWI abnormality in A. Therefore, all DWI lesions (A, arrows and arrowheads) had matched PWI abnormalities (B). DWI/PWI mismatch was present in the right frontal lobe as a mild hypoperfusion defect (yellow right frontal cortex compared with the red left frontal cortex; asterisk, B). Follow-up MR (C) showed that not all DWI lesions appearing as DWI/PWI matching lesions (arrows, A and C) proceeded to infarction. In addition, other DWI/PWI matching foci (arrowheads, A and C) even recovered without becoming infarction; these foci may represent either penumbra that was reversed with spontaneous reperfusion or oligemia that recovered without treatment. Contrary to the general belief that DWI/PWI mismatching is suggestive of penumbra, the right frontal lobe lesion (asterisk, B) developed into a small infarction (asterisk, C) despite spontaneous resolution of the right MCA occlusion. (From Yuh WT, Alexander MD, Ueda T, et al. Revisiting current golden rules in managing acute ischemic stroke: evaluation of new strategies to further improve treatment selection and outcome. AJR Am J Roentgenol 2017;208(1):40; with permission.)

SUMMARY

Although the treatment of AIS has recently shown encouraging progress with improved endovascular devices and technique, the current clinical paradigm remains mostly a one-size-fits-all time-based approach. Typically, the principle of "time is brain" triggers a cascade of emergency steps including searching for arterial occlusion and initiating emergent intervention toward reperfusion under the assumption that ischemic tissue consists mostly of penumbral tissue, in the absence of an available reliable method to differentiate among oligemia, penumbra, and infarction core. Even with the recent exciting results that further extended the therapeutic window up to 24 hours after symptom onset, it remains a daily predicament to select proper patients for reperfusion and to avoid treating patients at risk for hemorrhagic complication. To truly optimize patient outcome in AIS, better patient selection is required to individualize inclusion/exclusion criteria including indication for prompt intervention for penumbra, contraindication for infarction core, and no indication for oligemia. This is best accomplished by more accurate imaging definitions of the previously mentioned hypoperfusion terminologies to correlate with actual pathophysiology and ischemic injury, not necessarily the occlusive vascular lesions or an arbitrary fixed time window. Thus, a shift from the current clinical paradigm (time is brain) to that of a more physiology-based approach (rCBF is brain) is indicated. Such evolution requires more research to refine imaging definitions by evaluating hypoperfusion changes in the brain parenchyma using currently available imaging techniques and potentially novel techniques to better quantify rCBF, before and after successful reperfusion. Lastly, by presenting these challenges, our intent is certainly not to discourage the current use of imaging in the management of AIS, but rather to increase the awareness of potential limitations of imaging and a potential new window of opportunity to further facilitate clinical translation of stroke imaging and advance research to further improve patient management and outcome.

ACKNOWLEDGMENTS

Images in **Fig. 2** were prepared by Dr Thien Huynh, University of Washington and University of Toronto.

REFERENCES

1. Carandang R, Seshadri S, Beiser A, et al. Trends in incidence, lifetime risk, severity, and 30-day mortality of stroke over the past 50 years. JAMA 2006;296(24):2939–46.
2. Fang MC, Coca Perraillon M, Ghosh K, et al. Trends in stroke rates, risk, and outcomes in the United States, 1988 to 2008. Am J Med 2014; 127(7):608–15.
3. Mozaffarian D, Benjamin EJ, Go AS, et al. Heart disease and stroke statistics-2016 update: a report from the American Heart Association. Circulation 2016;133(4):e38–360.
4. Lees KR, Bluhmki E, von Kummer R, et al. Time to treatment with intravenous alteplase and outcome in stroke: an updated pooled analysis of ECASS, ATLANTIS, NINDS, and EPITHET trials. Lancet 2010;375(9727):1695–703.
5. Saver JL, Fonarow GC, Smith EE, et al. Time to treatment with intravenous tissue plasminogen activator and outcome from acute ischemic stroke. JAMA 2013;309(23):2480–8.
6. Wardlaw JM, Murray V, Berge E, et al. Recombinant tissue plasminogen activator for acute ischaemic stroke: an updated systematic review and meta-analysis. Lancet 2012;379(9834):2364–72.
7. Berkhemer OA, Fransen PS, Beumer D, et al. A randomized trial of intraarterial treatment for acute ischemic stroke. N Engl J Med 2015;372(1): 11–20.
8. Campbell BC, Mitchell PJ, Kleinig TJ, et al. Endovascular therapy for ischemic stroke with perfusion-imaging selection. N Engl J Med 2015;372(11): 1009–18.
9. Goyal M, Demchuk AM, Menon BK, et al. Randomized assessment of rapid endovascular treatment of ischemic stroke. N Engl J Med 2015;372(11): 1019–30.
10. Saver JL, Goyal M, Bonafe A, et al. Stent-retriever thrombectomy after intravenous t-PA vs. t-PA alone in stroke. N Engl J Med 2015;372(24):2285–95.
11. Jovin TG, Chamorro A, Cobo E, et al. Thrombectomy within 8 hours after symptom onset in ischemic stroke. N Engl J Med 2015;372(24): 2296–306.
12. Ueda T, Sakaki S, Yuh WT, et al. Outcome in acute stroke with successful intra-arterial thrombolysis and predictive value of initial single-photon emission-computed tomography. J Cereb Blood Flow Metab 1999;19(1):99–108.
13. Nogueira RG, Jadhav AP, Haussen DC, et al. Thrombectomy 6 to 24 hours after stroke with a mismatch between deficit and infarct. N Engl J Med 2018; 378(1):11–21.
14. National Institute of Neurological Disorders and Stroke rt-PA Stroke Study Group. Tissue plasminogen activator for acute ischemic stroke. N Engl J Med 1995;333(24):1581–7.
15. Tsivgoulis G, Zand R, Katsanos AH, et al. Safety of intravenous thrombolysis in stroke mimics:

prospective 5-year study and comprehensive meta-analysis. Stroke 2015;46(5):1281–7.

16. Jauch EC, Saver JL, Adams HP Jr, et al. Guidelines for the early management of patients with acute ischemic stroke: a guideline for healthcare professionals from the American Heart Association/American Stroke Association. Stroke 2013; 44(3):870–947.

17. Hacke W, Kaste M, Bluhmki E, et al. Thrombolysis with alteplase 3 to 4.5 hours after acute ischemic stroke. N Engl J Med 2008;359(13):1317–29.

18. Yuh WT, Alexander MD, Ueda T, et al. Revisiting current golden rules in managing acute ischemic stroke: evaluation of new strategies to further improve treatment selection and outcome. AJR Am J Roentgenol 2017;208(1):32–41.

19. Yuh WT, Alexander MD, Beauchamp NJ. Intraarterial treatment for acute ischemic stroke. N Engl J Med 2015;372(12):1176.

20. Jones TH, Morawetz RB, Crowell RM, et al. Thresholds of focal cerebral ischemia in awake monkeys. J Neurosurg 1981;54(6):773–82.

21. Kandel ER. Principles of neural science. 5th edition. New York: McGraw-Hill; 2013.

22. Kheradmand A, Fisher M, Paydarfar D. Ischemic stroke in evolution: predictive value of perfusion computed tomography. J Stroke Cerebrovasc Dis 2014;23(5):836–43.

23. Rivers CS, Wardlaw JM, Armitage PA, et al. Do acute diffusion- and perfusion-weighted MRI lesions identify final infarct volume in ischemic stroke? Stroke 2006;37(1):98–104.

24. Hakimelahi R, Vachha BA, Copen WA, et al. Time and diffusion lesion size in major anterior circulation ischemic strokes. Stroke 2014;45(10):2936–41.

25. Miteff F, Levi CR, Bateman GA, et al. The independent predictive utility of computed tomography angiographic collateral status in acute ischaemic stroke. Brain 2009;132(Pt 8):2231–8.

26. Aiyagari V, Gorelick PB. Management of blood pressure for acute and recurrent stroke. Stroke 2009; 40(6):2251–6.

27. Vlcek M, Schillinger M, Lang W, et al. Association between course of blood pressure within the first 24 hours and functional recovery after acute ischemic stroke. Ann Emerg Med 2003;42(5): 619–26.

28. Schwarz S, Georgiadis D, Aschoff A, et al. Effects of body position on intracranial pressure and cerebral perfusion in patients with large hemispheric stroke. Stroke 2002;33(2):497–501.

29. Wojner-Alexander AW, Garami Z, Chernyshev OY, et al. Heads down: flat positioning improves blood

30. Favilla CG, Mesquita RC, Mullen M, et al. Optical bedside monitoring of cerebral blood flow in acute ischemic stroke patients during head-of-bed manipulation. Stroke 2014;45(5):1269–74.

31. Hillis AE, Wityk RJ, Beauchamp NJ, et al. Perfusion-weighted MRI as a marker of response to treatment in acute and subacute stroke. Neuroradiology 2004; 46(1):31–9.

32. Hussain MS, Lin R, Cheng-Ching E, et al. Endovascular treatment of carotid embolic occlusions has a higher recanalization rate compared with cardioembolic occlusions. J Neurointerv Surg 2010; 2(1):71–3.

33. Rebello LC, Bouslama M, Haussen DC, et al. Stroke etiology and collaterals: atheroembolic strokes have greater collateral recruitment than cardioembolic strokes. Eur J Neurol 2017;24(6):762–7.

34. Huisman MC, van Golen LW, Hoetjes NJ, et al. Cerebral blood flow and glucose metabolism in healthy volunteers measured using a high-resolution PET scanner. EJNMMI Res 2012;2(1):63.

35. Heiss WD, Zaro Weber O. Validation of MRI determination of the penumbra by PET measurements in ischemic stroke. J Nucl Med 2017;58(2):187–93.

36. Sobesky J. Refining the mismatch concept in acute stroke: lessons learned from PET and MRI. J Cereb Blood Flow Metab 2012;32(7):1416–25.

37. Werner P, Saur D, Zeisig V, et al. Simultaneous PET/MRI in stroke: a case series. J Cereb Blood Flow Metab 2015;35(9):1421–5.

38. Guadagno JV, Warburton EA, Aigbirhio FI, et al. Does the acute diffusion-weighted imaging lesion represent penumbra as well as core? A combined quantitative PET/MRI voxel-based study. J Cereb Blood Flow Metab 2004;24(11):1249–54.

39. Sobesky J, Zaro Weber O, Lehnhardt FG, et al. Does the mismatch match the penumbra? Magnetic resonance imaging and positron emission tomography in early ischemic stroke. Stroke 2005; 36(5):980–5.

40. Heiss WD, Sobesky J, Smekal U, et al. Probability of cortical infarction predicted by flumazenil binding and diffusion-weighted imaging signal intensity: a comparative positron emission tomography/magnetic resonance imaging study in early ischemic stroke. Stroke 2004;35(8):1892–8.

41. de Havenon A, Haynor DR, Tirschwell DL, et al. Association of collateral blood vessels detected by arterial spin labeling magnetic resonance imaging with neurological outcome after ischemic stroke. JAMA Neurol 2017;74(4):453–8.

Clot Pathophysiology
Why Is It Clinically Important?

Patrick A. Brouwer, MD, MSc[a],*, Waleed Brinjikji, MD[b,c,d], Simon F. De Meyer, PhD[e]

KEYWORDS

• Thrombectomy • Cerebral ischemic stroke • Blood clot • Pathophysiology • Etiology

KEY POINTS

• Clot composition has a major effect on the result of thrombectomy with the current devices.
• Thrombectomy allows us to further analyse clots and therefore understand the underlying pathophysiology.
• Understanding clot pathophysiology may help us getting to new (supportive) therapies to potentially enhance efficacy.
• The combination of pathophysiological knowledge in combination with related clot imaging properties may lead to adaptation of treatment strategies.

Conventional treatment of cerebral ischemic stroke was based on recanalizing arteries by use of thrombolytic agents and, if indicated, hemicraniectomy. The results of this approach, with only 10% of patients receiving the drug and only 50% thereof responding postively,[1,2] have led to the continued search for alternative treatments. Since 2015, the first-line treatment for ischemic stroke has changed dramatically with the publication of the so-called positive trials,[3–7] which showed a benefit to endovascular stroke treatment. The neurointerventional field has started to implement this new strategy in a rapid pace in conjunction with, and sometimes even replacing, traditional medical stroke therapy.

With the development of newer devices and the extensive research that is being done, we are confronted with previously unknown hurdles in our endovascular procedures. One of the most important obstacles is the fact that clots tend to differ in consistency and removability. We can face a clot that comes out with simple proximal aspiration or thrombectomy, but in the next case we may be faced with a clot that is too resilient to be removed by any of the devices we have at hand. The case examples presented herein show the high

Disclosures: P.A. Brouwer is consultant for Cerenovus/Neuravi, Medtronic, Stryker. W. Brinjikji is consultant for Cerenovus, Superior Medical Editing and CEO of Marblehead Medical LLC. He is funded by NIH grant R01NS105853. S.F. De Meyer was supported by the FWO (Fonds voor Wetenschappelijk Onderzoek Vlaanderen G.0A86.13 and 1509216N to S.F. De Meyer), by an 'Onderzoekstoelage' grant from KU Leuven (OT/14/099, to S. F. De Meyer) and by a research grant from the Queen Elisabeth Medical Foundation (S.F. De Meyer). S.F. De Meyer has received funding from the European Union's Horizon 2020 research and innovation programme under grant agreement No 77072.
[a] Neuroradiology Department, Neurointervention Section, Karolinska University Hospital, Eugeniavägen 3, Stockholm, 171 64 Solna, Sweden; [b] Department of Radiology, Mayo Clinic, 1216 2nd St SW, Rochester, MN 55902, USA; [c] Department of Neurosurgery, Mayo Clinic, 1216 2nd St SW, Rochester, MN 55902, USA; [d] Joint Department of Medical Imaging, Toronto Western Hospital, 399 Bathurst St, Toronto, ON M5T 2S8, Canada; [e] Laboratory for Thrombosis Research, KU Leuven Campus Kulak Kortrijk, E. Sabbelaan 53, 8500 Kortrijk, Belgium
* Corresponding author.
E-mail address: patrickbrouwermd@gmail.com

variability and, so far, unpredictable nature of the clots in the stroke cases we face on a daily basis.

CASE 1

A 67-year-old woman presented with sudden onset right-sided hemiparesis and aphasia. Thrombectomy was performed after computed tomography (CT) and CT angiography (CTA) showed an M1 occlusion without hyperdense vessel sign. Four passes with a Solitaire 4x40 (Medtronic, Minneapolis, MN) were needed to achieve full recanalization (Fig. 1).

CASE 2

A 40-year-old woman, previously known for an occipital infarct 1 month earlier, came to the hospital for cardiac complications owing to her anorexia nervosa. During her stay in the ward, she developed new strokelike symptoms that, based on the CTA and CT perfusion images, was caused by a thrombus in the left middle cerebral artery (MCA) bifurcation. Thrombectomy was attempted, but the clot seemed very sticky and only after the sixth pass with several devices (Solitaire, Medtronic; Capture

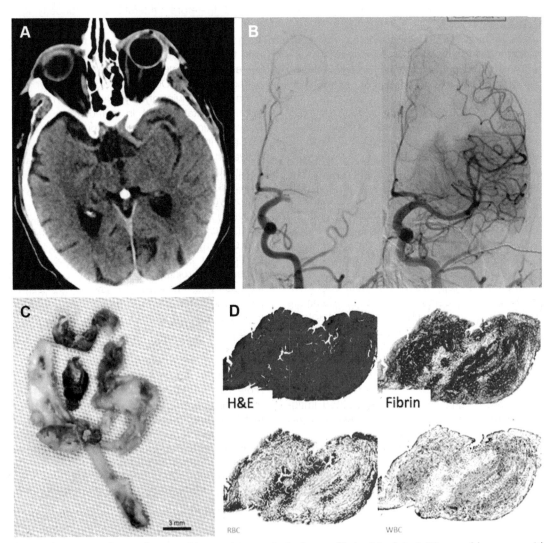

Fig. 1. Clot attenuation and composition and revascularization: a fibrin-rich clot. A 67-year-old woman with acute onset right-sided hemiparesis and aphasia. (A) Noncontrast computed tomography scan using thin section 1 mm reconstruction shows no hyperdense vessel. (B) Left internal carotid artery cerebral angiogram shows occlusion of the left middle cerebral artery. Four passes with a Solitaire 4x40 were needed to open the vessel. (C) Gross photo of the retrieved clot shows white clot consistent with fibrin-rich thrombus. (D) Hematoxylin and eosin (H&E) staining shows that a majority of the clot was composed of fibrin; the overall clot composition was 90% fibrin and 7% red blood cells (RBCs). WBC, white blood cells.

Mindframe/Medtronic) was the clot removed. As a complication, a small amount of blood and contrast were seen in the subarachnoid space. The image of the clot shows how the texture is totally different from other clots we normally encounter and that have a more heterogenous appearance (Fig. 2).

CASE 3

A 72-year-old woman with progressive dyspnea, a smoking history of 60 pack-years, and a malignant melanoma in the face 3 years earlier was found lying on the floor showing a full hemiplegia and aphasia. Thrombectomy of a nonhyperdense MCA trifurcation clot, performed within 3 hours from onset, resulted in a 10-pass procedure using 3 different devices (Solitaire, Medtronic; Capture Mindframe/Medtronic; Embotrap Neuravi/Cerenovus, Galway, Ireland). The clot could not be removed and seemed to be firmly attached to the wall of the artery. The size and shape of

the clot changed owing to manipulations and the rounded structure can be seen as a filling defect in the artery. After the futile thrombectomy the patient was further analyzed for increasing dyspnea. She died of previously undiagnosed lung cancer within the next 3 weeks after only moderately recovering from her stroke (Fig. 3).

CASE 4

A 24-year-old woman who underwent an aortic root replacement did not wake up after the surgery. She underwent noncontrast CT scanning, which showed a long hyperdense clot on the left side reaching from the carotid termination into the left MCA trifurcation. She was immediately taken to the angiosuite and underwent successful thrombectomy with full flow restoration. The clot had a dark appearance, which is consistent with a high red blood cell (RBC) content, subsequently supported by the histologic imaging using hematoxylin and eosin staining (Fig. 4).

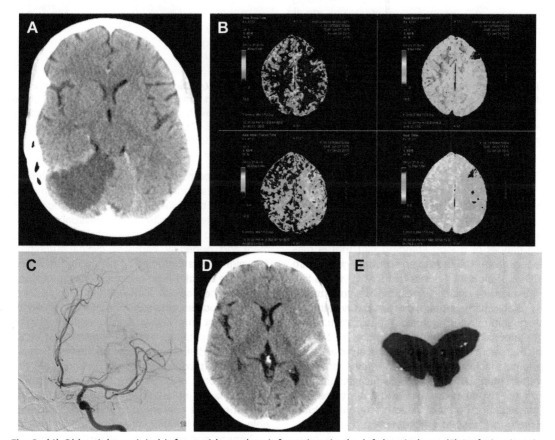

Fig. 2. (A) Older right occipital infarct with no clear infarct signs in the left hemisphere. (B) Perfusion imaging showing tissue at risk in the left hemisphere and a frontal manifest infarction. (C) Resilient clot taken out after 6 attempts. (D) Subarachnoid hemorrhage owing to thrombectomy. (E) The clot seems to be relatively homogeneous, glazy, reddish-purple and of an uncommon consistency.

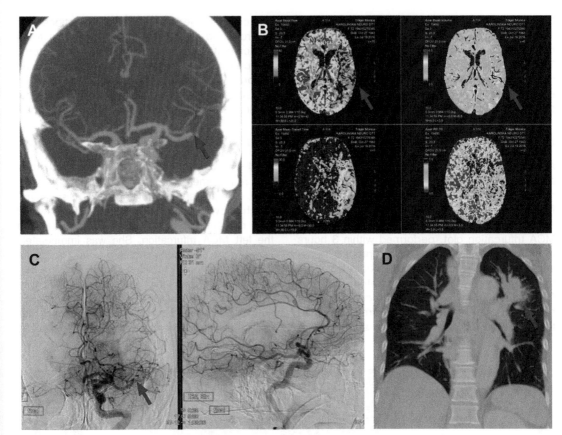

Fig. 3. (*A*) Computed tomography angiography showing the occlusion (*red arrow*) in the middle cerebral artery trifurcation and good collaterals. (*B*) Perfusion imaging showing a defect in the blood flow but maintained blood volume (*red arrows*). (*C*) Persistent occlusion (*red arrow*) after 10 passes with multiple devices. Procedure stopped because of futile attempts and moderate to good collateral circulation. (*D*) Tumor in the left apical segment of the lung (*red arrow*).

These 4 examples show that both the efficacy of treatment and the appearance of the clot can be highly variable across patients. In our own experience, thrombectomies are more likely to be difficult in patients with conditions such as lung cancer or a long-standing clot that is dislodged from the aortic arch, than the fresh RBC-rich clots. The mechanisms behind this remain largely unclear, and one can only postulate that paraneoplastic clots have a different composition and, therefore, behavior compared with atherosclerotic clots or clots of cardiac origin. Benchtop observations showed that fibrin-rich clots are more sticky than pure RBC clots on thrombectomy. This further finding supports the hypothesis that, beside patient related factors, clot properties influence thrombectomy failure or success to a large extent.

The problems owing to clot variations are, however, not specific to endovascular therapies. For both pharmacologic thrombolysis and mechanical thrombectomy, the culprit thrombus itself is indeed the primary target of therapy. Therefore, a better understanding of clot composition, physical properties, behavior, and how these occlusive thrombi interact with their environment will contribute to future advancements in patient treatment and, hopefully, improved clinical outcomes. The clot analysis studies of Liebeskind and colleagues,[8] Boeckh-Behrens and colleagues,[9] and Cline and colleagues[10] showed the distribution of fibrin, leukocytes, and RBCs in clots harvested after thrombectomy. The spread in content of each of the components, between the different clots, is striking and a composite of the results of these 3 cohorts is presented in **Fig. 5**. Because the clot analysis could only be performed on clots that were actually retrieved, it remains a question what the exact content of the resilient, unremovable, clots has been.

Gunning and colleagues[11] recently published a study looking into the friction coefficient in relation to the RBC and fibrin content of the clot. The study showed that the fibrin-rich clots had a significantly

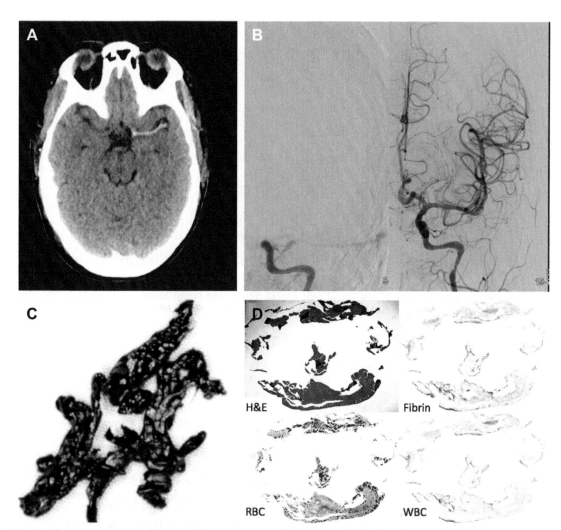

Fig. 4. Clot attenuation and composition and revascularization: red blood cell (RBC)–rich clot. A 24-year-old woman status post aortic root replacement who was not waking up 2 hours after surgery. (A) Noncontrast computed tomography scanning shows a long, hyperdense thrombus of the left middle cerebral artery. (B) The patient was taken straight to angiography, which confirmed the left middle cerebral artery occlusion. One pass with a 6-cm Solitaire was needed to revascularize the occlusion. (C) Gross photo of the clot shows dark red clot consisted with a RBC-rich thrombus. (D) Hematoxylin and eosin (H&E) staining shows that a majority of the clot was composed of red blood cells (94% RBC density). WBC, white blood cells.

higher friction than the clots with a high RBC content. In the same study, clots were tested after compression simulating "repeated stent retriever manipulation." The increase in the friction coefficient after manipulation was dramatic, suggesting that there may well be a potential increase in friction after multiple thrombectomy attempts in real life. This finding would explain why a resilient clot seems to be responding even less and less to subsequent thrombectomy attempts.

Previous studies indicate that thrombus composition can provide insights into stroke etiology, recanalization outcomes, and guide the development of newer technologies in stroke treatment.[8,12–16] A number of recently published studies have even demonstrated that clot composition can impact the choice of revascularization techniques owing to differences in clot–device interactions.[17,18] The ability to retrieve and study fresh thrombi in patients with acute stroke has opened a whole new door in the study of stroke pathogenesis and treatment. In this section, we review the current state-of-the-art literature in the study of clot in stroke.

CLOT COMPOSITION ANALYSIS

As seen in other vascular beds, the typical composition of a clot in stroke is a mixture of

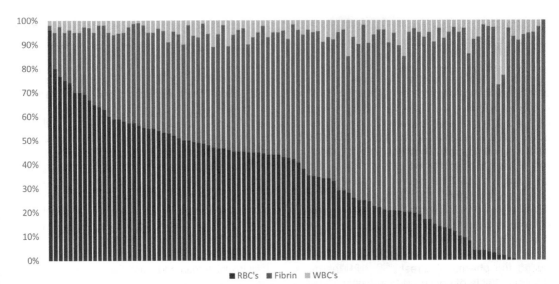

Fig. 5. Composition distribution of red blood cells (RBCs), fibrin, and white blood cells (WBCs) in 100 clots retrieved from patients with a cerebral ischemic stroke. (*Courtesy of* M. Mirza, MD, Neuravi/Cerenovus, Galway, Ireland.)

fibrin, platelets, white blood cells, and RBCs. Various histologic stains have been applied in the study of clot, including standard hematoxylin and eosin, Elastic van Gieson, Mallory's trichrome, and Martius scarlet blue, which allow for a detailed analysis of these clot components. Most of the current studies in the literature report quantitative values for each of these components when studying clot phenotype.[9] The most commonly used terms in describing clot composition are RBC rich or poor and fibrin rich or poor, because these components make up a majority of the composition of clots seen in patients with acute ischemic stroke.[19]

More recently, there has been growing interest in molecular markers of clot composition, including the evaluation of von Willebrand factor (VWF), T cells (CD3), neutrophils, macrophages, and endothelial cells. There is growing interest in electron microscopy as a tool in clot characterization; however, it is not yet widely applied.[19] For the purposes of clarity, this section focuses primarily on the basics of clot composition: fibrin, platelets, white blood cells, and RBCs. We cover VWF and neutrophils in Potential Pharmacologic Thrombus Targets for Treatment elsewhere in this article.

Clot Composition and Stroke Etiology

There is a growing body of literature examining the association between clot composition and stroke etiology. To date, a majority of published studies have failed to identify an association between RBC and fibrin composition and stroke etiology. Thus, to better identify clot characteristics associated with stroke etiology, some investigators have turned to the study of components including white blood cell composition and characteristics.[20] T cells have been an interesting target in some studies; these cells have been shown to be a major component of atherosclerotic lesions. In a study of 54 consecutive thrombi retrieved during mechanical thrombectomy, 1 group found that the number of T cells was significantly higher in thrombi from atherosclerotic plaques than those from a cardioembolic source.[21] Because the final step in plaque destabilization and rupture includes the release of elastase and metalloproteinases from activated T cells, the idea that T-cell composition would be higher in atheroembolic clots seems to be logical.[21] Ultimately, larger studies are needed to determine if indeed there is a consistent association between clot composition, both cellular and molecular, and stroke etiology.

Clot Composition and Recanalization

Studies examining the association between clot composition and recanalization rates have more or less consistently found a strong association between RBC density and ease of recanalization with both fibrinolytic therapies and endovascular techniques. The improved recanalization rates of RBC-rich clots over those that are composed of fibrin is likely due to a combination of decreased stiffness of

RBC-rich clots, thus, allowing for improved clot–device interaction and decreased friction of RBC-rich clots with the vessel wall, thus, allowing for easier clot extraction and increased permeability of RBC-rich clots, and thus, allowing improved permeability of thrombolytic agents.[20]

To date there have been no in vivo studies comparing the recanalization rates of various techniques and devices in the revascularization of fibrin-rich or RBC-rich clots. However, there are some in vitro data suggesting the benefit of unique stent–retriever designs for the treatment of stiffer, fibrin-rich thrombi. In a study comparing the Geometric Clot Extractor, a stent–retriever with a curved spiral configuration, with the Solitaire stent–retriever, Fennell and colleagues[22] found that the Geometric Clot Extractor had a success rate of 100% for retrieving fibrin-rich thrombi compared with just 8% for the Solitaire device. There are also data to suggest that RBC-rich thrombi are more prone to fragmentation, highlighting the need for proximal flow arrest with balloon guide catheters when revascularizing these types of clots.[23,24]

Clot Imaging Techniques

CT and MR imaging are the mainstay of stroke imaging in North America and Europe. Both noncontrast CT and CTA are useful in the process of clot characterization. When evaluating a clot on noncontrast CT, the use of thin slice CT (<2.5 mm) is strongly recommended, because several studies have shown that thin slice CT is more sensitive and specific in identifying hyperdense thrombus and more accurately measures thrombus length owing to the fact that thin slice CT minimizes partial volume averaging with the adjacent brain parenchyma and cerebrospinal fluid[25] (Fig. 6). Characteristics that can be easily discerned on thin slice CT include thrombus density (in Hounsfield units), clot location, and clot length—variables that have been shown to be strongly correlated with angiographic outcomes after mechanical thrombectomy.

CTA (also using thin section CT) is a very useful tool in clot imaging. The identification of the contrast gap between the proximal and distal ends of the clot is useful in assessing clot length and thus aiding in device choice, especially stent–retriever type and length.[26] CTA can also be useful in assessing the clot burden score, a semiquantitative method of measuring the extent of thrombus on CTA.[27] Delayed phase CTA is particularly useful in assessing clot burden and thrombus length because it can take time for

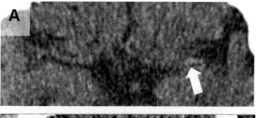
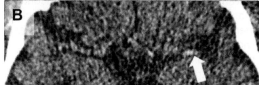
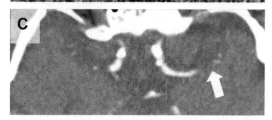

Fig. 6. Usefulness of thin-slice computed tomography (CT) in identifying hyperdense artery sign. A 75-year-old man with acute onset right-sided hemiparesis and aphasia. (A) Noncontrast CT with 5-mm slice thickness shows no evidence of a hyperdense artery sign on the left (arrow). (B) An 0.5-mm slice thickness reconstruction shows a hyperdense left middle cerebral artery (arrow). (C) The occlusion was confirmed on CT angiography (arrow).

contrast to make it to the distal face of the clot. There has been growing interest in the assessment of clot perviousness/permeability to iodinated contrast because increasing density/enhancement of clot on CTA has been shown to be associated with revascularization outcomes.[28]

MR imaging has substantial theoretic advantages over CT. The use of multicontrast MR imaging allows one to assess multiple different elements of thrombus composition. Although there are currently some in vitro data supporting the use T1-weighted, T2-weighted, and fluid-attenuated inversion recovery imaging in clot evaluation, susceptibility-weighted imaging is the mainstay of clot imaging on MR imaging owing to the consistent presence of blooming artifact associated with most clots. Susceptibility-weighted imaging can also allow for the evaluation of tiny distal emboli that may have showered in the initial ictus. One disadvantage of MR imaging in clot evaluation is the inability to assess clot length on noncontrast MR imaging.[29] The presence of blooming artifact on susceptibility-weighted imaging results in the overestimation of clot length. This problem can be obviated by using postcontrast

MR angiography. Evaluation of maximum intensity projection images in postcontrast MR angiography for the presence of a contrast gap has been shown be a useful tool in assessment of clot length.[29]

Association Between Imaging Findings and Clot Composition

Conventional imaging techniques (ie, noncontrast CT and MR imaging) are fairly accurate in the characterization of clot composition. Studies examining the association between noncontrast CT findings and clot composition are very consistent in demonstrating that the proportion of RBCs is strongly correlated with clot density. In general, hyperdense thrombi on CT are RBC rich across all X-ray energy ranges. There are some preliminary in vitro data to suggest that dual energy CT may have some added usefulness in distinguishing between RBC and fibrin-rich clots; however, this finding has yet to be studied in vivo.[30] In terms of MR imaging, hypointense thrombi on T2* imaging have been shown to have higher RBC content.[31] This finding is secondary to the increased iron density in the RBC-rich thrombi, which results in blooming artifact.[8]

Association Between Clot Imaging Findings and Recanalization

A number of studies have reported the association between imaging findings and recanalization rates. In a systematic review and metaanalysis, one group found that patients with good angiographic outcomes had a higher mean clot density than those with poor angiographic outcomes, both with tissue plasminogen activator (tPA) and mechanical thrombectomy.[20] In addition, patients with a hyperdense artery sign were more likely to have a good angiographic outcome than those without. This finding is logical, given that the hyperdense artery sign is associated with RBC-rich thrombi, and RBC-rich thrombi are more amenable to removal by thrombectomy.[20] Increasing clot length has also been shown to be associated with poorer angiographic outcomes.[32]

Studies of clot perviousness have generally demonstrated a consistent association between clot perviousness and revascularization outcomes. In a study of 221 patients receiving thin slice multiphase CTA, Santos and colleagues[28] found that increased attenuation of thrombus during the arterial phase of CTA was strongly associated with favorable functional and angiographic outcomes, whereas delayed phase imaging added no value. A similar finding was demonstrated by the publication by the entire MR CLEAN group.[33] In a study examining clot perviousness and tPA outcomes, the DUST investigators found that permeable thrombi were more responsive to tPA than those that were impermeable to contrast.[34]

It is likely that knowledge about clot consistency before treatment would influence the choice of the most effective thrombectomy device. The medical management of stroke may, however, benefit to a similar extent. If the target is clear, the therapy can be adapted accordingly by using the right pharmacologic agents.

POTENTIAL PHARMACOLOGIC THROMBUS TARGETS FOR TREATMENT

Given the limitations of current fibrinolytic therapy, there is an unmet need for alternative and improved thrombolytic agents. Depending on local guidelines, tPA can only be administered in the limited time window of 4.5 to 6.0 hours after the onset of stroke owing to the unacceptable risk of cerebral bleeding when treatment is delayed. As a consequence, tPA treatment is available to fewer than 10% of patients.[1] Remarkably, tPA results in recanalization only in less than one-half of the patients who receive it.[2] Factors that contribute to this so-called tPA resistance are not well-understood, but thrombus composition is a likely candidate determining fibrinolytic success rates. Various studies demonstrated that arterial platelet-rich clots in particular are more resistant to thrombolysis with tPA.[35–38] By studying stroke thrombi, our understanding of fibrin clot composition has much improved over the last years and other new potential targets for thrombolytic therapy have been identified. Some of those are discussed in the next section.

Fibrin

Since its approval in 1996 by the US Food and Drug Administration, tPA has become the standard pharmacologic intervention for thrombolysis in acute ischemic stroke. As part of the plasminogen activator system, tPA promotes the proteolytic activation of plasminogen to plasmin, which in turn is responsible for the enzymatic degradation of the fibrin mesh in a thrombus. Histologic studies of ischemic stroke thrombi typically revealed a heterogenous pattern of fibrin-rich areas in thrombi, with a wide range of fibrin amounts.[9,39,40] Various preclinical studies have demonstrated that, in particular, arterial platelet-rich and fibrin-rich clots are more resistant to thrombolysis with tPA compared with erythrocyte-rich thrombi.[35,36,38] Interestingly, Choi and colleagues[40] recently found that patients with higher amounts of fibrin and platelets in their thrombi were less responsive to intravenous thrombolysis. The fibrin structure is controlled by the environment in which the thrombus has been formed. In particular, stroke thrombi of cardioembolic origin are associated with a higher content of fibrin.[9,39,41–43] More research on human thrombus material is needed to investigate how fibrin characteristics determine success rates of tPA treatment. In this context, it will also be interesting to investigate the relative presence of potential inhibitors of fibrinolysis, such as α2-antiplasmin, plasminogen activator inhibitor-1, and thrombin activatable fibrinolysis inhibitor.

Von Willebrand Factor

In the past decade, VWF has been gaining increasing attention as an important factor in stroke pathology.[44] VWF is a large, multimeric plasma glycoprotein that mediates thrombus formation by recruiting platelets at sites of vascular injury. Together with fibrin(ogen), VWF links platelets together, further stabilizing the platelet thrombus.[44,45] Besides its thromboinflammatory role in cerebral ischemia/reperfusion injury,[46–49] recent findings point toward VWF as an attractive novel target to enhance thrombolysis. Via immunohistochemical staining for VWF, a recent study revealed that stroke thrombi retrieved from stroke patients contained significant amounts of VWF (Fig. 7A, B).[50] VWF was present in all thrombi, with amounts ranging from 5% to 50% of the thrombus content.

VWF can be cleaved by the metalloprotease ADAMTS13 (a disintegrin and metalloproteinase with a thrombospondin type 1 motif, member 13). By cleaving the Y1605-M1606 bond in the VWF A2 domain, ADAMTS13 digests VWF into smaller, less thrombogenic multimers. Following the hypothesis that ADAMTS13 can exert a thrombolytic effect in the setting of stroke, a mouse model was used in which the MCA was occluded by VWF-rich thrombi.[50] Interestingly, infusion of tPA did not lyse these MCA occlusions, but the administration of ADAMTS13 dose-dependently dissolved these tPA-resistant thrombi without bleeding side effects (Fig. 7C). As a result, fast restoration of MCA patency was achieved, which was associated with reduced cerebral infarct sizes 24 hours after the initial occlusion.[50] These results indicate that VWF could become a new target for improved thrombolytic activity in stroke. Beside cleaving by ADAMTS13, VWF can also be targeted to promote thrombolysis by blockade of the VWF–platelet interaction or by reducing the VWF monomer–monomer disulfide bonds by N-acetylcysteine.[51–53] Targeting VWF could prove particularly helpful in cases in which tPA is ineffective.

VWF content was significantly higher in thrombi retrieved after intravenous recombinant tPA use, compared with thrombi retrieved in primary thrombectomy, supporting the idea that thrombi resistant to intravenous thrombolysis may indeed be rich in VWF.[54] Of note, an inverse correlation was found between the amount of VWF and the amount of RBC content in stroke thrombi.[50] Because radiologic imaging upon patient admission is able to predict thrombus red cell content,[8,55] such information could become helpful to identify those patients who particularly benefit from ADAMTS13 treatment.

Neutrophil Extracellular Traps

Despite the large general variability in clot composition, leukocytes have been found to be consistently present in ischemic stroke thrombi.[8,9,41] Via specific immunostaining of stroke patient thrombi, Laridan and colleagues[56] showed that neutrophils are a commonly found leukocyte in these thrombi. Furthermore, this study also revealed the presence of neutrophil extracellular traps (NETs). Initially described as a novel form of neutrophil-mediated immunity, NETs form through the release of decondensated chromatin that is lined with granular components, creating fibrous structures.[57] It has become clear that, apart from their antimicrobial properties, NETs are also implicated in thrombus formation.[58] NETs form a scaffold for platelets and RBCs and influence the coagulation cascade.[59]

Histologic hematoxylin and eosin analysis of stroke thrombi revealed prominent extracellular nucleic acid-rich areas that were located in neutrophil-rich zones.[56] Selected immunostainings showed the presence of specific NETs markers on these extracellular DNA strands, demonstrating their neutrophilic origin (Fig. 8). Such extensive DNA networks were found in all thrombi, indicating that NETs are a common component of ischemic stroke thrombi. Leukocytes, but also NETs, are reported to be more abundant in stroke thrombi of cardioembolic origin.[9,56] This observation suggests that NETs might be specifically involved in thrombi formed in conditions of stasis, which is in agreement with results from Savchenko and colleagues,[60] who found NET accumulation in human venous thrombi. These new insights led to the hypothesis that NETs could also become a new target for thrombolysis. Serving as a thrombotic scaffold, NETs most likely contribute to overall thrombus stability and might confer resistance to fibrinolytic therapy as recently shown by Ducroux and colleagues.[61] DNA is known to be degraded by

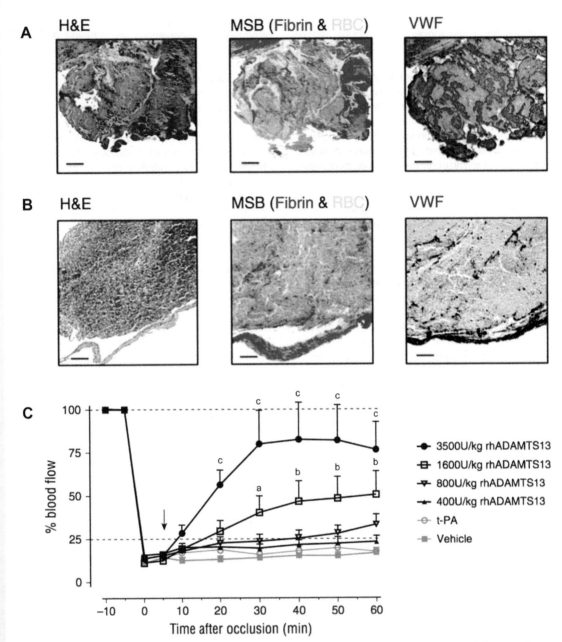

Fig. 7. von Willebrand factor (VWF) in ischemic stroke thrombi. Intracranial thrombi retrieved from stroke patients who underwent a thrombectomy were collected for histologic analysis. Consecutive thrombi sections were stained with hematoxylin and eosin (H&E), Martius Scarlet Blue (MSB) and anti-VWF antibodies. H&E staining show overall thrombus composition and organization. On MSB staining, red areas shows the presence of fibrin whereas red blood cells appear yellow. Varying amounts of VWF (*brown color*) were found in all the thrombi, Two representative patient thrombi are shown illustrating a VWF-rich thrombus (*A*) and an RBC-rich, VWF-poor thrombus (*B*). Scale bar: 50 μm. (*C*) An occlusive thrombus was generated in the right middle cerebral artery of C57Bl/6J mice. Five minutes after occlusion, vehicle, tissue plasminogen activator (tPA), or different doses of rhADAMTS13 were intravenously administered (*arrow*) and middle cerebral artery blood flow was monitored for 60 minutes. Average blood flow profiles show that rhADAMTS13 restored middle cerebral artery blood flow in a dose-dependent manner, whereas tPA was unable to restore blood vessel patency (n = 10 and 8 mice, respectively, for vehicle and 3500 U/kg rhADAMTS13; n = 5 for the lower doses of rhADAMTS13 and tPA). [a] $P<.05$; [b] $P<.01$; [c] $P<.001$ compared with vehicle. (*Adapted from* Denorme F, Langhauser F, Desender L, et al. ADAMTS13-mediated thrombolysis of t-PA–resistant occlusions in ischemic stroke in mice. Blood 2016;127(19):2337–45; with permission.)

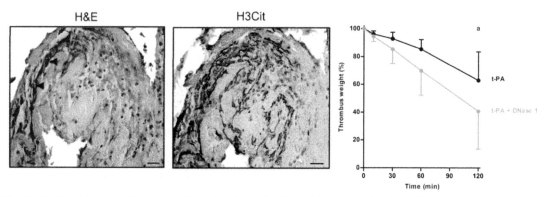

Fig. 8. Neutrophil extracellular traps in ischemic stroke thrombi. Intracranial thrombi retrieved from patients with a stroke who underwent thrombectomy procedure were collected for histologic analysis. Consecutive thrombus sections were stained with hematoxylin and eosin (H&E) and antibodies against citrullinated histones (H3Cit), a marker of neutrophil extracellular trap formation. Extracellular zones of nuclear material were often observed on H&E stainings (*left*), which were also positive for H3Cit (*right*). Scale bars: 10 μm. Right: Fresh thrombi (n = 8) retrieved from patients with an ischemic stroke were used for ex vivo lysis experiments. The thrombus parts were incubated for 120 minutes at 37°C in the presence of either tissue plasminogen activator (tPA) alone (*black*) or tPA plus DNase 1 (*gray*). Thrombus weight (percentage of original weight) was measured at time points 0, 10, 30, 60, and 120 minutes. Data are represented as mean with standard deviation. [a] $P<.01$. (*Adapted from* Laridan E, Denorme F, Desender L, et al. Neutrophil extracellular traps in ischemic stroke thrombi. Ann Neurol 2017;313:1451–10; with permission.)

DNases, which were recently shown to prevent vascular occlusion.[62] Interestingly, the addition of DNase 1 significantly improved tPA-mediated ex vivo dissolution of thrombi freshly retrieved from stroke patients (see **Fig. 8**).[56,61] DNase 1 was similarly shown to improve thrombolytic activity of coronary thrombi[63] and, in addition, it also reduces ischemic brain injury in mice.[64]

DNase 1 already is a safe, low-cost, drug approved by the US Food and Drug Administration and routinely used for cystic fibrosis to clear extracellular DNA in the lungs. Additional studies are needed to further assess the prothrombolytic potential of DNase 1 in the setting of stroke.

SUMMARY

Stroke thrombi are complex targets, containing various amounts of different cellular and molecular components. Emerging insights on thrombus composition provide valuable information that can stimulate the development of alternative and better strategies to efficiently remove the occluding thrombus. Promising new approaches are under development to improve mechanical thrombectomy as well as for improved pharmacologic approaches, including targeting VWF and NETs by ADAMTS13, and DNase 1. The combination of these new strategies with standard tPA could potentially allow decreasing the dose of tPA used, limiting its side effects and potentially increasing the therapeutic time

window. Especially in light of current limitations in stroke therapy, it will be interesting to follow future research in this area.

REFERENCES

1. Hacke W, Kaste M, Bluhmki E, et al. Thrombolysis with alteplase 3 to 4.5 hours after acute ischemic stroke. N Engl J Med 2008;359(13): 1317–29.
2. Rha J-H, Saver JL. The impact of recanalization on ischemic stroke outcome: a meta-analysis. Stroke 2007;38(3):967–73.
3. Berkhemer O, Beumer F, van den Berg L, et al. A randomized trial of intraarterial treatment for acute ischemic stroke (MR CLEAN). N Engl J Med 2015; 372:11–20.
4. Goyal M, Demchuk A, Menon B. Randomized assessment of rapid endovascular treatment of ischemic stroke (ESCAPE). N Engl J Med 2015; 372:1019–30.
5. Campbell B, Mitchell P, Kleinig T, et al. Endovascular therapy for ischemic stroke with perfusion-imaging selection (EXTEND-IA). N Engl J Med 2015;372:1009–18.
6. Saver J, Goyal M, Bonafe A, et al. Stent-retriever thrombectomy after intravenous t-PA vs. t-PA alone in stroke (SWIFT-PRIME). N Engl J Med 2015;372: 2285–95.
7. Jovin T, Chamorro A, Cobo E, et al. Thrombectomy within 8 hours after symptom onset in ischemic stroke (REVASCAT). N Engl J Med 2015;372: 2296–306.

8. Liebeskind DS, Sanossian N, Yong WH, et al. CT and MRI early vessel signs reflect clot composition in acute stroke. Stroke 2011;42:1237–43.

9. Boeckh-Behrens T, Schubert M, Förschler A, et al. The impact of histological clot composition in embolic stroke. Clin Neuroradiol 2016;26(2):189–97.

10. Cline B, Vos J, Carpenter J, et al. Pathological analysis of extracted clots in embolectomy patients with acute ischemic stroke. J Neurointerv Surg 2013;5(Suppl 2): A15–6. https://doi.org/10.1136/neurintsurg-2013-010870.27.

11. Gunning GM, McArdle K, Mirza M, et al. Clot friction variation with fibrin content; implications for resistance to thrombectomy. J Neurointerv Surg 2018; 10(1):34–8.

12. Ahn SH, Choo IS, Hong R, et al. Hyperdense arterial sign reflects the proportion of red blood cells in the thromboemboli of acute stroke patients. Cerebrovasc Dis 2012;33:236.

13. Chueh JY, Wakhloo AK, Hendricks GH, et al. Mechanical characterization of thromboemboli in acute ischemic stroke and laboratory embolus analogs. AJNR Am J Neuroradiol 2011;32:1237–44.

14. Froehler MT, Tateshima S, Duckwiler G, et al. The hyperdense vessel sign on CT predicts successful recanalization with the merci device in acute ischemic stroke. J Neurointerv Surg 2013;5: 289–93.

15. Guthrie S, Huang X, Moreton F, et al. The significance of the hyperdense vessel sign (HVS). Int J Stroke 2012;7:3.

16. Mehta BP, Nogueira RG. Should clot composition affect choice of endovascular therapy? Neurology 2012;79:S63–7.

17. van der Marel K, Chueh JY, Brooks OW, et al. Quantitative assessment of device-clot interaction for stent retriever thrombectomy. J Neurointerv Surg 2016;8(12):1278–82.

18. Nogueira RG, Levy EI, Gounis M. The Trevo device: preclinical data of a novel stroke thrombectomy device in two different animal models of arterial thrombo-occlusive disease. J Neurointerv Surg 2012;4:295–300.

19. De Meyer SF, Andersson T, Baxter B, et al. Analyses of thrombi in acute ischemic stroke: a consensus statement on current knowledge and future directions. Int J Stroke 2017;12:606–14.

20. Brinjikji W, Duffy S, Burrows A, et al. Correlation of imaging and histopathology of thrombi in acute ischemic stroke with etiology and outcome: a systematic review. J Neurointerv Surg 2017;9:529–34.

21. Dargazanli C, Rigau V, Eker O, et al. High cd3+ cells in intracranial thrombi represent a biomarker of atherothrombotic stroke. PLoS One 2016;11:e0154945.

22. Fennell VS, Setlur Nagesh SV, Meess KM, et al. What to do about fibrin rich 'tough clots'? Comparing the solitaire stent retriever with a novel Geometric clot extractor in an in vitro stroke model. J Neurointerv Surg 2018. [Epub ahead of print].

23. Chueh JY, Kuhn AL, Puri AS, et al. Reduction in distal emboli with proximal flow control during mechanical thrombectomy: a quantitative in vitro study. Stroke 2013;44:1396–401.

24. Brinjikji W, Starke RM, Murad MH, et al. Impact of balloon guide catheter on technical and clinical outcomes: a systematic review and meta-analysis. J Neurointerv Surg 2017. https://doi.org/10.1136/neurintsurg-2017-013179.

25. Riedel CH, Zoubie J, Ulmer S, et al. Thin-slice reconstructions of nonenhanced CT images allow for detection of thrombus in acute stroke. Stroke 2012; 43:2319–23.

26. Heo JH, Kim K, Yoo J, et al. Computed tomography-based thrombus imaging for the prediction of recanalization after reperfusion therapy in stroke. J Stroke 2017;19:40–9.

27. Kaschka IN, Kloska SP, Struffert T, et al. Clot burden and collaterals in anterior circulation stroke: differences between single-phase CTA and multi-phase 4d-CTA. Clin Neuroradiol 2016;26:309–15.

28. Santos EMM, d'Esterre CD, Treurniet KM, et al. Added value of multiphase CTA imaging for thrombus perviousness assessment. Neuroradiology 2018;60:71–9.

29. Ganeshan R, Nave AH, Scheitz JF, et al. Assessment of thrombus length in acute ischemic stroke by post-contrast magnetic resonance angiography. J Neurointerv Surg 2018;10(8):756–60.

30. Brinjikji W, Michalak G, Kadirvel R, et al. Utility of single-energy and dual-energy computed tomography in clot characterization: an in-vitro study. Interv Neuroradiol 2017;23:279–84.

31. Kim SK, Yoon W, Kim TS, et al. Histologic analysis of retrieved clots in acute ischemic stroke: correlation with stroke etiology and gradient-echo MRI. AJNR Am J Neuroradiol 2015;36:1756–62.

32. Jindal G, Miller T, Shivashankar R, et al. Relationship of thrombus length to number of stent retrievals, revascularization, and outcomes in acute ischemic stroke. J Vasc Interv Radiol 2014;25: 1549–57.

33. Borst J, Berkhemer OA, Santos EMM, et al. Value of thrombus CT characteristics in patients with acute ischemic stroke. AJNR Am J Neuroradiol 2017;38: 1758–64.

34. Santos EMM, Dankbaar JW, Treurniet KM, et al. Permeable thrombi are associated with higher intravenous recombinant tissue-type plasminogen activator treatment success in patients with acute ischemic stroke. Stroke 2016;47:2058–65.

35. Jang IK, Gold HK, Ziskind AA, et al. Differential sensitivity of erythrocyte-rich and platelet-rich arterial thrombi to lysis with recombinant tissue-type plasminogen activator. A possible explanation for

resistance to coronary thrombolysis. Circulation 1989;79(4):920–8.

36. Booth NA, Robbie LA, Croll AM, et al. Lysis of platelet-rich thrombi: the role of PAI-1. Ann N Y Acad Sci 1992;667:70–80.

37. Rusak T, Piszcz J, Misztal T, et al. Platelet-related fibrinolysis resistance in patients suffering from PV. Impact of clot retraction and isovolemic erythrocytapheresis. Thromb Res 2014;134(1):192–8.

38. Tomkins AJ, Schleicher N, Murtha L, et al. Platelet rich clots are resistant to lysis by thrombolytic therapy in a rat model of embolic stroke. Exp Transl Stroke Med 2015;7(1):1317.

39. Simons N, Mitchell P, Dowling R, et al. Thrombus composition in acute ischemic stroke: a histopathological study of thrombus extracted by endovascular retrieval. J Neuroradiol 2015;42(2):86–92.

40. Choi MH, Park GH, Lee JS, et al. Erythrocyte fraction within retrieved thrombi contributes to thrombolytic response in acute ischemic stroke. Stroke 2018. https://doi.org/10.1161/STROKEAHA.117.019138.

41. Boeckh-Behrens T, Kleine JF, Zimmer C, et al. Thrombus histology suggests cardioembolic cause in cryptogenic stroke. Stroke 2016;47(7):1864–71.

42. Sporns PB, Hanning U, Schwindt W, et al. Ischemic stroke: what does the histological composition tell us about the origin of the thrombus? Stroke 2017;48(8):2206–10.

43. Niesten JM, van der Schaaf IC, van Dam L, et al. Histopathologic composition of cerebral thrombi of acute stroke patients is correlated with stroke subtype and thrombus attenuation. PLoS One 2014;9(2):e88882.

44. De Meyer SF, Stoll G, Wagner DD, et al. von Willebrand factor: an emerging target in stroke therapy. Stroke 2012;43(2):599–606.

45. De Meyer SF, Deckmyn H, Vanhoorelbeke K. von Willebrand factor to the rescue. Blood 2009;113(21):5049–57.

46. De Meyer SF, Denorme F, Langhauser F, et al. Thromboinflammation in stroke brain damage. Stroke 2016;47(4):1165–72.

47. Verhenne S, Denorme F, Libbrecht S, et al. Platelet-derived VWF is not essential for normal thrombosis and hemostasis but fosters ischemic stroke injury in mice. Blood 2015;126(14):1715–22.

48. Kleinschnitz C, De Meyer SF, Schwarz T, et al. Deficiency of von Willebrand factor protects mice from ischemic stroke. Blood 2009;113(15):3600–3.

49. De Meyer SF, Schwarz T, Deckmyn H, et al. Binding of von Willebrand factor to collagen and glycoprotein Ibalpha, but not to glycoprotein IIb/IIIa, contributes to ischemic stroke in mice– brief report. Arterioscler Thromb Vasc Biol 2010;30(10):1949–51.

50. Denorme F, Langhauser F, Desender L, et al. ADAMTS13-mediated thrombolysis of t-PA–resistant occlusions in ischemic stroke in mice. Blood 2016;127(19):2337–45.

51. Momi S, Tantucci M, Van Roy M, et al. Reperfusion of cerebral artery thrombosis by the GPIb-VWF blockade with the Nanobody ALX-0081 reduces brain infarct size in guinea pigs. Blood 2013;121(25):5088–97.

52. Le Behot A, Gauberti M, de Lizarrondo SM, et al. GpIbα-VWF blockade restores vessel patency by dissolving platelet aggregates formed under very high shear rate in mice. Blood 2014;123(21):3354–63.

53. Martinez de Lizarrondo S, Gakuba C, Herbig BA, et al. Potent thrombolytic effect of N-acetylcysteine on arterial thrombi. Circulation 2017;136(7):646–60.

54. López-Cancio E, Millán M, Pérez de la Ossa N, et al. Immunohistochemical study of clot composition in thrombi retrieved from MCA with mechanical thrombectomy. Cerebrovasc Dis 2013;35(Suppl. 3):255.

55. Niesten JM, van der Schaaf IC, van der Graaf Y, et al. Predictive value of thrombus attenuation on thin-slice non-contrast CT for persistent occlusion after intravenous thrombolysis. Cerebrovasc Dis 2014;37(2):116–22.

56. Laridan E, Denorme F, Desender L, et al. Neutrophil extracellular traps in ischemic stroke thrombi. Ann Neurol 2017;82(2):223–32.

57. Brinkmann V, Reichard U, Goosmann C, et al. Neutrophil extracellular traps kill bacteria. Science 2004;303(5663):1532–5.

58. Fuchs TA, Brill A, Duerschmied D, et al. Extracellular DNA traps promote thrombosis. Proc Natl Acad Sci U S A 2010;107(36):15880–5.

59. Martinod K, Wagner DD. Thrombosis: tangled up in NETs. Blood 2014;123(18):2768–76.

60. Savchenko AS, Martinod K, Seidman MA, et al. Neutrophil extracellular traps form predominantly during the organizing stage of human venous thromboembolism development. J Thromb Haemost 2014;12(6):860–70.

61. Ducroux C, Di Meglio L, Loyau S, et al. Thrombus neutrophil extracellular traps content impair tPA-induced thrombolysis in acute ischemic stroke. Stroke 2018;49(3):754–7.

62. Jiménez-Alcázar M, Rangaswamy C, Panda R, et al. Host DNases prevent vascular occlusion by neutrophil extracellular traps. Science 2017;358(6367):1202–6.

63. Mangold A, Alias S, Scherz T, et al. Coronary neutrophil extracellular trap burden and deoxyribonuclease activity in ST-elevation acute coronary syndrome are predictors of ST-segment resolution and infarct size. Circ Res 2015;116(7):1182–92.

64. De Meyer SF, Suidan GL, Fuchs TA, et al. Extracellular chromatin is an important mediator of ischemic stroke in mice. Arterioscler Thromb Vasc Biol 2012;32(8):1884–91.

Neuro-Interventional Management of Acute Ischemic Stroke

Lotfi Hacein-Bey, MD[a,b,*], Jeremy J. Heit, MD, PhD[c], Angelos A. Konstas, MD[d]

KEYWORDS

• Acute stroke • Ischemia • Neuro-interventional management • Thrombectomy • Endovascular

KEY POINTS

• Mechanical thrombectomy is now standard of care in stroke from large-vessel occlusion with Class IA evidence.
• Treatment paradigms will likely evolve from time limits toward personalized physiology-based patient evaluation.
• Although a number of effective devices are available, techniques will continue to evolve.
• Increasingly better outcomes are obtained, with possible future enhancements through neuroprotection.
• Increasing numbers of patients will be treated, requiring workforce adjustments.

INTRODUCTION

Approximately 795,000 strokes occur each year in the United States alone,[1] the vast majority (87%) ischemic (as opposed to hemorrhagic) in nature.[2] Many patients survive, left with major limitations of daily life from neurologic prejudice,[1] resulting in an estimated annual financial cost to treat stroke survivors currently estimated at approximately $40 billion and rising.[3]

Currently known stroke risk factors include aging, hypertension, diabetes, obesity (increased waist-to-hip ratio), dyslipidemia, smoking, chronic kidney disease, and chronic cardiac disease.[4] Therefore, although prevention may play a significant role in addressing modifiable risk factors, the prevalence and severity of stroke are such that effective treatment strategies are necessary.

The first important breakthrough was the demonstration of improved outcomes after intravenous administration of the thrombolytic rt-PA (recombinant tissue plasminogen activator) within the appropriate time window. The process was, however, slow, taking almost 10 years to reach consensus on a 4.5-hour time window to offset the risk of symptomatic intracranial hemorrhage.[5–7]

During that period, the effectiveness of interventional transarterial thrombolytic administration within the clot within 6 hours of stroke onset was also being demonstrated.[8] Although never approved by the Food and Drug Administration (FDA), such treatment option soon became commonplace in most major centers.[9]

Early interventional experience contributed to the realization that clots could be disrupted and

Disclosure Statement: The authors have no disclosures to declare in relation with this article.
[a] Interventional Neuroradiology and Neuroradiology, Department of Medical Imaging, Sutter Health, Sacramento, CA 95815, USA; [b] Radiology Department, University of California Davis Medical School of Medicine, 4860 Y Street, Sacramento, CA 95817, USA; [c] Division of Neuroimaging and Neurointervention, Stanford Healthcare, 300 Pasteur Drive, Grant S047, Stanford, CA 94305, USA; [d] Interventional Neuroradiology and Neuroradiology, Department of Radiology, Huntington Memorial Hospital, 100 West California Boulevard, Pasadena, CA 91105, USA
* Corresponding author. Interventional Neuroradiology and Neuroradiology, Department of Medical Imaging, Sutter Health, Sacramento, CA 95815.
E-mail address: lhaceinbey@yahoo.com

neuroimaging.theclinics.com

possibly retrieved by direct mechanical methods, including catheters, guidewires, balloons, and snares, which led to the development of the Mechanical Embolus Removal in Cerebral Ischemia (MERCI) and Multi MERCI trials.[10–12] Following these trials, the FDA approved the MERCI device (initially dubbed the Concentric Retriever), which is made of Nickel-Titanium loops arranged in a corkscrew configuration, which are advanced past the clot and pulled back for retrieval to treat ischemic stroke within a 6-hour time window.

The relatively low performance of the MERCI device was one of the factors resulting in the publication in 2013 of 3 consecutive failed randomized trials comparing medical with endovascular stroke therapy, which was discouraging news for the stroke community at large at the time.[13–15]

Another suggested cause for these failed trials was inadequate patient selection, leading to the establishment of vascular imaging before triage for endovascular treatment, and a maximum infarct core threshold value measured with diffusion-weighted imaging magnetic resonance imaging (DWI-MRI) of 60 to 70 mL in favor of intervention.[16] It also became clear that the decision to deliver endovascular therapy had to be carefully made, as successful or not, intervention could be a major source of morbidity and death.[16]

Major revival of mechanical thrombectomy soon thereafter followed, with the advent of a new class of devices, that is, stent retrievers.

MECHANICAL THROMBECTOMY BECOMES STANDARD OF CARE

The Multicenter Randomized Clinical trial of Endovascular treatment for Acute ischemic stroke in the Netherlands (MR CLEAN) trial,[17] published in early 2015, was a landmark study that heralded a major and irreversible turn in stroke therapy. The study involved 26 centers throughout the Netherlands, in which 500 patients were enrolled prospectively and randomized to either standard, conventional noninterventional treatment that included intravenous (IV) thrombolysis (n = 267) or IV and intra-arterial treatment (n = 233). Patients were included who presented within 6 hours of a stroke after confirmation of large-vessel occlusion (LVO): internal carotid artery (ICA), M1, M2, A1 or A2 by either computed tomography angiography (CTA) or magnetic resonance angiography (MRA). The vast majority of patients who received interventional care (97%) were treated with Solitaire or Trevo stent retrievers. Recanalization, defined as thrombolysis in cerebral infarction (TICI) 2b-3 reperfusion scores (Table 1), was obtained in 59% of patients. Positive primary outcomes (modified Rankin score [mRs] at 90 days 0–2) were achieved in 32.6% of the treated group versus 19.1% in the untreated group; mortality and symptomatic hemorrhagic transformation were similar in both groups. The MR CLEAN study yielded an absolute 13.5% difference in the rate of functional independence in the treated group (95% confidence interval, 5.9 vs 21.2), the first major advancement in stroke treatment since IV-tPA thrombolysis in 1995. Interestingly, although those findings were valid for interventions performed within 6 hours of stroke onset, statistical significance was no longer present after 6 hours and 19 minutes of stroke onset.

A number of studies were published in the following months, all but one using stent retrievers, all confirming superiority of mechanical thrombectomy over standard management or IV thrombolysis alone.

The Endovascular Treatment for Small Core and Anterior Circulation Proximal Occlusion with Emphasis on Minimizing CT to Recanalization Times (ESCAPE) trial involved patients seen up to 12 hours after anterior circulation stroke onset.[18] Patients

Table 1
Comparison of reperfusion grade scales used in stroke trials

Grade	TIMI Score	TICI Score	Modified TICI Score
0	Absence of perfusion	Absence of perfusion	Absence of perfusion
1	Contrast penetration without perfusion	Minimal perfusion	Minimal perfusion: limited distal artery filling
2	Partial reperfusion	2a. Partial reperfusion to < two-thirds occluded territory 2b. Complete reperfusion with however slow filling	2a. Reperfusion of < half occluded territory 2b. Reperfusion > half occluded territory 2c. Reperfusion of > three-fourths occluded territory but not total
3	Complete reperfusion	Complete reperfusion	Complete reperfusion

Abbreviations: TICI, thrombolysis in cerebral infarction; TIMI, thrombolysis in myocardial infarction.

were evaluated by CT techniques, inclusion criteria were small infarct volume, occlusion of the ICA, M1 or at least 2 M2 branches, and CTA evidence of good arterial collaterals (>50% of ipsilateral collateral convexity collaterals). Patients were prospectively randomized to either IV t-PA within 4.5 hours of ictus (n = 150) or standard treatment plus mechanical thrombectomy. In the latter group, adequate reperfusion (TICI 2b-3) was achieved in 72.4%. The group of patients treated within 6 to 12 hours of stroke onset was too small, obviating useful statistical results. Clinical outcomes in patients treated with mechanical thrombectomy were better than in the MR CLEAN trial: mRs scores at 90 days were 53% versus 29.3% for IV t-PA only.

The Solitaire with the Intention for Thrombectomy as Primary Endovascular Treatment (SWIFT PRIME) study, which was prematurely halted on ethical grounds, was published at the same time.[19] The SWIFT PRIME trial, sponsored by industry (Covidien/Medtronic Neurovascular Clinical Affairs, Irvine, CA), was therefore primarily designed to evaluate the efficacy of the Solitaire device. Patients (n = 196) were included if they showed evidence by CTA or MRA of ICA or M1 occlusion, a core infarction of 50 mL or less on CT perfusion or diffusion-weighted imaging (DWI), evidence of a target mismatch between the core infarction and perfusion imaging, and were randomized to either IV t-PA within 4.5 hours of stroke onset (n = 98) or IV t-PA plus mechanical thrombectomy (n = 98). Reperfusion (TICI 2b-3) was achieved in 88% with the Solitaire device. Favorable outcomes (mRs 0–2 at 3 months) were 60.2% in the thrombectomy group versus 35.5% in the t-PA group.

The Extending the Time for Thrombolysis in Emergency Neurologic Deficits–Intra-Arterial (EXTEND-IA),[20] also industry sponsored, was aimed at assessing the efficacy of the Solitaire device (Covidien/Medtronic Neurovascular Clinical Affairs). Patients were evaluated by anatomic and perfusion imaging using either CT or MR modalities, and had to fulfill the following criteria: core infarct size less than 70 mL, LVO of the ICA, M1 or M2 branches, perfusion mismatch greater than 1.2 (absolute mismatch >10 mL). A total of 70 patients were randomized to either IV t-PA within 4.5 hours of stroke onset (n = 35) or IV t-PA plus Solitaire mechanical thrombectomy (n = 35). Reperfusion (TICI 2b-3) was achieved in 86% with the Solitaire device. Favorable outcomes (mRs 0–2 at 3 months) were 71% in the thrombectomy group versus 40% in the t-PA group.

The Randomized Trial of Revascularization with Solitaire FR Device versus Best Medical Therapy in the Treatment of Acute Stroke Due to Anterior Circulation Large Vessel Occlusion Presenting within

Eight Hours of Symptom Onset (REVASCAT) was published at the same time.[21] The REVASCAT study, jointly sponsored by the Spanish government and Covidien/Medtronic, was aimed at evaluating the Solitaire device, and conducted in 4 medical centers in and around Barcelona, Spain. Patients (n = 206) had to have no evidence of a large infarction, determined as an ASPECTS (Alberta Stroke Program Early CT Score) score greater than 6 on noncontrast CT, CTA, or MRA or angiographic evidence of ICA or M1 occlusion, and, again were randomized to either IV t-PA within 4.5 hours of stroke onset (n = 103) or IV t-PA plus Solitaire device mechanical thrombectomy (n = 103). Reperfusion (TICI 2b-3) was achieved in 66% with the Solitaire device. Favorable outcomes (mRs 0–2 at 3 months) were 43.7% in the thrombectomy group versus 28.2% in the thrombolysis group. This trial was also prematurely closed for clinical evidence of superiority of mechanical thrombectomy.

The THERAPY trial was a prospective randomized study that evaluated the Penumbra aspiration system compared with IV t-PA. The results of the THERAPY trial were published after the 5 studies comparing stent retrievers with medical therapy.[22] The major inclusion criterion was the presence of an intracranial arterial clot measuring 8 mm or longer. A total of 102 patients were included before early cessation of the trial due to evidence provided by other mechanical thrombectomy trials. Final primary analysis in this study failed to demonstrate a statistical benefit of endovascular therapy, although efficacy of thrombectomy was strongly suggested on secondary analyses.[22]

The THRACE trial, which was conducted in France, was also halted prematurely after the inclusion of 404 patients.[23]

Comparative effectiveness of thrombectomy using either first-line aspiration catheters or first-line stent retrievers was evaluated in the large Contact Aspiration versus Stent Retriever for Successful Revascularization (ASTER) study of 381 patients treated in 8 large centers in France.[24] Similar recanalization rates were found with both techniques: TICI 2b-3 scores of 85.4% for aspiration versus 83.1% for stent retrievers; clinical outcomes at 3 months were also similar in both groups. Interestingly, in patients with M2 occlusion (n = 79), aspiration thrombectomy showed a modest, non–statistically significant advantage (TICI 2b-3 rate of 89.6% vs 83.9%).[25]

A meta-analysis of 1287 patients enrolled in the 5 major trials concluded to absence of benefit from thrombectomy if performed after 7.3 hours of stroke onset.[26]

Table 2 summarizes the findings of recent major trials

Table 2
Summary of recent large randomized stroke trials supporting endovascular treatment

Trial	Inclusion Criteria	Imaging Criteria	Time from Onset	Device	Device Usage, %	Reperfusion Rate, mTICI 2b-3, %	Outcome, mRs 0–2 at 90 d, %	Intervention vs IV t-PA (Except ARISE II and DAWN Trials)
MR CLEAN	NIHSS ≥2	LVO on CTA, MRA, DSA, TCD	<6 h	Trevo/Solitaire	81.5	59	32.6 vs 19.0	500 (233 vs 267)
ESCAPE	NIHSS ≥5	LVO on CT/CTA Small infarct core (ASPECTS 6–10) Good collaterals on multiphase CTA	<12 h	Solitaire/Trevo	86	72	53.0 vs 29.3	315 (165 vs 150)
SWIFT PRIME	NIHSS 8–29	LVO on CT/CTA or MRI/MRA Infarct core ≤50 mL Target mismatch on Perfusion MR	<6 h	Solitaire	100	88	60.2 vs 35.5	196 (98 vs 98)
EXTEND-IA	Prestroke mRS≤0–1	LVO on CTA/CTP/MRA/MRP Infarct core ≤70 mL Target mismatch on Perfusion MR	<6 h	Solitaire	100	86	71 vs 40	70 (35 vs 35)
REVASCAT	NIHSS≥6	LVO on CTA/MRA/DSA ASPECTS score≥6	<8 h	Solitaire	100	66	43.7 vs 28.2	206 (103 vs 103)
THRACE	NIHSS 10–25	LVO on CT/CTA/MRA	<5 h	Solitaire	100		53.0 vs 42.1	404 (200 vs 202)
THERAPY	NIHSS≥8	Clot length on CT ≥8 mm Infarct core ≤1/3 MCA	<8 h	Penumbra (Aspiration)	100	70	38 vs 30	108 (55 vs 53)
ARISE II	NIHSS 8–25	LVO on CTA/MRA/DSA	<8 h	EmboTrap	100	79.5	70	228 vs literature on Solitaire and Trevo
DAWN	NIHSS≥10 (groups A-B) NIHSS≥20 (group C)	DWI-MRI/CTP (RAPID software) Small infarct core (≤51 mL)	6–24 h	Trevo	100	84	49 vs 13	206 (107 vs 99 standard care)
DEFUSE 3	NIHSS≥10 (13 patients NIHSS<10)	DWI-MRI/CTP (RAPID software) infarct core <70 mL (median 35 mL)	6–16 h	Any FDA approved device	98	76	45 vs 17	182 (92 vs 90 standard care)

Abbreviations: ASPECTS, Alberta Stroke Program Early CT Score; CTA, computed tomography angiography; CTP, computed tomography perfusion; DSA, digital subtraction angiography; DWI, diffusion-weighted imaging; IV, intravenous; LVO, large-vessel occlusion; MCA, middle cerebral artery; MRA, magnetic resonance angiography; MRP, magnetic resonance perfusion; mRs, modified Rankin score; mTICI, modified treatment in cerebral ischemia; NIHSS, National Institutes of Health Stroke Scale; t-PA, tissue plasminogen activator.

CURRENT DEVICES USED IN MECHANICAL THROMBECTOMY

The Solitaire stent retriever (**Fig. 1**), initially marketed by eV3 Endovascular (Irvine, CA) as the Solitaire Flow Restoration (FR) device, was the first of its kind to be granted FDA clearance in 2012. The dedicated study, which evaluated the Solitaire device against the MERCI Retriever (the only FDA-cleared device before that) was the Solitaire FR with the Intention for Thrombectomy (SWIFT) study.[27] The study (n = 113), which time window for intervention was 8 hours, showed TICI 2 to 3 reperfusion rates of 61% for the Solitaire FR versus 24% for the MERCI device, outcomes at 90 days (mRs 0–2) of 58% versus 33%, and reduction in mortality at 3 months from 28% to 17%.

Later the same year, the Trevo stent retriever (**Fig. 2**), initially marketed as the Trevo ProVue Retriever by Stryker Neurovascular (Kalamazoo, MI), was also evaluated in a study that was designed similarly to the SWIFT trial, and was also found to be superior to the MERCI device. In the 178 study patients, TICI 2 to 3 recanalization rates were 86% (Trevo) versus 60%, good clinical outcomes (mRs 0–2 at 3 months) were 33% versus 24%, and mortality at 3 months was 33% versus 24%.[28]

The EmboTrap stent retriever (Neuravi-Codman Neuro, Fremont, CA) has an interesting design of 2 channels, the inner allowing immediate flow restoration, the outer granting clot trapping (**Fig. 3**). This device, which was granted CE mark approval (European FDA equivalent) in September 2016, was evaluated in the Analysis of Revascularization in Ischemic Stroke With EmboTrap (ARISE II) Study, which enrolled 228 patients in 19 centers in Europe and the United States. Study results showed a recanalization rate of 79.5% and a high rate of functional independence (mRs 0–2 at 3 months) of 70%. Mortality was 9% and symptomatic hemorrhage 5%.[29]

In parallel, newer generation, large-bore aspiration catheters led to refinements of the ADAPT (A Direct-Aspiration first-Pass) technique, which allows the en bloc extraction of the entire intracranial arterial thrombus.[30–33] The Penumbra aspiration device, which is attached to a negative-pressure electrical pump (**Fig. 4**) (Alameda, CA) benefited from several upgrades in luminal size and improvements in navigability, and was evaluated in the THERAPY trial against IV t-PA. Despite recanalization rates of 70% and good clinical outcomes (mRs 0–2 at 3 months) of 38% versus 30%, it fell short of demonstrating superiority.[22]

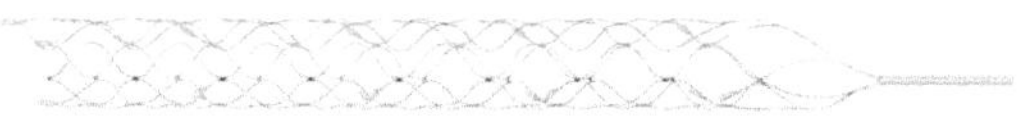

A hybrid interventional technique based on the concomitant use of a stent retriever advanced in the thrombus and a large-bore catheter advanced at the clot base was soon reported, dubbed SOLUMBRA (the combination of the 2 brand names Solitaire and Penumbra). This technique was reported to yield recanalization rates in the 90% to 95% range.[34]

Another large-bore catheter, the Sofia (Soft torqueable catheter Optimized For Intracranial Access; Microvention, Tustin, CA), with a unique design of coil and braid reinforcement (**Fig. 5**) conferring a high navigability profile, was reported to show high effectiveness and ultra-short working times with both the ADAPT and SOLUMBRA techniques.[35,36] The Sofia catheter can be safely advanced into the intracranial circulation without a guidewire or guiding microcatheter owing to a soft tip and a flexible construct,[36] which permits prompt and highly effective thrombo-aspiration (**Fig. 6**), and facilitates combined intervention with a stent retriever (**Fig. 7**) owing to large inner diameters (0.056-inch and 0.070-inch, respectively, for the currently available 5-French and 6-French sizes).[36,37]

TIME METRICS AND PRACTICAL ASPECTS OF INTERVENTIONAL CARE

The Brain Attack Coalition, which comprises more than 15 professional societies under the National Institute of Neurologic Disorders and Stroke with the National Institutes of Health (NIH) has generated treatment benchmarks. In 2011, a 2-hour door to endovascular treatment benchmark was recommended.[38,39]

The Rapid Reperfusion Registry, which was initiated based on those guidelines to evaluate the time performance at 7 stroke centers in the United States and Canada demonstrated in 2012 that in no more than 52% of patients was the 2-hour target door-to-puncture time achieved.[40]

In 2015, the Society of Neurointerventional Surgery (SNIS), which is part of the Brain Attack Coalition, suggested a number of time metrics to guide the management of patients at institutions that had been granted comprehensive stroke center status.[41] Guidelines recommended by SNIS include the following times: (1) door-to–CTA interpretation less than 20 minutes, (2) door-to–first femoral puncture less than 60 minutes, and (3) door-to–intracranial recanalization less than 90 minutes.

Successful application of such metrics requires several strategies for the optimization of workflow, including parallel processing, team building,

Fig. 1. The Solitaire device. (*Courtesy of* Covidien/Medtronic Neurovascular Clinical Affairs, Irvine, CA; with permission).

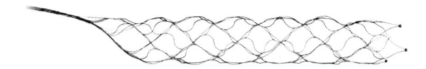

Trevo® XP ProVue Retriever 6x25 mm

Fig. 2. The Trevo stent retriever. (*Courtesy of* Stryker Neurovascular, Fremont, CA; with permission).

training, and standardization of procedures.[42] Adequate training of all team members and maintenance of skills require constant attention and a proactive approach.[43]

A high level of efficiency is necessary in triaging patients in emergency rooms,[44] prioritizing radiological studies and interpretation,[45] and expediting the process of preparing patients for intervention.[46] Procedural consent may be a potential cause for delay; this issue was successfully addressed in some clinical trials with a smartphone application that allows for obtaining an electronic informed consent (e-consent).[47]

In the United States, current average times from stroke onset to femoral puncture are 6 hours, and recanalization takes an average additional hour.[48] Streamlining and parallel processing of tasks involved in patient preparation for procedures have been shown to significantly reduce door-to-puncture times.[49] The simultaneous (not sequential) performance of tasks involved in high-level, time-sensitive processes was shown to be key.[41,46] Short femoral puncture-to-recanalization times (<30 minutes) may be achieved in most patients.[41]

SUMMARY OF CURRENT EVIDENCE AND REMAINING QUESTIONS

Despite potential concerns for relationship with industry concerning several of the positive, industry-sponsored trials published in 2015 and 2016, management of acute ischemic stroke due to LVO using IV t-PA followed by mechanical thrombectomy was granted Class IA clinical practice guideline status in 2016 (the highest recommendation) in Europe and the United States.[50] Class I recommendation is a strong indication with demonstrated high effectiveness, high benefit/risk ratio or high comparative effectiveness, whereas level A designates high-level evidence, usually derived from several well-conducted randomized, prospective controlled trials.

At this time, although the recommended window for intervention remains 6 hours from ictus, some centers are extending the time window to 8 hours or longer provided infarct size and collateral status are favorable, and there is a strong demand and a clear understanding of risk on the part of the patient's family.

Beyond 6 Hours

The DAWN (DWI or CTP Assessment With Clinical Mismatch in the Triage of Wake Up and Late Presenting Strokes Undergoing Neurointervention With Trevo) trial has generated significant interest by suggesting that some patients with ischemic stroke could be treated up to 24 hours after the last time they were seen healthy.[51] This trial, also industry sponsored (Trevo stent retriever; Stryker

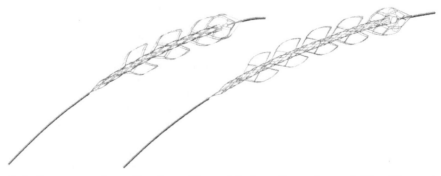

Fig. 3. The EmboTrap stent retriever. (*Courtesy of* Neuravi-Codman Neuro, Fremont, CA; with permission).

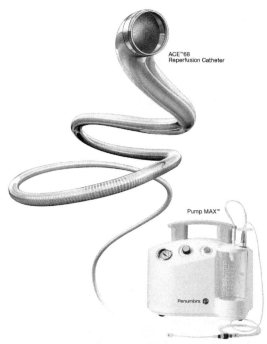

Fig. 4. The Penumbra aspiration device comes with a negative-pressure electrical pump. (*Courtesy of* Penumbra, Alameda, CA; with permission.)

Neurovascular, Fremont, CA) enrolled 206 patients (107 treated with thrombectomy vs 99 with standard therapy). In the DAWN trial, patients were carefully selected, primarily based on small core infarct volume (less than 51 mL in all patients, and <31 mL for most) measured primarily with DWI-MRI (virtually gold standard) or perfusion CT using a validated, FDA-cleared, automated software (RAPID; iSchemaView, Menlo Park, CA). Patients were offered thrombectomy only if major mismatch between small infarct volume and severity of neurologic deficit was clearly demonstrated. Intervention resulted in recanalization in 84%, and functional independence was 49% for

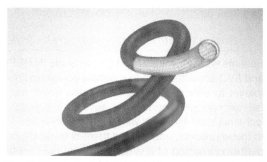

Fig. 5. The Sofia (soft torqueable catheter optimized for intracranial access). (*Courtesy of* Microvention, INC, Tustin, CA; with permission.)

thrombectomy versus 13%. Mortality at 3 months was similar in both groups: 19% versus 18% (thrombectomy vs standard therapy, and symptomatic hemorrhage 6% in the thrombectomy group vs 3% in the control group, considered beneath statistical significance).

The Endovascular Therapy Following Imaging Evaluation for Ischemic Stroke 3 (DEFUSE 3) trial enrolled 182 patients (92 in the thrombectomy group vs 90 in the medical treatment group) within 6 to 16 hours of the time last known to be well, and with evidence of significant residual noninfarcted tissue. Again, infarct size had to be <70 mL, measured either with DWI-MRI or perfusion CT using the RAPID software (iSchemaView). Functional independence was 45% for thrombectomy versus 17% for medical treatment. Ninety-day mortality was 14% in the thrombectomy group versus 26% in the medical treatment group, and symptomatic hemorrhage 7% in the thrombectomy group versus 4% in the control group, considered not statistically significant.[52]

At the time of this review, although the recommended time window for intervention based on national guidelines in the United States and Europe remains 6 hours, the results of the DAWN and DEFUSE 3 trials have triggered the easing of guidelines past the 6-hour window in properly selected patients. Adequate identification of candidates (mainly those with small-core infarcts and highly developed collateral networks) for delayed intervention will likely be a major topic of investigation in years to come (**Fig. 8**).

Beyond First Order Branches (M1)

Retrospective data analysis from 6 trials, including the Solitaire Flow Restoration Thrombectomy for Acute Revascularization (STAR), SWIFT, and SWIFT PRIME studies, and 3 large multicenter prospective studies identified 50 patients with M2 occlusions, whose outcomes were similar to those with more proximal occlusions.[53] A retrospective review of 288 patients treated at 10 US institutions by mechanical thrombectomy for M2 occlusions also suggested a reasonable safety profile and similar clinical benefit as for more proximal occlusions.[54]

Retrospective review of data from the IMS-III trial showed benefit of mechanical thrombectomy in patients with M2 trunk occlusion, especially when arterial territory harbors highly eloquent function (ie, language). Benefit was not demonstrated for more distal M2 occlusions.[55] Risk/benefit assessment should be made, as arterial branches distal to the anterior cerebral fissure run untethered in the subarachnoid space,

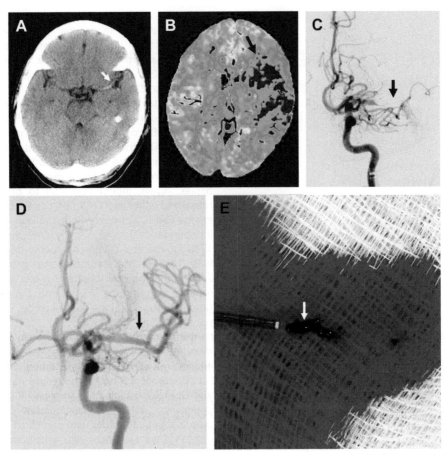

Fig. 6. A 45-year-old woman with cardiomyopathy 2 hours after acute aphasia and right hemiparesis (NIHSS 21). CT shows dense left MCA (*A, arrow*). Large MCA territory at risk on perfusion CT (Tmax map) (*B, arrow*). Angiogram shows occluded left M1 MCA (*C, arrow*). Thromboaspiration with the 6-French Sofia catheter (*D, arrow*) allows total revascularization in 9 minutes. Immediate full clinical recovery. Note that retrieved red thrombus maintains shape of MCA bifurcation (*E, arrow*).

therefore at higher risk for rupture, whereas clinical benefit from distal branch reperfusion may not be significant.

Posterior Circulation

Although posterior circulation strokes account for only approximately 20% of all ischemic strokes, they account for significant morbidity and fatality. Evidence is currently lacking as to effectiveness and risk of endovascular intervention in this patient group, despite anecdotal reports of success stories. Registries and trials are under way that will hopefully result in evidence-based guidelines.

The Basilar Artery International Cooperation Study (BASICS) is an international registry that was initiated in 2013, and aimed at evaluating endovascular therapy (vs medical management including IV t-PA) in acute basilar artery occlusion treated within 6 hours of stroke onset. The primary outcome measure is mRs less than 3.[56]

The Acute Basilar artery occlusion: Endovascular interventions versus Standard medical Treatment (BEST) trial, currently ongoing, aims at enrolling 344 patients in China, treated within 8 hours of acute basilar artery occlusion with mechanical thrombectomy versus standard medical treatment. The primary outcome measure is mRs less than 3.[57]

Low National Institutes of Health Stroke Scale

Patients with a low initial NIH Stroke Scale (NIHSS) and LVO are often able to maintain adequate flow thanks to effective arterial collaterals, which may fail secondarily, leading to severe, irreversible ischemia past the time window for intervention.[58] In those patients, especially if there is evidence on perfusion imaging of a large territory at risk, acute intervention may be the appropriate option (Fig. 9), although this group remains to be evaluated in a prospective, randomized trial. A recent meta-analysis,

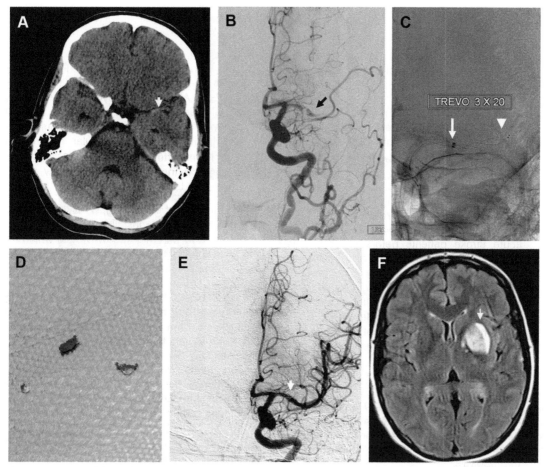

Fig. 7. A 38-year-old 24 hours after transthoracic mitral valve repair, with acute aphasia and right hemiparesis (NIHSS 18). CT (within 1 hours of onset) shows dense left MCA (*A, arrow*). Angiographic confirmation of left M1 MCA occlusion (*B, arrow*). After multiple failed passes with stent retriever alone, stent retriever is deployed across left M1-M2 MCA (*C, arrowhead*), whereas 5-French Sofia catheter is advanced at thrombus base (*C, arrow*). Fragmented fibrin-rich clot is retrieved (*D*), resulting in left MCA recanalization (*E, arrow*); fibrin-rich thrombi respond generally poorly to thrombectomy. Groin to recanalization = 65 minutes. MRI at 24 hours shows subcortical fluid-attenuated inversion recovery changes with no cortical injury (*F, arrow*). NIHSS 0 at 72 hours.

however, identified 5 studies that focused on mechanical thrombectomy in patients with LVO and mild strokes at presentation (NIHSS ≤5); these patients had better 90-day functional outcomes than those receiving medical therapy alone.[59]

Occluded Carotid Artery

In patients with anterior circulation strokes and an acutely occluded carotid artery, intracranial access may require intervention on the carotid artery. Although emergent carotid stenting before intracranial access was reported to be an acceptable maneuver,[60] valid concern is present for significant hemorrhagic risk in relation to necessary dual-antiplatelet therapy.[61] Currently, there is no consensus regarding the management of tandem extracranial carotid occlusions due to

atherosclerotic disease. The disparity in practices is reflected in the subgroup analysis of the ESCAPE trial. Of the 30 intervention-arm subjects, 17 (57%) underwent emergency endovascular extracranial stent-assisted revascularization (10 before and 7 on completion of mechanical thrombectomy). Although the use of antiplatelet agents after acute carotid stenting was variable, no symptomatic intracranial hemorrhage was reported in those receiving emergency stenting.[62] Until further data are available, when feasible, angioplasty seems a safer strategy to gain emergent intracranial access.

Stroke from Cervicocephalic Arterial Dissection

Dissections account for up to 20% of strokes in adults 45 years old and younger, and more than

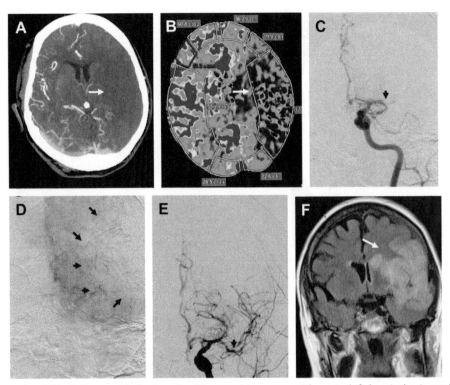

Fig. 8. Example of "futile" revascularization. An 83-year-old woman with acute left hemispheric stroke (NIHSS 22). CTA/CTP (within 45 minutes of onset) shows large hypoperfused left MCA area (*A, arrow*) and large, matching penumbra (*B, arrow*). Angiogram obtained within 90 minutes of stroke onset shows occluded left M1 MCA stem (*C, arrow*), and large nonperfused area on late capillary phase (*D, arrows*), consistent with poor collateral status on CTA. Despite left MCA recanalization (*E, arrow*) within less than 2 hours of stroke onset, progression to total left MCA territory infarction (*F, arrow*) from poor collaterals and poor cerebrovascular reserve.

2% of strokes in the general population. Patients with steno-occlusive lesions due to arterial dissections and intracranial thrombus should be treated the same way as patients with atherosclerotic lesions. The assessment of circle of Willis collaterals following thrombectomy is crucial in assisting decision making as to the need for carotid revascularization. Again, if carotid artery recanalization is necessary for intracranial access, angioplasty is recommended over stenting for fear of increased hemorrhagic risk from antiplatelet therapy.[63]

Anesthesia: With or Without?

Conflicting data currently exist as to whether general anesthesia in thrombectomy procedures may lead to worse outcomes compared with thrombectomy with or without intravenous sedation. Early studies suggested poorer outcomes in patients receiving general anesthesia,[64–66] whereas others suggested no difference in outcomes between patients who received anesthesia and those who did not,[67,68] including the Swedish randomized Sedation vs Intubation for Endovascular Stroke TreAtment Trial (SIESTA) trial, which, however, reported

a higher incidence of pneumonia and other minor anesthesia-related complications.[69]

More recently, Campbell and colleagues[70] performed a meta-analysis of 7 trials including 1764 patients, 871 whom were treated by mechanical thrombectomy out of a large European database (HERMES) in which stent retrievers were used in anterior circulation strokes, and found, after adjusting for possible biases, including baseline prognostic variables, worse outcomes in patients who underwent thrombectomy with general anesthesia compared with those treated with/without sedation. However, patients who received general anesthesia fared better than those treated with IV thrombolysis only, leading to the recommendation to not withhold anesthesia in those for whom it is considered medically necessary.

Mechanisms by which anesthesia may contribute to worsening of ischemia include hypotension at the time of anesthesia induction, delay in treatment, a higher risk of aspiration pneumonia, alterations in CO_2 reactivity, and arterial steal from "reverse Robin Hood syndrome."[71]

A mechanism dubbed cortical spreading depression (CSD) has so far received little

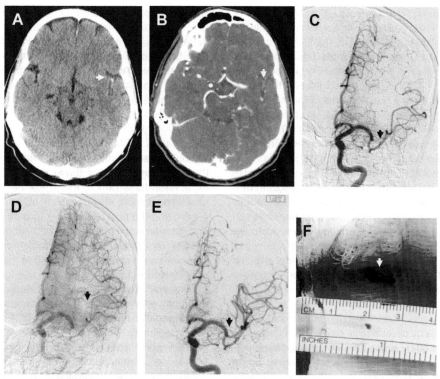

Fig. 9. A 59-year-old man 3 hours within stroke onset with NIHSS fluctuating between 0 and 3. CT shows dense left M2 MCA (*A, arrow*). CTA shows occluded proximal left M2 MCA superior division (*B, arrow*). Angiographic evidence of occluded left M2 MCA (*C, arrow*) and good collaterals (*D, arrow*) is present. Prompt recanalization is obtained (groin to recanalization = 16 minutes) (*E, arrow*), after retrieval of long red thrombus (*F, arrow*).

attention, although it is likely responsible for significant early worsening of ischemia in patients with stroke in whom brain energy metabolism is compromised. CSD can induce phenomena referred to as "peri-infarct depolarization" and "anoxic depolarization," both related to transient local increases of neurotransmitters, that is, glutamate and extracellular K^+.[72] Such depolarization further compromises ischemic tissue not only by exhausting energy, but also by causing active paradoxic vasoconstriction, referred to as "inverse coupling," which does further compromise tissue integrity. Experimental evidence of gradual increase in hypoperfused brain volumes following each peri-infarct depolarization has been demonstrated.[72,73] Interestingly, some sedatives used in anesthesia (ie, ketamine) have been shown to reduce the severity of cortical spreading depolarizations in patients with stroke.[74] One important implication of this phenomenon is potential benefit from neuroprotective drugs such as N-methyl-D-aspartate receptor antagonists, nitric oxide donors, or other molecules, some of which could be delivered intra-arterially during interventional procedures.[75]

SUMMARY

Major advances have been made in recent years in the acute medical and interventional management of ischemic stroke. A shift from "time is brain" to more focused individual physiologic assessment toward acute intervention is currently taking place, which is mainly imaging driven. As a result, increasingly larger numbers of patients with intracranial LVO, estimated to represent approximately 10% of ischemic strokes[76] will become eligible for acute intervention, likely requiring significant worldwide workforce and public health policy adjustments.

REFERENCES

1. Benjamin EJ, Blaha MJ, Chiuve SE, et al. Heart disease and stroke statistics-2017 update: a report from the American Heart Association. Circulation 2017;135:e146–603.
2. Mozaffarian D, Benjamin EJ, Go AS, et al. Heart disease and stroke statistics-2015 update: a report from the American Heart Association. Circulation 2015;131:e29–322.

3. Skolarus LE, Freedman VA, Feng C, et al. Care received by elderly US stroke survivors may be underestimated. Stroke 2016;47:2090–5.

4. Feigin VL, Lawes CM, Bennett DA, et al. Stroke epidemiology: a review of population-based studies of incidence, prevalence, and case-fatality in the late 20th century. Lancet Neurol 2003;2:43–53.

5. Hacke W, Kaste M, Fieschi C, et al. Intravenous thrombolysis with recombinant tissue plasminogen activator for acute hemispheric stroke. The European Cooperative Acute Stroke Study (ECASS). JAMA 1995;274(13):1017–25.

6. Steiner T, Bluhmki E, Kaste M, et al. The ECASS 3-hour cohort. Secondary analysis of ECASS data by time stratification. ECASS Study Group. European Cooperative Acute Stroke Study. Cerebrovasc Dis 1998;8(4):198–203.

7. Hacke W, Kaste M, Bluhmki E, et al. Thrombolysis with alteplase 3 to 4.5 hours after acute ischemic stroke. N Engl J Med 2008;359(13):1317–29.

8. del Zoppo GJ, Higashida RT, Furlan AJ, et al. PROACT: a phase II randomized trial of recombinant pro-urokinase by direct arterial delivery in acute middle cerebral artery stroke. PROACT Investigators. Prolyse in acute cerebral thromboembolism. Stroke 1998;29(1):4–11.

9. Furlan AJ, Abou-Chebl A. The role of recombinant pro-urokinase (r-pro-UK) and intra-arterial thrombolysis in acute ischaemic stroke: the PROACT trials. Prolyse in acute cerebral thromboembolism. Curr Med Res Opin 2002;18(Suppl 2):s44–7.

10. Gobin YP, Starkman S, Duckwiler GR, et al. MERCI 1: a phase 1 study of mechanical embolus removal in cerebral ischemia. Stroke 2004;35(12):2848–54.

11. Smith WS, Sung G, Starkman S, et al. Safety and efficacy of mechanical embolectomy in acute ischemic stroke: results of the MERCI trial. Stroke 2005;36(7):1432–8.

12. Shi ZS, Loh Y, Walker G, et al. Clinical outcomes in middle cerebral artery trunk occlusions versus secondary division occlusions after mechanical thrombectomy: pooled analysis of the Mechanical Embolus Removal in Cerebral Ischemia (MERCI) and Multi MERCI trials. Stroke 2010;41(5):953–60.

13. Broderick JP, Palesch YY, Demchuk AM, et al. Endovascular therapy after intravenous t-PA versus t-PA alone for stroke. N Engl J Med 2013;368:893–903.

14. Ciccone A, Valvassori L, Nichelatti M, et al. Endovascular treatment for acute ischemic stroke. N Engl J Med 2013;368:904–13.

15. Kidwell CS, Jahan R, Gornbein J, et al. A trial of imaging selection and endovascular treatment for ischemic stroke. N Engl J Med 2013;368:914–23.

16. Wisco D, Uchino K, Saqqur M, et al. Addition of hyperacute MRI AIDS in patient selection, decreasing the use of endovascular stroke therapy. Stroke 2014;45(2):467–72.

17. Berkhemer OA, Fransen PS, Beumer D, et al. A randomized trial of intraarterial treatment for acute ischemic stroke. N Engl J Med 2015;372:11–20.

18. Goyal M, Demchuk AM, Menon BK, et al. Randomized assessment of rapid endovascular treatment of ischemic stroke. N Engl J Med 2015;372:1019–30.

19. Saver JL, Goyal M, Bonafe A, et al. Stent-retriever thrombectomy after intravenous t-PA vs. t-PA alone in stroke. N Engl J Med 2015;372:2285–95.

20. Campbell BC, Mitchell PJ, Kleinig TJ, et al. Endovascular therapy for ischemic stroke with perfusion-imaging selection. N Engl J Med 2015;372:1009–18.

21. Jovin TG, Chamorro A, Cobo E, et al. Thrombectomy within 8 hours after symptom onset in ischemic stroke. N Engl J Med 2015;372:2296–306.

22. Mocco J, Zaidat OO, von Kummer R, et al. Aspiration thrombectomy after intravenous alteplase versus intravenous alteplase alone. Stroke 2016;47(9):2331–8.

23. Bracard S, Ducrocq X, Mas JL, et al. Mechanical thrombectomy after intravenous alteplase versus alteplase alone after stroke (THRACE): a randomised controlled trial. Lancet Neurol 2016;15(11):1138–47.

24. Lapergue B, Blanc R, Gory B, et al. Effect of endovascular contact aspiration vs stent retriever on revascularization in patients with acute ischemic stroke and large vessel occlusion: the ASTER randomized clinical trial. JAMA 2017;318(5):443–52.

25. Gory B, Lapergue B, Blanc R, et al. Contact aspiration versus stent retriever in patients with acute ischemic stroke with M2 occlusion in the ASTER randomized trial (Contact Aspiration Versus Stent Retriever for Successful Revascularization). Stroke 2018;49(2):461–4.

26. Saver JL, Goyal M, van der Lugt A, et al. Time to treatment with endovascular thrombectomy and outcomes from ischemic stroke: a meta-analysis. JAMA 2016;316(12):1279–88.

27. Saver JL, Jahan R, Levy EI, et al. Solitaire flow restoration device versus the Merci Retriever in patients with acute ischaemic stroke (SWIFT): a randomised, parallel-group, non-inferiority trial. Lancet 2012;380(9849):1241–9.

28. Nogueira RG, Lutsep HL, Gupta R, et al. Trevo versus Merci retrievers for thrombectomy revascularization of large vessel occlusions in acute ischaemic stroke (TREVO 2): a randomised trial. Lancet 2012;380(9849):1231–40.

29. Anderson T. Communication at the 9th Annual Meeting of the European Society for Minimally Invasive Neurological Therapy. Nice, France, September 7–9, 2017.

30. Turk AS, Spiotta A, Frei D, et al. Initial clinical experience with the ADAPT technique: a direct aspiration first pass technique for stroke thrombectomy. J Neurointerv Surg 2014;6(3):231–7.

31. Turk AS, Frei D, Fiorella D, et al. ADAPT FAST study: a direct aspiration first pass technique for acute

stroke thrombectomy. J Neurointerv Surg 2014;6(4): 260–4.

32. Frei D, Gerber J, Turk A, et al. The SPEED study: initial clinical evaluation of the Penumbra novel 054 Reperfusion Catheter. J Neurointerv Surg 2013; 5(Suppl 1):i74–6.

33. Turk AS, Turner R, Spiotta A, et al. Comparison of endovascular treatment approaches for acute ischemic stroke: cost effectiveness, technical success, and clinical outcomes. J Neurointerv Surg 2015;7(9):666–70.

34. Delgado Almandoz JE, Kayan Y, Young ML, et al. Comparison of clinical outcomes in patients with acute ischemic strokes treated with mechanical thrombectomy using either Solumbra or ADAPT techniques. J Neurointerv Surg 2016;8(11):1123–8.

35. Wong JHY, Do HM, Telischak NA, et al. Initial experience with SOFIA as an intermediate catheter in mechanical thrombectomy for acute ischemic stroke. J Neurointerv Surg 2017;9(11):1103–6.

36. Möhlenbruch MA, Kabbasch C, Kowoll A, et al. Multicenter experience with the new SOFIA Plus catheter as a primary local aspiration catheter for acute stroke thrombectomy. J Neurointerv Surg 2017;9(12):1223–7.

37. Heit JJ, Wong JH, Mofaff AM, et al. Sofia intermediate catheter and the SNAKE technique: safety and efficacy of the Sofia catheter without guidewire or microcatheter construct. J Neurointerv Surg 2018; 10(4):401–6.

38. Alberts MJ, Latchaw RE, Jagoda A, et al. Revised and updated recommendations for the establishment of primary stroke centers: a summary statement from the Brain Attack Coalition. Stroke 2011; 42:2651–65.

39. Leifer D, Bravata DM, Hinchey JA, et al. Metrics for measuring quality of care in comprehensive stroke centers: detailed follow-up to Brain Attack Coalition comprehensive stroke center recommendations. A statement for healthcare professionals from the American Heart Association/American Stroke Association. Stroke 2011;42:849–77.

40. Sun CHJ, Ribo M, Goyal M, et al. Door-to-puncture: a practical metric for capturing and enhancing system processes associated with endovascular stroke care, preliminary results from the rapid reperfusion registry. J Am Heart Assoc 2014;3:e000859.

41. McTaggart RA, Ansari SA, Goyal M, et al. Initial hospital management of patients with emergent large vessel occlusion (ELVO): report of the standards and guidelines committee of the Society of NeuroInterventional Surgery. J Neurointerv Surg 2017;9(3): 316–23.

42. Saver JL, Smith EE, Fonarow GC, et al, GWTG-Stroke Steering Committee and Investigators. The "golden hour" and acute brain ischemia presenting features and lytic therapy in >30,000 patients arriving within 60 minutes of stroke onset. Stroke 2010;41:1431–9.

43. Jones SP, Miller C, Gibson JME, et al. The impact of education and training interventions for nurses and other health care staff involved in the delivery of stroke care: an integrative review. Nurse Educ Today 2017;61:249–57.

44. Jauch EC, Holmstedt C, Nolte J. Techniques for improving efficiency in the emergency department for patients with acute ischemic stroke. Ann N Y Acad Sci 2012;1268:57–62.

45. Goyal M, Menon BK, Hill MD, et al. Consistently achieving computed tomography to endovascular recanalization < 90 minutes solutions and innovations. Stroke 2014;45:e252–6.

46. Frei D, McGraw C, McCarthy K, et al. A standardized neurointerventional thrombectomy protocol leads to faster recanalization times. J Neurointerv Surg 2017;9(11):1035–40.

47. Haussen DC, Doppelheuer S, Schindler K, et al. Utilization of a smartphone platform for electronic informed consent in acute stroke trials. Stroke 2017;48(11):3156–60.

48. Zaidat OO, Castonguay AC, Gupta R, et al. North American Solitaire Stent Retriever Acute Stroke registry: post-marketing revascularization and clinical outcome results. J Neurointerv Surg 2014;6: 584–8.

49. Mehta BP, Leslie-Mazwi TM, Chandra RV, et al. Reducing door-to-puncture times for intra-arterial stroke therapy: a pilot quality improvement project. J Am Heart Assoc 2014;3:e000963.

50. Asadi H, Williams D, Thornton J. Changing management of acute ischaemic stroke: the new treatments and emerging role of endovascular therapy. Curr Treat Options Neurol 2016;18(5):20.

51. Nogueira RG, Jadhav AP, Haussen DC, et al. Thrombectomy 6 to 24 hours after stroke with a mismatch between deficit and infarct. N Engl J Med 2018; 378(1):11–21.

52. Albers GW, Marks MP, Kemp S. Thrombectomy for stroke at 6 to 16 hours with selection by perfusion imaging. N Engl J Med 2018;378(8):708–18.

53. Coutinho JM, Liebeskind DS, Slater LA, et al. Mechanical thrombectomy for isolated M2 occlusions: a post hoc analysis of the STAR, SWIFT, and SWIFT PRIME Studies. AJNR Am J Neuroradiol 2016;37(4): 667–72.

54. Sarraj A, Sangha N, Hussain MS, et al. Endovascular therapy for acute ischemic stroke with occlusion of the middle cerebral artery M2 segment. JAMA Neurol 2016;73(11):1291–6.

55. Tomsick TA, Carrozzella J, Foster L, et al. Endovascular therapy of M2 occlusion in IMS III: role of M2 segment definition and location on clinical and revascularization outcomes. AJNR Am J Neuroradiol 2017;38(1):84–9.

56. van der Hoeven EJ, Schonewille WJ, Vos JA, et al. The Basilar Artery International Cooperation Study (BASICS): study protocol for a randomised controlled trial. Trials 2013;14:200.

57. Liu X, Xu G, Liu Y, et al. Acute basilar artery occlusion: endovascular interventions versus standard medical treatment (BEST) trial-design and protocol for a randomized, controlled, multicenter study. Int J Stroke 2017;12(7):779–85.

58. Haussen DC, Lima FO, Bouslama M, et al. Thrombectomy versus medical management for large vessel occlusion strokes with minimal symptoms: an analysis from STOPStroke and GESTOR cohorts. J Neurointerv Surg 2018;10(4):325–9.

59. Griessenauer CJ, Medin C, Maingard J, et al. Endovascular mechanical thrombectomy in large vessel occlusion ischemic stroke presenting with low NIHSS: a systematic review and meta-analysis. World Neurosurg 2018;110:263–9.

60. Malik AM, Vora NA, Lin R, et al. Endovascular treatment of tandem extracranial/intracranial anterior circulation occlusions: preliminary single-center experience. Stroke 2011;42(6):1653–7.

61. Heck DV, Brown MD. Carotid stenting and intracranial thrombectomy for treatment of acute stroke due to tandem occlusions with aggressive antiplatelet therapy may be associated with a high incidence of intracranial hemorrhage. J Neurointerv Surg 2015;7(3):170–5.

62. Assis Z, Menon BK, Goyal M, et al. Acute ischemic stroke with tandem lesions: technical endovascular management and clinical outcomes from the ESCAPE trial. J Neurointerv Surg 2018;10(5):429–33.

63. Gory B, Piotin M, Haussen DC, et al. Thrombectomy in acute stroke with tandem occlusions from dissection versus atherosclerotic cause. Stroke 2017; 48(11):3145–8.

64. Abou-Chebl A, Lin R, Hussain MS, et al. Conscious sedation versus general anesthesia during endovascular therapy for acute anterior circulation stroke: preliminary results from a retrospective, multicenter study. Stroke 2010;41(6):1175–9.

65. John N, Mitchell P, Dowling R, et al. Is general anaesthesia preferable to conscious sedation in the treatment of acute ischaemic stroke with intra-arterial mechanical thrombectomy? A review of the literature. Neuroradiology 2013;55(1):93–100.

66. Abou-Chebl A, Zaidat OO, Castonguay AC, et al. North American SOLITAIRE Stent-Retriever Acute Stroke Registry: choice of anesthesia and outcomes. Stroke 2014;45:1396–401.

67. Slezak A, Kurmann R, Oppliger L, et al. Impact of anesthesia on the outcome of acute ischemic stroke after endovascular treatment with the solitaire stent retriever. AJNR Am J Neuroradiol 2017;38(7): 1362–7.

68. Löwhagen Hendén P, Rentzos A, Karlsson JE, et al. General anesthesia versus conscious sedation for endovascular treatment of acute ischemic stroke: The AnStroke Trial (Anesthesia During Stroke). Stroke 2017;48(6):1601–7.

69. Schönenberger S, Uhlmann L, Hacke W, et al. Effect of conscious sedation vs general anesthesia on early neurological improvement among patients with ischemic stroke undergoing endovascular thrombectomy: a randomized clinical trial. JAMA 2016;316:1986–96.

70. Campbell BCV, van Zwam WH, Goyal M, et al. Effect of general anaesthesia on functional outcome in patients with anterior circulation ischaemic stroke having endovascular thrombectomy versus standard care: a meta-analysis of individual patient data. Lancet Neurol 2018;17(1):47–53.

71. van den Berg LA, Koelman DL, Berkhemer OA. Type of anesthesia and differences in clinical outcome after intra-arterial treatment for ischemic stroke. Stroke 2015;46(5):1257–62.

72. Shin HK, Dunn AK, Jones PB, et al. Vasoconstrictive neurovascular coupling during focal ischemic depolarizations. J Cereb Blood Flow Metab 2006;26(8): 1018–30.

73. Woitzik J, Hecht N, Pinczolits A, et al. Propagation of cortical spreading depolarization in the human cortex after malignant stroke. Neurology 2013;80(12): 1095–102.

74. Hertle DN, Dreier JP, Woitzik J, et al. Effect of analgesics and sedatives on the occurrence of spreading depolarizations accompanying acute brain injury. Brain 2012;135(Pt 8):2390–8.

75. Dreier JP. The role of spreading depression, spreading depolarization and spreading ischemia in neurological disease. Nat Med 2011;17(4): 439–47.

76. Campbell BCV, Donnan GA, Lees KR, et al. Endovascular stent thrombectomy: the new standard of care for large vessel ischaemic stroke. Lancet Neurol 2015;14(8):846–54.

Noninterventional Treatment Options for Stroke

Andreas Hartmann, MD[a],*, Jay P. Mohr, MD[b]

KEYWORDS

- Acute stroke • Thrombolysis • Early management • Noninterventional treatment • Neuroprotection
- Anticoagulants

KEY POINTS

- Noninterventional treatment strategies in ischemic stroke aim at rapid restoration of blood flow and protection against further brain cell damage.
- Systemic thrombolysis within 3.0 (4.5) hours of onset is the method of choice after exclusion of contraindications. Administration of thrombolysis should be as early as possible.
- Rapid assessment of the clinical syndrome and initiation of treatment may serve to modify collateral blood flow and facilitate compensatory mechanisms of the brain. Door-to-needle times should be well under 1 hour.
- Prior use of anticoagulants, hemorrhagic transformation, management of parenchymal hematoma, and restarting oral anticoagulation are complex issues affecting long-term outcome.

INTRODUCTION

In the 6th edition of *Harrison's Textbook of Medicine* published in 1970, thrombosis was implied to be the principal cause of ischemic stroke.[1] Stroke registries,[2,3] improved diagnostic categories,[4,5] and major advances in brain imaging (computed tomography [CT] and especially MR imaging) led to a dramatic increase in awareness that embolism is the leading cause of ischemic stroke.[5] No longer justified in assuming the majority of ischemic stroke were from chronic and fixed wall lesions, attention turned to ways the embolus could be dissolved or dislodged. Treatment for acute ischemic stroke has developed to a degree that there are now standards of practice guidelines. Centers large and small follow the emergency management pattern earlier limited to cardiac and peripheral vascular diseases.

These methods fall into 2 major categories: (1) restoration of, or improvement in, blood flow and substrate delivery (eg, oxygen and other nutrients) before major brain injury has occurred and (2) protection against ischemia or preservation of partially damaged brain cells. These categories are complementary and overlapping, with some therapies achieving both goals.

ACUTE PHASE ASSESSMENT
Need for Speed in Diagnosis and Therapy

The most commonly used agent to attempt recanalization of arterial occlusion in acute ischemic stroke is recombinant tissue plasminogen activator (tPA). Patients are now ideally treated as early as possible, preferably not later than 3.0 to 4.5 hours after stroke, and at a dose of 0.9 mg/kg. Although no differences favoring

Disclosure Statement: The authors have no disclosures to declare in relation with this article.
[a] Department of Neurology, Klinikum Frankfurt (Oder), Müllroser Chaussee 7, Frankfurt (Oder) 15236, Germany; [b] Doris & Stanley Tananbaum Stroke Center, Neurological Institute of New York, Columbia University Medical Center, 710 West 168th Street, New York, NY 10032, USA
* Corresponding author.
E-mail address: andreas.hartmann@charite.de

Neuroimag Clin N Am 28 (2018) 639–648
https://doi.org/10.1016/j.nic.2018.06.006
1052-5149/18/© 2018 Elsevier Inc. All rights reserved.

treatment are typically evident within 24 hours (few "on-the-table" recoveries), faith in its use has been driven by the 3-month outcome in the initial study, which showed an absolute benefit for the modified Rankin scale of 16.2% compared with placebo. To meet these guidelines, efforts must not be delayed. A major metaanalysis focusing on disabling stroke and death, noted that for those who "achieved substantial reperfusion, ... each 1-h delay to reperfusion was associated with a less favorable degree of disability."[6] The time-dependent probability of reaching a good functional outcome is shown in **Fig. 1** as a result of a pooled analysis of several large thrombolysis trials.[7]

Prestroke Antithrombotic Agents

Drawing on data from Get With The Guidelines—Stroke, a recent literature of 540,993 cases of acute stroke from 1661 American hospitals indicates prior antithrombotic therapy has a favorable effect on outcome from acute ischemic stroke.[8] Such publication can only add to the increased use of antithrombotics in ischemic stroke prevention. In a major review in the American Stroke Association Get With The Guidelines registry of 85,071 patients,[9] an unadjusted risk of

symptomatic intracranial hemorrhage was higher in those having received prior antiplatelet therapy (5.0% vs 3.7%), the number needed to harm was 147. However, that group had a greater risk-adjusted likelihood of independent ambulation, with a number needed to treat of 43.

One consequence of the need for speed is a reliance on CT alone in the decision for the use of intravenous tPA; this decision based mainly on the clinical syndrome of acute stroke and the exclusion of patients with hemorrhagic lesions. Although an efficient approach, it does not document whether the tPA achieves recanalization, nor whether it achieved the presumed rescue of the ischemic process. CT angiography, perfusion studies, and MR imaging sequences to depict stroke early after onset and to determine brain tissue at risk are now often used and are described in another part of this publication set. Centers lacking these technologies undertake tPA and endovascular treatments at an unknown risk. It should come as no surprise that 25% of the 61,598 tPA-eligible patients arriving within 2 hours in a large survey failed to receive tPA.[10] The failures were attributed to older age, female sex, non-white race, diabetes mellitus, prior stroke, atrial fibrillation, prosthetic heart valve, National Institutes of Health Stroke Scale (NIHSS) score of less than 5,

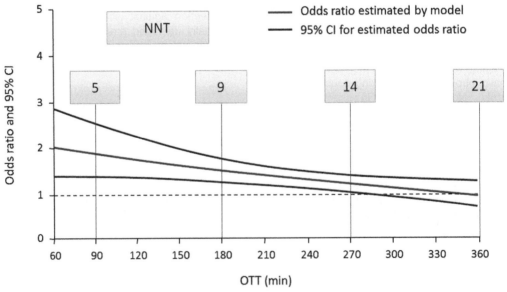

Analysis from NINDS, ECASS 1-3, ATLANTIS, EPITHET: mRS0-1 over time

Fig. 1. Number needed to treat (NNT) to reach functional independence after systemic thrombolysis of ischemic stroke over time. CI, confidence interval; mRS, modified Rankin scale; OTT, onset to treatment time. (*Adapted from* Lees KR, Bluhmki E, von Kummer R, et al. Time to treatment with intravenous alteplase and outcome in stroke: an updated pooled analysis of ECASS, ATLANTIS, NINDS, and EPITHET trials. Lancet 2010;375:1699; with permission.)

arrival during off-hours and not via emergency medical services, longer onset-to-arrival and door-to-CT times, earlier calendar year, and arrival at rural, nonteaching, nonstroke center hospitals.

The National Institutes of Health Stroke Scale

The most frequently used clinical assessment tool is the NIHSS, which is heavily weighted to the motor elements of the syndrome. An example of its use is analysis of 44,331 patients with a reported modified Rankin scale at 3 months. Of these, 11,632 had shown artery occlusion with CT or MR angiography. NIHSS scores of 12 or less were considered to be optimal threshold values for functional independency after intravenous thrombolysis.[11]

Recent analysis has further shown that the best gaze item in the NIHSS alone is strongly associated with large artery anterior occlusion (internal carotid, carotid–terminus, M1-segment of the middle cerebral artery). Increased sensitivity was noted when the best gaze response was added to all 3 items in the face-arm-speech-time (FAST) test.[12]

This emphasis on motor and best gaze is not a reliable marker for lesion volume; despite a graded relationship found between the NIHSS and the median diffusion-weighted imaging lesion volume in cubic centimeters, the lesion volume in another recent study was significantly higher in those with neglect, language disorder, and visual field impairment.[13] This bias toward the motor deficit makes it difficult to estimate how much rescue therapy influences the nonmotor components.

Thrombolysis for Restoration of Blood Flow

Modern imaging also offered the opportunity to determine the time frame for the development of tissue changes reflecting infarction. In 1988 an National Institutes of Health–supported dose-escalation study of tPA reported 21 patients treated within the 90-minute time frame drawn from coronary artery thrombolysis experience.[14] In a parallel study of 68 patients imaged within 4 hours by CT and MR imaging (magnets then only 0.5 T) 8 of 26 showed changes within 1 hour, reaching an asymptote at 2 to 3 hours from known clinical event, with a marginally significant correlation with syndrome severity.[5] By 1993, the feasibility of treatment within 90 minutes was demonstrated.[15] In the years since, there has been no lack of tPA clinical trials and of tPA against other clot-lysing agents,[16] including streptokinase, urokinase, prourokinase, and even Ancrod (derived from the venom of the Malayan pit viper).[17]

This initial success prompted plans to test larger doses and extend the time window, hoping to identify those most favorable response. The initial European trials (ECASS I) attempted higher dosage (1.1 mg/kg) with disappointing results, and ECASS-II tested an extension of the time window (≤6 hours) for the 0.9 mg/kg dose for those with less severe strokes. The International Stroke Trial #3 (IST-3) randomized 3035 patients in an open-label design using the same dosing 0.9 mg/kg but in an extended window up to 6 hours from onset.[18] A review of these trials in 2017 noted a 2% fatal hemorrhagic risk, but better long-term outcome for the patients treated with 0.9 mg/kg tPA within 4.5 hours.[19]

This dose of tPA has achieved the most wide acceptance and dominates the literature. The initial concerns for cost effectiveness[20] and calls in the United States for resisting such therapy faded after approval by the US Food and Drug Administration for use within the 3-hour time window from symptom onset.[21] Despite these formal limitations, current guidelines recommend intravenous alteplase treatment in the 3.0- to 4.5-hour time window with rigorous adherence to thrombolysis protocols regarding contraindications such as age 80 years or older, history of diabetes, prior stroke, NIHSS score of 25 or greater, prior medication of any oral anticoagulants, and imaging evidence of ischemic injury involving more than one-third of the middle cerebral artery territory. As of January 2018, PubMed shows 1975 references for the subjects tPA and stroke. Based largely on the accumulating information, new US Food and Drug Administration prescribing information for alteplase treatment has decreased the number of contraindications within the 3-hour time window somewhat. Among others, this concerns treatment of severe stroke, mild stroke, neuroimaging findings, and seizure at onset.

Guidelines on the early management of stroke also recommend mechanical thrombectomy in eligible patients with causative internal cerebral artery or proximal (M1) middle cerebral artery occlusion within 6 hours after stroke onset.[22] This procedure and the possible extension of the time window to 16 hours or even 24 hours in certain eligible patients based on the results of the most recently published studies[23,24] is the subject of another publication in this journal.

Ischemia-Modifying Effects of Collateral Blood Flow

Before the availability of acute thrombolytic therapy, angiographically based documentation of intracranial occlusion had already the potential for an ischemia-modifying effect from retrograde collateral flow into the affected territory via flow through the border zones shared by the major arterial territories.[25] Recent publications indicate the degree of collateral flow (documented by angiography and matched against the infarct site and size revealed by MR imaging) can have a dramatically favorable effect on the initial brain injury, even from large proximal occlusions.[26,27]

It has long been known that there is a highly variable degree of direct collateral availability for individual branches shared across the border zones of the major arterial territories.[28] For many, only 1 or perhaps 2 branches are actually of a size large enough to mediate immediate retrograde collateral to spare the individual branch from infarction. One example showed anterior cerebral branch retrograde collateral over the border zone spared an entire territory of the middle cerebral branch down to the site of original occlusion, infarction affecting those branches not salvaged by such collateral.[29] This unpredictable collateral explains the frequent irregular topographic infarct appearance in MR imaging. Little is known about what promotes the acute response of border zone collaterals or what mediated improvement in the collateral and over what period of time.

Thus far, no specific therapy has appeared that produces immediate dilation of the branch by branch collaterals sufficient to provide beneficial effects for an evolving infarct. The calcium antagonist nimodipine has been demonstrated to have such effects, although they are somewhat modest.[14] Its manufacture has been as a racemic mixture that, used in intravenous form, has led to systemic hypotension at doses sufficiently high to have suitable brain penetration.[15] The oral form is conjugated in the liver to generate the suitable the D:L ratio for good brain penetration, which has limited its value in acute ischemic stroke. Should it be manufactured in the correct D:L ratio, its use might be suitably retested. Another calcium antagonist, verapamil, a potent cerebral vasodilator, seems promising based on animal models,[16] but has had only limited use in acute ischemic stroke.[30]

Functional Compensatory Mechanisms

Inferred recanalization has been the proposed mechanism for those showing a spectacular shrinking deficit with middle cerebral territory occlusion.[31] However, another effect that is often underappreciated is that of functional compensatory mechanisms attributed to surviving adjacent territories.[32] Such effects have been documented with infarcts generally a gyrus in size and with little

depth into the centrum semiovale. Long-standing assumptions that such infarcts were predictive of permanent sequelae have been blunted by dramatic improvements within hours to days for dominant hemisphere infarction affecting Broca's area,[33] posterior insula,[34,35] Wernicke's area,[36] and Rolandic infarct affecting the hand knob,[37] among others. That the process seems to begin almost immediately has been demonstrated by transcranial stimulation mapping of cortical areas after limb removal and stroke[38] and in response to transient deafferentation in the forearm.[39] Independent studies with midazolam have also shown relapse of clinical syndromes of transient ischemic attack up to a week after the event, no abnormalities found on MR imaging of the brain.[40]

Neuroprotection

Neuroprotective therapy is intended to maintain or rescue damaged nerve cells suffering ischemia. The basis for this approach has been hope or belief that surrounding an actual infarct is a graduated area of ischemia, those cells deepest or furthest away from satisfactory blood flow presumably the most affected, whereas those on the borders are less so. These latter regions comprise a so-called ischemic penumbra, possibly amenable to neuroprotective therapy.

Animal models (mainly rodents) have documented a large number of agents that decrease the size of the infarction with preischemic therapy, some even given after middle cerebral artery occlusion. For these models, most of the sparing has been along the upper rim of the cerebral convexity, reflecting retrograde collateral flow into the infarct zone, carrying with it any neuroprotective effects of the agent. Far less benefit is seen in the core of the infarct affecting the basal ganglia, vascular territories not subject to retrograde collateral flow because most of these vessels are endarteries. There may be some importance in the border zone collaterals for most rodents, being rather large loops over the lissencephalic hemispheres, showing little of the network of small vessels typical to those found in humans.

Calcium channel antagonists are the largest group of neuroprotective agents. The American nimodipine trial found no effect on outcome after ischemic stroke when the data were analyzed to include all patients treated within a 48-hour period, but a subset analysis found a clinical benefit tested by the Toronto and Mathew Stroke Scales for those treated within 12 hours.[41] These results provided support that time would prove a vital factor in all therapies. However, subsequent trials for the 120-mg oral dose proved disappointing.[42]

Other forms of neuroprotection involve antioxidants, receptor agonists, and cell membrane substrates. Of the few trials undertaken, the results have been negative or not strongly enough positive to ensure their approval by most of the regulatory agencies.[43] These include tirilazad clomethiazole, fosphenytoin, lifarizine, GM1, citicoline, enlimomab and others.

Despite the disappointments, investigators with strong animal laboratory experience recommend renewed efforts with more sensitive imaging and clinical methods to find the translational link between animal and human outcomes.[44,45]

ACUTE INPATIENT MANAGEMENT
Respiration

In acute stroke, pathologic respiration patterns and risk of aspiration may occur, and patients with unstable airway situations require intubation and mechanical ventilation. For all others, data remain sparse if the routine insufflation of oxygen is of clinical use. In the recently published study with 8003 acute stroke patients, oxygen was administered continuously for 72 hours, nocturnally (9.00 PM to 7.00 AM), or only if indicated in each arm. Functional outcome was determined at 90 days after stroke. There was no significant difference between the groups (odds ratio of 0.97 for oxygen vs control; odds ratio of 1.03 for continuous vs nocturnal oxygen) and no subgroup was identified that benefited from the administration of oxygen. The findings did not support the routine administration of low-dose oxygen (2–3 L/min) in nonhypoxic patients.[46]

Blood Glucose

Many patients who have a stroke also have diabetes, but hyperglycemia is also found in up to 60% of stroke patients without known prior diabetes. In-hospital hyperglycemia during the first 24 hours is associated with a worse outcome. Values of greater than 90 mg/dL are sufficient to fuel the cell-damaging lactate, and the higher the value the more the lactate. Therefore, hyperglycemia should be treated with the goal to achieve blood glucose levels of 140 to 180 mg/dL. Subcutaneous application of insulin is usually sufficient unless excessive glucose levels require intravenous treatment. Especially the latter needs to monitored closely. Hypoglycemia (blood glucose of <60 mg/dL) should be corrected as well.

Blood Pressure

The ideal blood pressure level after ischemic stroke is not known. With possibly impaired cerebrovascular autoregulation, aggressive lowering of blood pressure in ischemic strokes should be avoided. In patients who are candidates for thrombolysis, blood pressure should be carefully lowered to less than 185/110 mm Hg, and thrombolysis should not be administered if blood pressure levels cannot be maintained below this threshold. Without current better data, similar levels are advised before instituting interventional therapy. Lacking comorbid conditions such as acute myocardial infarction, heart failure, renal failure, or hypertensive encephalopathy, to name a few, the blood pressure can be allowed to remain high, and only persistently excessive levels should carefully be lowered. In many patients with initial hypertension, blood pressure levels decrease spontaneously after the first few days. After thrombolysis, registry data suggest the lowest complication rates for systolic blood pressure levels between 140 and 150 mm Hg.

Body Temperature

Increased body temperature after stroke led to increased infarct volume in the animal model and was described to be associated with poor outcomes.[47,48] Although lacking controlled clinical trials, the recommendation is to attempt normothermia. The effect of prophylactic acetaminophen after stroke even in normothermic patients only showed nonsignificant trends toward better outcome and cannot be recommended.[49]

Prophylactic Antibiotics

The same can be said for prophylactic antibiotic treatment. One earlier study was stopped after a negative association of clinical outcome was observed with the standard application of levofloxacin.[50] Another study, investigating moxifloxacin, also failed to demonstrate the advantage of prophylactic antibiotic therapy for aspiration pneumonia regarding outcome or survival at 6 months.[51] However, this trial confirmed the poor outcome associated with infections after acute nonlacunar middle cerebral artery stroke. Prevention of the much feared aspiration pneumonia plays a large role for functional outcome and warrants careful dysphagia management.

Anticoagulants

The efficacy of heparin, the earliest and best-known of the oral anticoagulants, has been a subject of few clinical trials. The International Stroke Trial (IST), the best-known and largest trial of heparin, enrolled nearly 20,000 patients treated within 48 hours of stroke onset with subcutaneous heparin in 2 different doses (5000 IU vs 10,000 IU), aspirin at 300 mg/d, both heparin and aspirin, or neither. Importantly, the treatment was with subcutaneous heparin in 2 doses, not with continuous intravenous infusion. The published findings suggested a benefit of aspirin with little additional benefit of subcutaneous heparin. However, the data indicated that the program of 5000 IU subcutaneous heparin given twice daily had a benefit in preventing stroke recurrence within 2 weeks (2.9% vs 3.8%), but when used at a dose of 12,500 IU subcutaneously twice daily the hemorrhagic complications in the latter offset the benefits.[52]

In the last few decades, other challenges to the use of heparin have appeared from low-molecular-weight heparinoid (nadroparin) also given by the subcutaneous route. The best-known of these, Trial of Acute Stroke Therapy (TOAST) found a favorable outcome in a post hoc subgroup analysis for those with high-grade large artery stenosis. Overall, the trial was unable to show benefits, in part because of the complication rates of hemorrhage.[20] A current review of 9 trials involving 3137 patient concluded that "treatment with a Low Molecular-Weight Heparin (LMWH) or heparinoid after acute ischemic stroke appears to decrease the occurrence of deep vein thrombosis (DVT) compared with standard unfractionated heparin (UFH), but there are too few data to provide reliable information on their effects on other important outcomes, including functional outcome, death and intracranial haemorrhage."[53]

Hemorrhagic Transformation and Parenchymatous Hematomas

For tPA administration, individual publications amply document the risk of hemorrhagic transformation after tPA administration.[54] Its rate reportedly varies from 2% to 20% in published clinical trials.[55,56] Pre-tPA use of antiplatelet agents, especially at double dose, adds to the risk.[57]

Stroke neurologists often despair that printed reports of observations from both CT and MR imaging commonly fail to discriminate between hemorrhagic infarction and parenchymatous hematoma,[58] even at times appearing as hemorrhage into an infarct.[59] This variation in definition has impacted on the reported incidence in the tPA treatment era.[60] In traditional neuropathologic practice, the discrimination was an easy one, the former involving hemorrhagic effects embedded in the territory of infarction most commonly in the cortical mantle, less so in the deep white matter, compared with parenchymatous hematoma, which was a varying size mass,

displacing adjacent otherwise normal cortical mantle, deep white matter, or deep nuclear structures.

Apart from imaging, close clinical monitoring for the first 24 hours, avoidance of antiplatelet agents and anticoagulants, and a recommendation of the blood pressure kept to less than 180/105 mm Hg are the major elements in the American Stroke Association guidelines. Common symptoms are headache, nausea, vomiting, or neurologic worsening. Asymptomatic hemorrhagic infarction is not often appreciated in clinical practice. One reason is that, in all but the largest examples, the transformation localized to the infarct site does not alter the acute syndrome.[25] Often deferred when the clinical picture seems to be stable or improved, uniform pursuit of evidence of hemorrhagic infarction is infrequently reported, yet its detection has been reported as high as 20% for those with MR imaging within 6 to 60 hours after admission.[61]

Management of Hemorrhagic Infarction

Hemorrhagic infarction associated with antithrombotics (antithrombotic agents, anticoagulants, and after tPA administration) relies mainly on correcting the coagulopathy.[62,63] Although criticized as to effectiveness, a long history exists with still-widely used fresh frozen plasma, dosed in adults at 1 to 2 U.[64] Preferred is the cryoprecipitate from fresh frozen plasma, used in a 10-U dose, to achieve fibrinogen levels of less than 150 mg/dL.[65] Other options, less successful but possibly more available, include platelet transfusion of 6 to 8 U; prothrombin complex concentrate[66] (this treatment carrying a risk of 1.5% thrombotic outcomes[67]); intravenous vitamin K with a small risk of anaphylactoid reaction); antifibrinolytic agents, the leading example being aminocaproic acid and tranexamic acid, with limited reports of use in brain hematomatherapy[55,68,69]; and activated factor VII. Approved by the US Food and Drug Administration for factor VIII-resistant hemophiliacs, it was superior to prothrombin complex concentrate in a retrospective analysis of 63 patients with warfarin-related intracranial hemorrhage.[70]

Management of Parenchymous Hematoma

Nonsurgical therapies
Therapies dating back decades attempted to control a developing hematoma by digital compression of the ipsilateral carotid artery. No studies were published and autopsy review of the hematoma mass prevented any useful insight into whether this attempt was successful. Modern

efforts include lowering the blood pressure, hoping the reduction might slow or stop the evolving mass. Reductions in hematoma growth occurred for those treated to lower the mean systemic blood pressure to less than 140 mm Hg within 6 hours (INTERACT2) in a cohort of 964 of 2839 patients (40%) with CT imaging. This group had a median baseline NIHSS 11, and Glasgow Coma Scale of 14 (interquartile range, 12–15). The decrease was compared with those whose blood pressure was less than 180 mm Hg. The growth and Rankin score were inversely correlated with the degree and duration of systolic blood pressure reduction.[71] A deep location affected 84%. In a similar study of 1000 patients, for whom deep location affected 90%, a median hematoma volume of greater than 10 and a Glasgow Coma Scale of 5 or greater (55% had scores of >15) did not show additional benefits for further reduction to levels 110 to 140 mm Hg.[72]

Neurosurgical management
Management algorithms are scant for outcomes for neurosurgical intervention for those failing to respond to medical therapy to correct the coagulopathy.[73,74] The interventional model is based on spontaneous hematomas not complicated by coagulopathy, where timely evacuation from lobar or cerebellum locations before the mass effect has irreversibly compressed major motor pathways justifies surgery.[75] Randomized clinical trials have shown less obvious benefits for hematomas in deeper regions.[76]

Resumption of Oral Anticoagulation

Formerly often assumed that resumption of vitamin K oral antagonists would risk recurrence of brain hemorrhage, a recent large survey of 1012 survivors found resumption of therapy for those with lobar and nonlobar locations actually decreased all-cause stroke incidence ($P<.01$). Resumption of therapy was within 3 months, with a lesser risk of thromboembolic complications and a similar risk of hemorrhage recurrence.[77]

Information on the newer oral anticoagulants remains limited, but hematomas tend to be somewhat smaller than from vitamin K antagonists, with slightly better outcomes, and possibly a similar risk of recurrence and ischemic stroke recurrence.[78]

Prestroke treatment with newer oral anticoagulants often presents a problem when the neurologist is faced with urgent thrombolysis decisions. Standard clotting tests (International Normalized Ratio and activated partial thromboplastin time) are not reliable to document a

clinically relevant anticoagulant effect. With dabigatran, there is a correlation between its plasma concentration and activated partial thromboplastin time results, but it is not linear. Thrombin time and ecarin clotting time are sensitive and show good plasma correlations, but are not widely used in the emergency room setting and often take long to measure. The same is true for measuring anti–factor Xa activity in patients on rivaroxaban, apixaban or edoxaban. Although they may cause a prolongation of the activated partial thromboplastin time or prothrombin time, these tests are also not reliable to document pharmacologic effects before thrombolysis. In these patients, taking the medical history of anticoagulant treatment and determining the time since last intake is crucial to combine with the results of standard coagulation parameters.[76]

To date, no studies have settled the clinical efficacy of nonspecific agents to reverse hemorrhage with the newer oral anticoagulant, but experience is beginning to accumulate for idarucizumad for dabigitran and andexanet-alfa for factor Xa inhibitor reversal.[63]

DISCHARGE PLANNING

Many institutions using electronic medical records start to assemble a discharge plan even on the day of admission. A recent literature search found predictions of discharge home are higher for those with an NIHSS of less than 5, those with scores 6 to 13 to institutionalized care including rehabilitation facility, and those with scores of 14 or greater likely to be institutionalized in skilled nursing facilities.[79]

REFERENCES

1. Fisher C, Mohr JP, Adams RD. Cerebrovascular diseases. Harrison's principles of internal medicine. [Chapter 29]. 6th edition. New York: McGraw-Hill; 1970. p. 172–85.
2. Mohr JP, Caplan LR, Melski JW, et al. The Harvard Cooperative Stroke Registry: a prospective registry. Neurology 1978;28:754–62.
3. Bamford J, Sandercock P, Dennis M, et al. A prospective study of acute cerebrovascular disease in the community: the Oxfordshire Community Stroke Project 1981-86. 1. Methodology, demography and incident cases of first-ever stroke. J Neurol Neurosurg Psychiatry 1988;51: 1373–80.
4. Leira EC, Adams HP Jr, Rosenthal GE, et al. Baseline NIH stroke scale responses estimate the probability of each particular stroke subtype. Cerebrovasc Dis 2008;26:573–7.

5. Kunitz SC, Gross CR, Heyman A, et al. The pilot Stroke Data Bank: definition, design, and data. Stroke 1984;15:740–6.

6. Sandercock P, Wardlaw JM, Lindley RI, et al. The benefits and harms of intravenous thrombolysis with recombinant tissue plasminogen activator within 6 h of acute ischaemic stroke (the third international stroke trial [IST-3]): a randomised controlled trial. Lancet 2012;379:2352–63.

7. Lees KR, Bluhmki E, von Kummer R, et al. Time to treatment with intravenous alteplase and outcome in stroke: an updated pooled analysis of ECASS, ATLANTIS, NINDS, and EPITHET trials. Lancet 2010;375:1695–703.

8. Myint PK, Hellkamp AS, Fonarow GC, et al. Prior antithrombotic use is associated with favorable mortality and functional outcomes in acute ischemic stroke. Stroke 2016;47:2066–74.

9. Xian Y, Federspiel JJ, Grau-Sepulveda M, et al. Risks and benefits associated with prestroke antiplatelet therapy among patients with acute ischemic stroke treated with intravenous tissue plasminogen activator. JAMA Neurol 2016;73:50–9.

10. Messe SR, Khatri P, Reeves MJ, et al. Why are acute ischemic stroke patients not receiving IV tPA? Results from a national registry. Neurology 2016;87:1565–74.

11. Cooray C, Fekete K, Mikulik R, et al. Threshold for NIH stroke scale in predicting vessel occlusion and functional outcome after stroke thrombolysis. Int J Stroke 2015;10:822–9.

12. Scheitz JF, Abdul-Rahim AH, MacIsaac RL, et al. Clinical selection strategies to identify ischemic stroke patients with large anterior vessel occlusion: results from SITS-ISTR (safe implementation of thrombolysis in stroke international stroke thrombolysis registry). Stroke 2017;48:290–7.

13. Yaghi S, Herber C, Boehme AK, et al. The association between diffusion MRI-defined infarct volume and NIHSS score in patients with minor acute stroke. J Neuroimaging 2017;27:388–91.

14. Brott T, Haley EC, Levy DE, et al. The investigational use of tPA for stroke. Ann Emerg Med 1988;17:1202–5.

15. Haley EC Jr, Brott TG, Sheppard GL, et al. Pilot randomized trial of tissue plasminogen activator in acute ischemic stroke. The TPA Bridging Study Group. Stroke 1993;24:1000–4.

16. Wardlaw JM, Murray V, Berge E, et al. Thrombolysis for acute ischaemic stroke. Cochrane Database Syst Rev 2014;(7):CD000213.

17. Levy DE, del Zoppo GJ, Demaerschalk BM, et al. Ancrod in acute ischemic stroke: results of 500 subjects beginning treatment within 6 hours of stroke onset in the Ancrod stroke program. Stroke 2009;40:3796–803.

18. Khatri P, Tayama D, Cohen G, et al. Effect of intravenous recombinant tissue-type plasminogen activator in patients with mild stroke in the third international stroke trial-3: post hoc analysis. Stroke 2015;46:2325–7.

19. Sandercock PAG, Ricci S. Controversies in thrombolysis. Curr Neurol Neurosci Rep 2017;17:60.

20. Fagan SC, Morgenstern LB, Petitta A, et al. Cost-effectiveness of tissue plasminogen activator for acute ischemic stroke. NINDS rt-PA Stroke Study Group. Neurology 1998;50:883–90.

21. Chapman SN, Mehndiratta P, Johansen MC, et al. Current perspectives on the use of intravenous recombinant tissue plasminogen activator (tPA) for treatment of acute ischemic stroke. Vasc Health Risk Manag 2014;10:75–87.

22. Powers WJ, Rabinstein AA, Ackerson T, et al. 2018 Guidelines for the Early Management of Patients With Acute Ischemic Stroke: a guideline for healthcare professionals from the American Heart Association/American Stroke Association. Stroke 2018;49. https://doi.org/10.1161/STR.0000000000000158.

23. Albers GW, Marks MP, Kemp S, et al. Thrombectomy for stroke at 6 to 16 hours with selection by perfusion imaging. New Eng J Med 2018. https://doi.org/10.1056/NEJMoa1713973.

24. Nogueira RG, Jadhav AP, Haussen DC. Thrombectomy 6 to 24 hours after stroke with a mismatch between deficit and infarct. N Engl J Med 2018;378:11–21.

25. Wolpert SM, Bruckmann H, Greenlee R, et al. Neuroradiologic evaluation of patients with acute stroke treated with recombinant tissue plasminogen activator. The rt-PA Acute Stroke Study Group. AJNR Am J Neuroradiol 1993;14:3–13.

26. Liebeskind DS. Collateral perfusion: time for novel paradigms in cerebral ischemia. Int J Stroke 2012;7:309–10.

27. Leng X, Fang H, Leung TW, et al. Impact of collateral status on successful revascularization in endovascular treatment: a systematic review and meta-analysis. Cerebrovasc Dis 2016;41:27–34.

28. Mohr JP. Neurologic complications of cardiac valvular disease and cardiac surgery. In: Vinken PJ, Bruyn GW, editors. Handbook of clinical neurology, 34. Amsterdam: North Holland Publ; 1979. p. 143–71.

29. Rostanski S, Lavine S, Mohr J. Collateral blood flow availability in acute ischemic stroke: a case report. Neurology 2016;86(16 Suppl):P4.360.

30. El-Zammar ZM, Latorre JG, Wang D, et al. Intra-arterial vasodilator use during endovascular therapy for acute ischemic stroke might improve reperfusion rate. Ann N Y Acad Sci 2012;1268:134–40.

31. Minematsu K, Yamaguchi T, Omae T. 'Spectacular shrinking deficit': rapid recovery from a major hemispheric syndrome by migration of an embolus. Neurology 1992;42:157–62.

32. Mohr JP. Historical observations on functional reorganization. Cerebrovasc Dis 2004;18:258–9.

33. Mohr JP. Rapid amelioration of motor aphasia. Arch Neurol 1973;28:77–82.

34. Mohr JP. Superficial and deep anterosuperior Sylvian syndromes. Neurologia, neurocirugia, psiquiatria 1977;18:27–33.

35. Mohr JP, Pessin MS, Finkelstein S, et al. Broca aphasia: pathologic and clinical. Neurology 1978; 28:311–24.

36. Yagata SA, Yen M, McCarron A, et al. Rapid recovery from aphasia after infarction of Wernicke's area. Aphasiology 2017;31:951–80.

37. de Medeiros FC, Viana DCR, Cunha MN, et al. Pure motor monoparesis due to infarction of the "hand knob" area: radiological and morphological features. Neurol Sci 2017;38:1877–9.

38. Hallett M. Functional reorganization after lesions of the human brain: studies with transcranial magnetic stimulation. Rev Neurol (Paris) 2001;157:822–6.

39. Brasil-Neto JP, Cohen LG, Pascual-Leone A, et al. Rapid reversible modulation of human motor outputs after transient deafferentation of the forearm: a study with transcranial magnetic stimulation. Neurology 1992;42:1302–6.

40. Lazar RM, Fitzsimmons BF, Marshall RS, et al. Midazolam challenge reinduces neurological deficits after transient ischemic attack. Stroke 2003;34:794–6.

41. Clinical trial of nimodipine in acute ischemic stroke. The American Nimodipine Study Group. Stroke 1992;23:3–8.

42. Kaste M, Fogelholm R, Erila T, et al. A randomized, double-blind, placebo-controlled trial of nimodipine in acute ischemic hemispheric stroke. Stroke 1994; 25:1348–53.

43. Sareen D. Neuroprotective agents in acute ischemic stroke. J Assoc Physicians India 2002;50:250–8.

44. Neuhaus AA, Couch Y, Hadley G, et al. Neuroprotection in stroke: the importance of collaboration and reproducibility. Brain 2017;140:2079–92.

45. Ginsberg MD. Expanding the concept of neuroprotection for acute ischemic stroke: the pivotal roles of reperfusion and the collateral circulation. Prog Neurobiol 2016;145-146:46–77.

46. Roffe C, Nevatte T, Sim J, et al. Effect of routine low-dose oxygen supplementation on death and disability in adults with acute stroke: the stroke oxygen study randomized clinical trial. JAMA 2017;318: 1125–35.

47. Greer DM, Funk SE, Reaven NL, et al. Impact of fever on outcome in patients with stroke and neurologic injury: a comprehensive meta-analysis. Stroke 2008;39:3029–35.

48. Hajat C, Hajat S, Sharma P. Effects of poststroke pyrexia on stroke outcome: a meta-analysis of studies in patients. Stroke 2000;31:410–4.

49. den Hertog HM, van der Worp HB, van Gemert HM. The Paracetamol (Acetaminophen) In Stroke (PAIS) trial: a multicentre, randomised, placebo-controlled, phase III trial. Lancet Neurol 2009;8: 434–40.

50. Chamorro A, Horcajada JP, Obach V, et al. The early systemic prophylaxis of infection after stroke study: a randomized clinical trial. Stroke 2005;36: 1495–500.

51. Harms H, Prass K, Meisel C, et al. Preventive antibacterial therapy in acute ischemic stroke: a randomized controlled trial. PLoS One 2008;3:e2158.

52. Adjusted-dose warfarin versus low-intensity, fixed-dose warfarin plus aspirin for high-risk patients with atrial fibrillation: stroke prevention in atrial fibrillation III randomised clinical trial. Lancet 1996;348: 633–8.

53. Sandercock PA, Leong TS. Low-molecular-weight heparins or heparinoids versus standard unfractionated heparin for acute ischaemic stroke. Cochrane Database Syst Rev 2017;(4):CD000119.

54. Stapf C, Mohr JP, Theallier-Janko A, et al. Cerebral hemorrhage after systemic fibrinolysis in a patient with severe carotid artery stenosis. Acta Neurol Scand 1999;100:407–10.

55. Goldstein JN, Marrero M, Masrur S, et al. Management of thrombolysis-associated symptomatic intracerebral hemorrhage. Arch Neurol 2010;67:965–9.

56. Stone JA, Willey JZ, Keyrouz S, et al. Therapies for Hemorrhagic Transformation in Acute Ischemic Stroke. Curr Treat Options Neurol 2017;19:1.

57. Cucchiara B, Kasner SE, Tanne D, et al. Factors associated with intracerebral hemorrhage after thrombolytic therapy for ischemic stroke: pooled analysis of placebo data from the Stroke-Acute Ischemic NXY Treatment (SAINT) I and SAINT II Trials. Stroke 2009;40:3067–72.

58. Lovelock CE, Anslow P, Molyneux AJ, et al. Substantial observer variability in the differentiation between primary intracerebral hemorrhage and hemorrhagic transformation of infarction on CT brain imaging. Stroke 2009;40:3763–7.

59. Trouillas P, von Kummer R. Classification and pathogenesis of cerebral hemorrhages after thrombolysis in ischemic stroke. Stroke 2006;37:556–61.

60. Seet RC, Rabinstein AA. Symptomatic intracranial hemorrhage following intravenous thrombolysis for acute ischemic stroke: a critical review of case definitions. Cerebrovasc Dis 2012;34:106–14.

61. Kablau M, Kreisel SH, Sauer T, et al. Predictors and early outcome of hemorrhagic transformation after acute ischemic stroke. Cerebrovasc Dis 2011;32: 334–41.

62. Yaghi S, Willey JZ, Cucchiara B, et al. Treatment and outcome of hemorrhagic transformation after intravenous alteplase in acute ischemic stroke: a scientific statement for healthcare professionals from the American Heart Association/American Stroke Association. Stroke 2017;48:e343–61.

63. Tornkvist M, Smith JG, Labaf A. Current evidence of oral anticoagulant reversal: a systematic review. Thromb Res 2017;162:22–31.

64. Puetz J. Fresh frozen plasma: the most commonly prescribed hemostatic agent. J Thromb Haemost 2013;11:1794–9.

65. Fenger-Eriksen C, Christiansen K, Laurie J, et al. Fibrinogen concentrate and cryoprecipitate but not fresh frozen plasma correct low fibrinogen concentrations following in vitro haemodilution. Thromb Res 2013;131:e210–3.

66. Fiore LD, Scola MA, Cantillon CE, et al. Anaphylactoid reactions to vitamin K. J Thromb Thrombolysis 2001;11:175–83.

67. Sorensen B, Spahn DR, Innerhofer P, et al. Clinical review: prothrombin complex concentrates–evaluation of safety and thrombogenicity. Crit Care 2011;15:201.

68. Sprigg N, Renton CJ, Dineen RA, et al. Tranexamic acid for spontaneous intracerebral hemorrhage: a randomized controlled pilot trial (ISRCTN50867461). J stroke Cerebrovasc Dis 2014;23:1312–8.

69. French KF, White J, Hoesch RE. Treatment of intracerebral hemorrhage with tranexamic acid after thrombolysis with tissue plasminogen activator. Neurocrit Care 2012;17:107–11.

70. Woo CH, Patel N, Conell C, et al. Rapid Warfarin reversal in the setting of intracranial hemorrhage: a comparison of plasma, recombinant activated factor VII, and prothrombin complex concentrate. World Neurosurg 2014;81:110–5.

71. Carcel C, Wang X, Sato S, et al. Degree and timing of intensive blood pressure lowering on hematoma growth in intracerebral hemorrhage: intensive blood pressure reduction in acute cerebral hemorrhage trial-2 results. Stroke 2016;47:1651–3.

72. Qureshi AI, Palesch YY, Barsan WG, et al. Intensive blood-pressure lowering in patients with acute cerebral hemorrhage. N Engl J Med 2016;375:1033–43.

73. Le Roux P, Pollack CV Jr, Milan M, et al. Race against the clock: overcoming challenges in the management of anticoagulant-associated intracerebral hemorrhage. J Neurosurg 2014;121(Suppl):1–20.

74. de Oliveira Manoel AL, Goffi A, Zampieri FG, et al. The critical care management of spontaneous intracranial hemorrhage: a contemporary review. Crit Care 2016;20:272.

75. Lopponen P, Tetri S, Juvela S, et al. A population based study of outcomes after evacuation of primary supratentorial intracerebral hemorrhage. Clin Neurol Neurosurg 2013;115:1350–5.

76. Mendelow AD, Gregson BA, Rowan EN, et al. Early surgery versus initial conservative treatment in patients with traumatic intracerebral hemorrhage (STITCH[Trauma]): the first randomized trial. J Neurotrauma 2015;32:1312–23.

77. Murthy SB, Gupta A, Merkler AE, et al. Restarting anticoagulant therapy after intracranial hemorrhage: a systematic review and meta-analysis. Stroke 2017;48:1594–600.

78. Wilson D, Charidimou A, Shakeshaft C, et al, CROMIS-2 Collaborators. Volume and functional outcome of intracerebral hemorrhage according to oral anticoagulant type. Neurology 2016;86:360–6.

79. Thorpe ER, Garrett KB, Smith AM, et al. Outcome measure scores predict discharge destination in patients with acute and subacute stroke: a systematic review and series of meta-analyses. J Neurol Phys Ther 2018;42:2–11.

What to Look for on Post-stroke Neuroimaging

Angelos M. Katramados, MD[a], Lotfi Hacein-Bey, MD[b,c],
Panayiotis N. Varelas, MD, PhD[d],*

KEYWORDS

• Acute ischemic stroke • Neuroimaging • Hemorrhagic transformation • Seizure

KEY POINTS

• Hemorrhage is a feared event that may follow ischemic stroke, treated and untreated. Modern neuroimaging plays an important role in predicting and managing hemorrhagic transformation.
• Several signs of active extravasation or hematoma expansion, such as the spot sign, have been reported, but most of these have been described or validated in spontaneous intracerebral hemorrhage and not for acute ischemic stroke hemorrhagic transformation.
• Seizures are rare after ischemic stroke but can also lead to confusion as stroke mimics. Perfusion parameters may be used to differentiate between the two conditions and allow adjustment of treatment.
• Malignant cerebral edema post-stroke, which could lead to herniation, may be predicted by neuroimaging allowing appropriate preventive treatment.
• Lastly, neuroimaging can help predict recovery potential, and guide rehabilitation efforts.

INTRODUCTION

In the postacute ischemic stroke period, hemorrhage, seizures, and malignant cerebral edema are major concerns for the treating team. The frequency of severity of such complications is influenced by the reperfusion method (fibrinolysis vs thrombectomy) and by the time course, leading to the need for additional neuroimaging studies, which play a major role in the prediction, detection, and management of post-stroke patients.

HEMORRHAGE

Hemorrhagic transformation (HT; bleeding within infarcted tissue) is part of the natural history of stroke: minor degrees of HT occur spontaneously in 4% to 70% of patients, and detection varies depending on the imaging technique used and the timing of imaging. Studies using MR imaging have demonstrated higher detection rates compared with those using computed tomography (CT). HT may be seen up to several weeks after the stroke.[1] Intravenous (IV) thrombolysis with alteplase (the only currently Food and Drug Administration–approved medical treatment of ischemic stroke) within 4.5 hours of onset increases the overall risk of HT by three-fold, and the risk of symptomatic HT by 10-fold.[2] Mechanical endovascular recanalization with older-generation devices was associated with a high rate of HT: in the multi-MERCI trial, asymptomatic

Disclosure Statement: P.N. Varelas has received speaker's honorarium from UCB Pharma, Belgium.
[a] Department of Neurology, Wayne State University, Henry Ford Hospital, K-11, 2799 West Grand Boulevard, Detroit, MI 48202, USA; [b] Interventional Neuroradiology and Neuroradiology, Department of Medical Imaging, Sutter Health, Sacramento, CA 95815, USA; [c] Radiology Department, University of California Davis Medical School of Medicine, 4860 Y Street, Sacramento, CA 95817, USA; [d] NeuroCritical Care Service, Neurosciences Intensive Care Unit, Departments of Neurology and Neurosurgery, Henry Ford Hospital, K-11, 2799 West Grand Boulevard, Detroit, MI 48202, USA
* Corresponding author. NeuroCritical Care Service, Neurosciences Intensive Care Unit, Department of Neurology, Henry Ford Hospital, K-11, 2799 West Grand Boulevard, Detroit, MI 48202.
E-mail address: varelas@neuro.hfh.edu

HT rate was 30.5%, and symptomatic intracerebral hemorrhage (sICH) was 9.8%. Newer generation endovascular devices (ie, stent-retrievers) seem to have a higher safety profile. A meta-analysis of the five major recent randomized controlled trials of ischemic stroke treatment (HERMES collaboration) revealed a rate of sICH of 4.4%, not significantly different from the control group.[3] Even with delayed intervention (up to 24 hours from onset), modern mechanical thrombectomy did not result in increased rates of sICH[4,5] as shown in recent reviews.[6,7] The SWIFT-DIRECT trial, currently underway, will prospectively address this question.

Pathophysiology of Hemorrhagic Transformation

Spontaneous HT results from reperfusion after the cerebral vasculature has been damaged by ischemia. Two different time windows for spontaneous HT have been suggested: early spontaneous HT (within 18–24 hours from stroke onset) seems to be related to early blood-brain barrier (BBB) disruption, and is promoted by matrix metalloproteinase (MMP)-9 and brain-derived MMP-2, whereas late spontaneous HT (past 18–24 hours) may be related to late BBB disruption, mediated by brain-derived MMP-9, vascular remodeling, and postischemic inflammation.[8] With either scenario, spontaneous revascularization plays a major role. Spontaneous recanalization of the occluded middle cerebral artery (MCA) within 2 hours, in the medical arm of the PROACT II intra-arterial thrombolysis trial, occurred in 18% of medically treated patients.[9] Similarly, a prospective study of recanalization after acute cardioembolic stroke showed early recanalization (within 6 hours) and delayed recanalization (6–48 hours) rates, respectively, of 18.8% and 52.8%.[10]

IV thrombolysis has been shown to increase the risk of HT compared with the natural history of ischemic stroke in the following ways: (1) increased recanalization rate by 46.2% shown in a study assessing the impact of recanalization on outcomes[11]; (2) bench demonstration that alteplase upregulates MMP-9 (previously noted to contribute in early HT), and conversely, coadministration of alteplase and MMP-inhibitors results in decrease of HT and reperfusion injury[12]; and (3) alteplase (despite its overall benefits) may promote excitotoxic cell death by adversely affecting the neurovascular matrix.[13]

Mechanical endovascular recanalization, particularly with older devices, results in increased hemorrhagic risk, presumably from increased risk of endothelial injury, mechanical endothelial cell denudement, and (presumably) secondary neuronal injury from deleterious cytokine cascades.[14] Newer devices (presumably responsible for lesser endothelial injury) do not incrementally elevate hemorrhagic risk when used in conjunction with IV thrombolysis, and increased recanalization rates with mechanical endovascular recanalization alone do not result in an increased risk of reperfusion injury in late recanalization up to 24 hours from stroke onset.[4,5]

Classification of Hemorrhagic Transformation

HT has been categorized using radiologic and clinical criteria. Radiologic criteria (ie, extent and size of HT) have been refined over time. The ECASS classification distinguished between hemorrhagic infarction (HI; HT of infarcted brain tissue) and parenchymal hematoma (PH; intracerebral hemorrhage [ICH]) within and extending beyond infarcted tissue.[15] However, extraischemic HT or other hemorrhagic complications (eg, subarachnoid hemorrhage (Fig. 1), intraventricular hemorrhage) and subdural hemorrhage were not considered. For that reason, a more recent iteration of radiologic criteria was developed, referred to as the Heidelberg Bleeding Classification (Table 1).[16]

Clinical criteria were required to distinguish between symptomatic HT (ie, resulting in neurologic deterioration, worse neurologic outcome or death) and asymptomatic HT. Several definitions of symptomatic HT (mostly sICH) have been advanced, leading to confusion,[17–23] which prompted the Heidelberg group to define sICH as hemorrhage that (1) occurs 24 hours after intervention; (2) can alone explain the neurologic deterioration; (3) results in an increase of greater than or equal to four points in the total National Institute of Health Stroke Scale (NIHSS) score from baseline (or ≥2 points in one NIHSS item); and (4) leads to intubation, hemicraniectomy, external ventricular drain placement, or other major medical/surgical intervention.[24]

Prediction of Hemorrhagic Transformation

Hemorrhage is a most feared complication of IV thrombolysis, which has contributed to a slow process of adoption of IV thrombolysis, particularly in the early years following Food and Drug Administration approval.[25] Unfortunately, even with complete compliance to the thrombolysis protocol, it is not entirely possible to predict the development of HT (Fig. 2). Such predictive ability at the time of initial presentation would potentially allow to minimize risk of HT and expand eligibility criteria and therapeutic window in patients not "destined" to

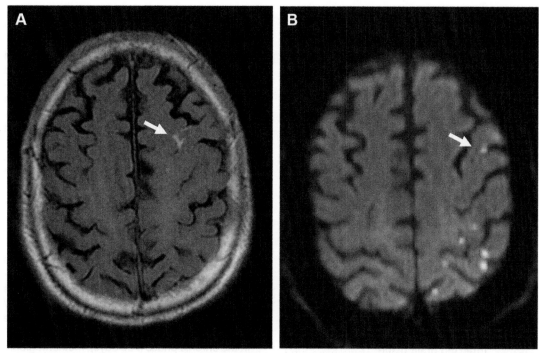

Fig. 1. A 74-year-old patient 3 days status post left anterior circulation ischemic stroke. The patient is on dual-antiplatelet therapy for a carotid stent. Sudden onset of dull left frontal headache. Axial FLAIR MR imaging shows discrete subarachnoid blood in left middle frontal gyrus (*A*, *arrow*), likely from hemorrhagic conversion of small left frontal ischemic injuries seen on diffusion-weighted imaging (*B*, *arrow*).

have HT.[26] In the absence of such predictive algorithms, various models/predictions scores have been applied, most using clinical (rather than radiologic criteria). A comprehensive list of these models is described in the recent American Heart Association Guidelines on treatment of post-thrombolysis HT.[24]

With regard to neuroimaging alone, CT on presentation may reveal factors that may predispose to HT. Extensive early ischemic signs on pretreatment CT, semiquantitively assessed by the Alberta Stroke Program Early CT Score (ASPECTS), were noted to have a significantly higher risk of thrombolysis-related PH.[27] Baseline hypoattenuation on noncontrast CT and low cerebral blood volume (CBV) on CT perfusion are associated with post-thrombolysis PH.[28] Despite strong theoretic and experimental foundation, there is currently unclear evidence as to whether imaging BBB permeability can improve the prediction of post-thrombolysis HT.[29,30] A recent study demonstrated that iodine extravasation on dual-energy CT performed after mechanical thrombectomy (defined as the presence of a parenchymal hyperdensity with a maximum iodine concentration of >1.35 mg/mL) can identify patients at risk for developing PH with high sensitivity (100%) and lower specificity (67.6%).[31]

MR imaging can reveal conditions associated with a higher risk of HT. Cerebral microbleeds on pretreatment MR imaging have been associated with a higher risk of sICH in a meta-analysis of 10 relevant studies.[32] A recent study attempted to apply machine learning to tackle the problem of HT prediction. The model would learn to extract imaging markers of HT directly from source perfusion-weighted imaging images rather than from pre-established metrics.[33] The combination of low (10th percentile) CBV and high (90th percentile) microvascular permeability on multiparametric MR imaging has been shown to be an independent predictor of PH.[34] The hyperintense acute reperfusion marker sign on MR imaging, a marker of early BBB disruption, has been associated with an increased risk of post-thrombectomy HT, particularly PH.[35,36]

Detection of Hemorrhagic Transformation

The appearance of hemorrhage on CT depends on the hematocrit, hemoglobin fraction, protein content, and degree of clot retraction (which does not typically occur immediately).[37] The initial clot seems to have similar attenuation to the adjacent brain parenchyma in the hyperacute phase (from minutes to 1 hour) and may be difficult to detect.

Table 1
Characteristics of intracranial hemorrhage patterns

Class	Type	Description
1		Hemorrhagic transformation of infarcted brain tissue
1a	HI1	Scattered small petechiae, no mass effect
1b	HI2	Confluent petechiae, no mass effect
1c	PH1	Hematoma within infarcted tissue, occupying <30%, no substantive mass effect
2		Intracerebral hemorrhage within and beyond infarcted brain tissue
	PH2	Hematoma occupying 30% or more of the infarcted tissue, with obvious mass effect
3		Intracerebral hemorrhage outside the infarcted brain tissue or intracranial-extracerebral hemorrhage
3a		Parenchymal hematoma remote from infarcted brain tissue
3b		Intraventricular hemorrhage
3c		Subarachnoid hemorrhage
3d		Subdural hemorrhage

Abbreviation: HI, hemorrhagic infarction.

From von Kummer R, Broderick JP, Campbell BC, et al. The Heidelberg bleeding classification: classification of bleeding events after ischemic stroke and reperfusion therapy. Stroke 2015;46(10):2981–6.

Subsequently, in the acute and early subacute phase (1 hour to 1 week), attenuation increases, particularly in the center of the hemorrhage, whereas a peripheral hypodense rim suggests the development of perilesional edema. In the late subacute phase (1 week to 1 month), attenuation again decreases and the hemorrhage becomes isodense and eventually hypodense (>1 month from onset). Ex vacuo hydrocephalus, focal atrophy, and dystrophic calcifications may be present in the chronic stage.[38]

MR imaging can detect hyperacute blood with greater accuracy and may establish the chronology of hemorrhage. MR imaging appearance of blood depends on the water content of the bleed and the magnetic properties of by-products of hemoglobin.[37–39]

In the hyperacute phase (<24 hours), red blood cells (RBCs) within the hemorrhage are intact and may contain high amounts of oxyhemoglobin (because of the arterial origin of the hemorrhage). Intracellular oxyhemoglobin, which is diamagnetic (has paired electrons in the heme iron), cannot result in T2 shortening and therefore appears T2 hyperintense, and T1 hypointense because of high water content.

In the acute phase (1–3 days), RBCs remain intact but oxyhemoglobin has mostly been oxidized to deoxyhemoglobin. Intracellular deoxyhemoglobin, which is paramagnetic (has unpaired electrons in the heme iron), causes T2 shortening (T2 hypointense) and is T1 hypointense or isointense because of relative decrease in water content.

In the early subacute phase (3–7 days), RBCs are still intact but oxyhemoglobin has become permanently oxidized to methemoglobin. Intracellular methemoglobin is also paramagnetic and is T1 hyperintense and T2 hypointense. The development of the T1 hyperintensity helps distinguish between the acute and subacute phase.

In the late subacute phase (7–30 days), RBCs have lyzed and methemoglobin is now extracellular, becoming T1 and T2 hyperintense. The development of T2 hyperintensity with already established T1 hyperintensity is a hallmark of the late subacute phase.

In the chronic phase (>30 days), methemoglobin is converted to extracellular hemosiderin, and becomes mostly hypointense on T1 and T2, with the exception of slight T2 rim hyperintensity.

Management of Hemorrhagic Transformation

Spontaneous hemorrhagic transformation

Asymptomatic HT is technically not associated with immediate deterioration, but may not be innocuous, because it may increase the risk of worsening outcome. A risk-benefit decision (depending on the underlying indication) needs to be made with regard to the resumption of chemical deep venous thromboembolism prophylaxis, antiplatelet, and anticoagulation treatment. The recent 2018 Guidelines of Early Management of Ischemic Stroke report that antithrombotic treatment has been noted to be safe in the setting of HT in multiple observational studies, and that anticoagulation for atrial fibrillation can typically be started within 4 to 14 days of stroke onset for most patients.[40] Patients with large hemispheric strokes, or with established PH, may start anticoagulation in a delayed fashion at the discretion of the treating physician. The overall care of spontaneous HT is otherwise directed by the American Heart Association guidelines on management of sICH,[41] with the understanding that the recommendation for blood pressure less than 140/90 for ICH needs to be balanced against the need to avoid critical hypoperfusion in the setting of an index acute ischemic stroke, particularly if there is known fixed intracranial or extracranial stenosis (Fig. 3).

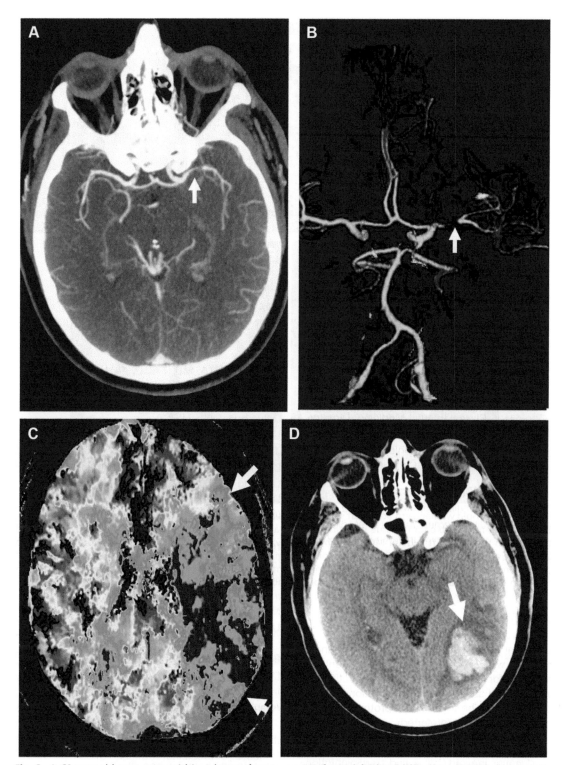

Fig. 2. A 69-year-old man seen within 1 hour of acute onset of word finding difficulty and right arm paresis; NIHSS 4. CT angiography shows small left M1 MCA thrombus (*A, arrow*), which is not completely occlusive as shown on three-dimensional rendering (*B, arrow*). Perfusion CT shows large MCA territory at risk (*C, arrows*). The patient is treated with IV tissue plasminogen activator, and improves initially. Within 2 hours, acute deterioration follows, caused by large left temporo-occipital hemorrhage (*D, arrow*), possibly in relation to amyloid angiopathy.

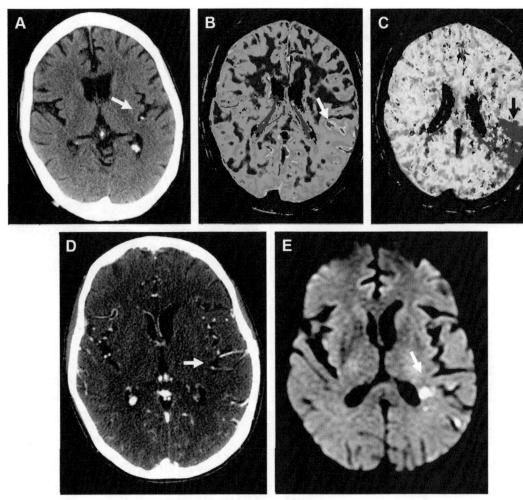

Fig. 3. A 75-year-old woman with acute left sensory aphasia and right arm paresis, which are fluctuating; NIHSS 6. The patient is not eligible for IV tissue plasminogen activator or mechanical thrombectomy. CT shows a calcified thrombus in the distal left angular MCA branch (*A, arrow*). Perfusion CT suggests small infarct core on CBV map (*B, arrow*), and relative large penumbra at risk on Tmax map (*C, arrow*). CT angiography suggests patent arterial circulation past the calcified clot (*D, arrow*). Management with blood pressure support, euvolemia, and aspirin results in good clinical recovery (NIHSS 1 at 72 hours), and small infarct size on MR imaging (*E, arrow*).

Thrombolysis-related symptomatic intracerebral hemorrhage

Universal potential for benefit has only been with reversal with cryoprecipitate. Other agents are reserved for specific circumstances. Patients on warfarin and subtherapeutic international normalized ratio may be treated with prothrombin complex concentrate (preferred), or fresh frozen plasma. Patients with thrombocytopenia may be treated with platelets. Antifibrinolytics may be used if the patient does not accept blood products, or if cryoprecipitate is not available.[24] Hematoma expansion is best prevented with meticulous blood pressure control, again while weighing the risks of hypoperfusion particularly in the setting of incomplete recanalization. Neurosurgical treatment (decompressive craniectomy or hematoma extraction) may be undertaken if there is suspicion of benefit, according to the principles described in the relevant guidelines (best for cerebellar sICH, or as a life-saving procedure in patients with supratentorial ICH who are in a coma, have large hematomas with significant midline shift, or have elevated intracranial pressure refractory to medical management[41]) with the understanding that alteplase-related coagulopathy may negate any potential benefit.

Hematoma Expansion

Active contrast extravasation has been described as the "spot sign" in patients with ICH and this has been associated with hematoma expansion (sensitivity, 91%; specificity, 89%).[42] In the PRE-DICT study, the presence of spot sign was additionally associated with worsening of the NIHSS within the first 24 hours and worse modified Rankin score and mortality in 3 months.[43] Other radiographic findings in ICH include the percentage change in Hounsfield units between early and late phase CT with contrast, which has led to the development of the leakage sign (cutoff >110%), with superior sensitivity and specificity than the spot sign.[44]

The "black hole" sign has been recently defined as an area of relative hypoattenuation that is well-demarcated, compared with the surrounding hyperattenuating hematoma. It has been reported to be a predictor of hematoma growth.[45] Other recently reported predictors of hematoma growth include the "island sign" (extremely irregular hematoma with surrounding multiple small hematomas),[46] the "satellite sign" (any smaller hematoma in the periphery of a larger hematoma),[47] and the "blend sign" (blending of a hypoattenuating area with adjacent hyperattenuating region within a hematoma, albeit with a well-defined border).[48] All of these signs, similar to the older "swirl sign" (regions of hypoattenuation or isoattenuation compared with the attenuation of brain parenchyma within the hyperattenuated ICH, initially defined for epidural hematomas but recently proposed for ICHs)[49] suggest that certain patterns of intrahematoma heterogeneity are predictive of short-term growth. All these signs have been described in spontaneous ICH and could be relevant in HT (especially in PH2-HBC 2) because it is typically captured in the hyperacute phase.

The management of ischemic hemorrhagic conversion versus primary ICH with spot sign is classically based on tight blood pressure control. The data supporting this, however, are not clear. In a recent analysis of the SCORE-IT trial (a nested substudy of the ATTACH II study), the sensitivity and specificity of the spot sign was much lower (54% and 63%, respectively) and its presence was not associated with hematoma size expansion decrease after intensive blood pressure control.[50]

SEIZURES

Early poststroke seizures, defined as seizures occurring between the first 24 hours to the first 4 weeks, usually occur at the stroke onset in 1.5% to 33% of patients and constitute most poststroke seizures.[51–55] Late poststroke seizures have an incidence of 2.5% to 67%, depending

on the definition and the duration of follow-up.[53,56–58] Early seizures are more likely partial and late seizures generalized.[59] The most common type of seizures is complex partial seizures (48.7%), followed by primary generalized (24.3%), simple partial (10.8%), and undetermined (16.2%) seizures.[60] Several factors have been associated with postischemic stroke seizures, such as younger age, higher stroke severity, acute nonneurologic infection, history of diabetes mellitus, cardioembolic cause, and history of preceding transient ischemic attack.[61,62] Location or extension of the stroke is another factor. Compared with deep infarcts, lobar infarcts confer up to 11 times an increased risk for seizures (95% confidence interval, 2.6–47.6)[60] and among cortical infarcts, watershed distribution confers a four-fold increased risk for early seizures.[63] HT is also a predictor of early poststroke seizures.[64] After endovascular treatment of acute anterior circulation ischemic stroke, HT is associated with a nearly five times higher rate of developing poststroke seizures within 2 years compared with patients without HT. The median time to first seizure was 111 days (interquartile range, 28–369 days).[65]

Seizures may not only be a consequence of acute ischemic stroke, they are also one of the most common stroke mimics, making up 1% to 30% of all stroke admissions.[66] Therefore, the clinician and the radiologist often face a dilemma in determining whether a neurologic deficit is caused by the stroke, a seizure as stroke mimic, or even a seizure superimposed on an acute stroke. The classic neuroimaging findings on CT of a new hypodensity within an arterial distribution, or on MR imaging (diffusion-weighted imaging [DWI]-apparent diffusion coefficient (ADC) changes of cytotoxic edema) are not always conclusive in sorting out these emergent situations, which mandate fast treatment decisions. Alternative neuroimaging studies may provide direct or indirect evidence for one or the other diagnosis. During seizures, perfusion CT shows increased or decreased mean transit time and increased CBV in areas that do not follow an arterial distribution, unlike what would be expected in stroke.[66] Postseizure focal tissue dysfunction presents clinically as a negative sign (ie, Todd paralysis) compared with a positive sign (ie, convulsion or contralateral head and eye turn during the ictal phase). However, unlike ischemic deficits, postictal changes are usually transient and improve within minutes to few hours (between one-half hour and 36 hours, with an average of 15 hours).[67] Postictal paresis associated with perfusion CT evidence of increased cerebral blood flow and CBV, and decreased mean transit time in the vascular territory corresponding to patient's symptom has also been reported.[68] In a recent prospective study aiming at differentiating between acute ischemic stroke and seizures as the cause of acute neurologic deficit in patients with normal routine CT of the head, the only significantly different variable on the CT perfusion was time-to-peak in the middle cerebral artery lateral territory.[69]

Similar to CT changes during seizures, MR imaging changes have also been described and named transient peri-ictal MR imaging abnormalities. These are usually not associated with brief seizures, however, but mostly with status epilepticus.[66] Recent evidence suggests that DWI restriction adjacent to ongoing seizure activity may result from local cortical metabolic disturbances and more widespread corticocortical and corticothalamic synchronization abnormalities.[70] Lesions that do not conform to vascular territories present as low-density changes on CT, high T2 signal on MR imaging, DWI-ADC changes consistent with cytotoxic edema (mainly in the cortical ribbon, with involvement of the ipsilateral thalamus), subcortical white matter DWI-ADC changes consistent with vasogenic edema, early leptomeningeal or gyral postcontrast enhancement, local hyperperfusion on MR angiography, and cerebral activation on functional MR imaging, all reversible; although those findings have strong associations with partial epilepsy and especially status epilepticus, they could help differentiate between ischemic stroke and seizure activity.[66,71–75] Therefore, combining DWI and perfusion on MR imaging examinations may result in higher diagnostic accuracy than ADC alone, and help distinguish the effect of seizures from that of oligemia or ischemia caused by stroke. Hypoperfusion may also be shown on postcontrast MR imaging or arterial spin labeling sequences.[76,77] MR spectroscopy may also be useful, showing lactate elevation and N-acetylaspartate decrease in the epileptic focus.[75] Response to antiepileptic treatment may also provide retrospective diagnostic information. A recent report on two patients with partial status epilepticus associated with an old infarction, who had two episodes each of left hemiparesis and hemisensory disturbance without convulsion, showed restricted diffusion on DWI in the peri-infarct cortex, mimicking a recurrent stroke. Despite failure of electroencephalogram to show ictal discharges or interictal paroxysmal activities in three of four episodes, perfusion imaging with arterial spin labeling clearly demonstrated ictal hyperperfusion in the area corresponding to the cortical hyperintense lesion on DWI; in both patients, full clinical recovery occurred after appropriate antiepileptic treatment.[78] By the

same token, postictal Todd paralysis may be associated with hypoperfusion on MR imaging perfusion, but in parallel with expected clinical improvement (as opposed to a permanent deficit after acute ischemic stroke), MR perfusion findings are expected to resolve with time,[79] although early or late postictal phase findings may differ with the area tested and reverse,[80] further complicating the interpretation in real-time.

Therefore, how these acute imaging findings evolve is not entirely clear and may depend on either short-lasting or repetitive, longer-lasting cellular injury from single seizure or from status epilepticus, respectively. For example, DWI changes are largely reversible, but if prolonged seizures are present, may be associated with laminar necrosis and irreversible deficits.[81] In a cohort of 26 patients with acute seizure-related MR imaging changes, residual gliosis or focal atrophy was found in 42%, whereas the remainder had reversible findings, which resolved between 15 and 150 days (average, 62 days). Partial simple and complex seizures were associated with hippocampal involvement. Status epilepticus, however, was associated with incomplete reversibility of MR imaging abnormalities.[82]

The treatment of acute seizures, regardless of cause, aims at prompt resolution of the ictal activity, and avoiding recurrence or escalation to status epilepticus, which still carries significant mortality and morbidity. Simple measures, such as the detection and correction of hypoglycemia or hypoxemia, placement of an IV line, quick evaluation of airway, and circulation for support, should always be entertained regardless of the suspicion being stroke or seizure. Antiepileptic medications after a first ever, single seizure is not indicated, but if the seizure is prolonged beyond 5 minutes, status epilepticus treatment algorithm should be initiated.[83]

CEREBRAL EDEMA

Cerebral edema that develops after ischemic stroke is cytotoxic because of reduced substrate delivery to the tissue, decreased ATP generation via aerobic or anaerobic pathways, and opening of sodium channels with intracellular sodium influx followed by water. The term malignant middle cerebral artery territory infarction or malignant edema was introduced in the 1990s to describe a severe stroke with malignant course ending in transtentorial herniation.[84]

Numerous efforts to use clinical and neuroimaging markers toward early prediction of a malignant course to treat accordingly before herniation occurs have taken place in recent years. CT- and

MR imaging–based prognostic factors have been developed.

Computed Tomography–Based Prognostication

In a prospective study of 53 angiographically proven MCA trunk occlusions treated with recombinant tissue plasminogen activator, hypodensity involving greater than 50% of the MCA territory had an 85% positive predictive value (PPV) for fatal outcome, with a sensitivity of 61% and a specificity of 94%. For local brain swelling, those values were 70%, 78%, and 83%, respectively.[85] In another prospective study of 55 patients with complete MCA territory infarction admitted to a neonatal intensive care unit, poor collateral blood flow, absence of recanalization, and distal internal carotid artery (ICA) or proximal MCA occlusion were markers of poor outcome.[84] A prospective multicenter study evaluating lubeluzole compared 23 patients (from the placebo arm) who died from brain edema with 112 patients (with a similar or higher NIHSS) who survived. Baseline brain CT (obtained within 187–153 minutes of stroke onset in the malignant and benign groups) variables that predicted death were greater than 50% MCA territory and hypodensity involving the temporal lobe or other territory. Logistic regression analysis, however, only retained greater than 50% MCA hypodensity as an independent predictor of fatal brain edema (odds ratio [OR], 6.1; 2.3–16.6).[86]

Several retrospective studies have tried to define predictive findings of evolution to malignant edema. The earliest reported study evaluated 74 patients with acute carotid artery distribution stroke, who received intra-arterial (n = 68) and IV recombinant tissue plasminogen activator (n = 6) and reported that angiographic confirmation of a carotid T occlusion was predictive of a fatal outcome (OR, 5.3; 1.7–16.2; PPV, 47%; negative predictive value [NPV], 85%; sensitivity, 53%; specificity, 83%), whereas cortical hypodensity greater than 33% of MCA territory was not.[87] In another multicenter case-control study of 201 patients with large MCA strokes, of which 94 eventually died from brain edema, greater than 50% MCA hypodensity, involvement of other arterial territories, and presence of early mass effect were predictive of poor outcome. Logistic regression adjusted by age and clustered by participating center showed greater than 50% MCA hypodensity (OR, 6.3; 3.5–11.6) and involvement of additional vascular territories, such as anterior cerebral artery, posterior cerebral artery, or anterior choroidal artery (OR, 3.3; 1.2–9.4) to be independent predictors of fatal brain edema.[88] Another

study of 55 patients with MCA infarction showed larger infarction volumes, HI, and angiographic recanalization to be predictors of malignant course in univariate analysis. Discriminant analysis revealed that an infarction volume of greater than 240 cm^3 and a shift of the midline structures greater than 8.5 mm was predictive of malignant infarction with 76.4% and 89.1% accuracy, respectively.[89] The timing of signs for prognostication was also examined: early (<12 hours) involvement of greater than 50% MCA territory (OR, 14.02; 1.04–189.42) and a hyperdense MCA sign at any time (OR, 21.6; 3.54–130.04) were independent predictors of neurologic deterioration. The positive predictive power for early involvement of greater than 50% MCA territory and hyperdense MCA was 0.75 and 0.91, respectively.[90] Subsequent retrospective studies suggested other prognostic variables of 30-day fatal outcome, such as anteroseptal shift greater than or equal to 5 mm (OR, 10.9; 3.2–37.6) and infarction beyond the MCA territory (OR, 4.9; 1.6–15.0)[91]; involvement of additional vascular territories was a marker of progressive and ongoing deterioration[92,93]; large hypoattenuation (>2/3 of MCA territory) predicted malignant evolution with a 100% specificity and PPV (sensitivity, 73%; NPV, 84%; accuracy, 89%).[94] Another study suggested that infarcted lesion volume greater than 220 mL and midline shift greater than 3.9 mm provided 100% sensitivity and 98% specificity for malignant evolution. For the subgroup of patients with bicaudate index less than 0.16 (implying absence of significant brain atrophy), a cutoff of 190 mL was also predictive of malignant edema (specificity, 89.7%; sensitivity, 100%).[95]

MR Imaging–Based Prognostication

In a prospective, multicenter, observational cohort study of 140 patients with MCA main stem occlusion studied within 6 hours of symptom onset, 27 developed malignant MCA infarction. Larger DWI lesion (per 1 mL OR was 1.04; 1.02–1.06) and combined MCA plus internal carotid artery occlusion (5.38; 1.55–18.68) were independent predictors of malignant infarction in a multivariate binary regression analysis. DWI volumes of 66 and 79 mL were identified as optimal thresholds in an receiver operating characteristic analysis with sensitivity 0.63 and 0.59 and specificity 0.98 and 0.95 respectively. A prespecified DWI volume of greater than 82 mL predicted malignant evolution with sensitivity of 0.52, specificity of 0.98, PPV of 0.88, and NPV of 0.90, and ICA and MCA occlusion, respectively, with 0.7, 0.63, 0.31, and 0.90.[96] A subsequent study of 135 patients from the same cohort with available 24-hour NIHSS data from symptom onset were included in a classification and regression trees analysis; the same number of patients (n = 27) developed malignant MCA infarct. DWI volume greater than or equal to 78 mL and NIHSS greater than or equal to 22 were identified as optimal cutoffs.[97]

Data from retrospective studies are also available. In a study of 37 patients with acute MCA infarction and proximal vessel occlusion (carotid-T, MCA main stem) who were imaged within 6 hours of symptom onset, the best predictor for malignant evolution was ADC less than 80% (denoting 80% threshold ADC values compared with the contralateral unaffected hemisphere) of greater than 82 mL, with a sensitivity of 87% and specificity of 91%.[98] In another study of 28 patients with an MCA infarct and proven MCA or carotid T occlusion on MR imaging angiography performed within 14 hours after onset, 10 developed malignant edema. Total MCA territory infarct, and DWI volume greater than 145 mL were univariate predictors of a malignant course. Infarct volume greater than 145 mL on DWI provided a sensitivity of 100%, specificity of 94%, PPV of 91%, and NPV of 100%. Additional bivariate models combining volume on DWI and ADC increased the sensitivity and specificity to 100%.[99] A subsequent study of 51 patients with proximal MCA occlusion suggested a cutoff infarct volume of 177 mL predictive of a malignant course with 0.82 accuracy (sensitivity, 0.88; specificity, 0.77; PPV, 0.64; NPV, 0.93).[100] Additional studies using various DWI infarct volume cutoffs greater than 145 mL showed a high probability to develop malignant edema requiring hemicraniectomy[101]; infarct volume greater than 160 mL on DWI achieved a 97% specificity and 76% sensitivity.[95]

Treatment of cerebral edema after acute ischemic stroke is medical and surgical. Induction of an osmolar gap between the serum and the brain may remove water out of the latter and allow more space within the tight, closed cranial cavity. Both mannitol and hypertonic saline seem to be safe, but osmolar gap (with mannitol) and sodium levels and serum osmolality (with hypertonic saline) should be frequently monitored to guide treatment of cerebral edema and tissue shifts.[102] Mannitol boluses decrease the volume of noninfarcted brain relative to infarcted areas.[103] Although emergent administration of hypertonic saline for transtentorial herniation can halt or reverse the process,[104] a systematic review of acute ischemic stroke management did not find enough evidence to support the use of mannitol use.[105] A small case series using PET to compare equiosmolar doses of mannitol with 23.4% saline in treating edema from stroke

showed no change in CBV, oxygen extraction fraction, and CMRO$_2$ (metabolic rate of oxygen consumption) after administration of either agent. However, the contralateral, healthy hemisphere demonstrated a significant correlation between cerebral blood flow change and baseline mean arterial pressure with either agent.[106] If medical treatment fails, or there is strong prognostication for malignant edema development (discussed previously), decompressive craniectomy, especially in patients less than 60 years of age should be entertained early (within 24–48 hours from stroke onset), and certainly before signs of transtentorial herniation appear.[102,107]

EARLY BIOMARKERS OF POST-STROKE RECOVERY

Stroke is a heterogeneous condition with regard to presentation, response to treatment, and recovery process. The development of biomarkers of stroke recovery is expected to improve the design of future clinical trials and help customize rehabilitative care for individual stroke patients. Various clinical, neurophysiologic, and neuroimaging markers have been proposed with regard to the recovery of motor function, somatosensory function, cognition, and language,[108] primarily relying on MR imaging techniques:

1. Diffusion tensor imaging has been particularly used in the study of the recovery of the corticospinal tract. Measures of disruption of the microstructural integrity of the brain or the descending white matter tracts (eg, axial diffusivity, or fractional anisotropy) were shown to be associated with worse motor outcomes.[109]
2. Resting state functional MR imaging helps assess resting state functional connectivity. This is particularly relevant in the study of interconnected remote areas within the language network, and, therefore, in the prognostication of recovery from post-stroke aphasia.[110]
3. Even routine MR imaging sequences during the hyperacute stroke phase (before thrombolysis) may provide valuable prognostic information.[111]

REFERENCES

1. Terruso V, D'Amelio M, Di Benedetto N, et al. Frequency and determinants for hemorrhagic transformation of cerebral infarction. Neuroepidemiology 2009;33(3):261–5.
2. Group Nt-PSS. Intracerebral hemorrhage after intravenous t-PA therapy for ischemic stroke. The NINDS t-PA Stroke Study Group. Stroke 1997;28(11):2109–18.

3. Goyal M, Menon BK, Van Zwam WH, et al. Endovascular thrombectomy after large-vessel ischaemic stroke: a meta-analysis of individual patient data from five randomised trials. Lancet 2016; 387(10029):1723–31.

4. Nogueira RG, Jadhav AP, Haussen DC, et al. Thrombectomy 6 to 24 hours after stroke with a mismatch between deficit and infarct. N Engl J Med 2018;378(1):11–21.

5. Albers GW, Marks MP, Kemp S, et al. Thrombectomy for stroke at 6 to 16 hours with selection by perfusion imaging. N Engl J Med 2018;378(8): 708–18.

6. Coutinho JM, Liebeskind DS, Slater L-A, et al. Combined intravenous thrombolysis and thrombectomy vs thrombectomy alone for acute ischemic stroke: a pooled analysis of the SWIFT and STAR studies. JAMA Neurol 2017;74(3):268–74.

7. Wang H, Zi W, Hao Y, et al. Direct endovascular treatment: an alternative for bridging therapy in anterior circulation large-vessel occlusion stroke. Eur J Neurol 2017;24(7):935–43.

8. Glen CJ, DaZhi L, Boryana S, et al. Hemorrhagic transformation after ischemic stroke in animals and humans. J Cereb Blood Flow Metab 2014; 34(2):185–99.

9. Furlan A, Higashida R, Wechsler L, et al. Intra-arterial prourokinase for acute ischemic stroke: the PROACT II study: a randomized controlled trial. JAMA 1999;282(21):2003–11.

10. Molina CA, Montaner J, Abilleira S, et al. Timing of spontaneous recanalization and risk of hemorrhagic transformation in acute cardioembolic stroke. Stroke 2001;32(5):1079–84.

11. Rha JH, Saver JL. The impact of recanalization on ischemic stroke outcome: a meta-analysis. Stroke 2007;38(3):967–73.

12. Wang W, Li M, Chen Q, et al. Hemorrhagic transformation after tissue plasminogen activator reperfusion therapy for ischemic stroke: mechanisms, models, and biomarkers. Mol Neurobiol 2015; 52(3):1572–9.

13. Lo EH, Broderick JP, Moskowitz MA. tPA and proteolysis in the neurovascular unit. Stroke 2004;35(2): 354–6.

14. Teng D, Pannell JS, Rennert RC, et al. Endothelial trauma from mechanical thrombectomy in acute stroke: in vitro live-cell platform with animal validation. Stroke 2015;46(4):1099–106.

15. Fiorelli M, Bastianello S, von Kummer R, et al. Hemorrhagic transformation within 36 hours of a cerebral infarct: relationships with early clinical deterioration and 3-month outcome in the European Cooperative Acute Stroke Study I (ECASS I) cohort. Stroke 1999;30(11):2280–4.

16. von Kummer R, Broderick JP, Campbell BC, et al. The Heidelberg Bleeding Classification:

classification of bleeding events after ischemic stroke and reperfusion therapy. Stroke 2015; 46(10):2981–6.

17. National Institute of Neurological Disorders and Stroke rt-PA Stroke Study Group. Tissue plasminogen activator for acute ischemic stroke. N Engl J Med 1995;333(24):1581–7.

18. Hacke W, Kaste M, Bluhmki E, et al. Thrombolysis with alteplase 3 to 4.5 hours after acute ischemic stroke. N Engl J Med 2008;359(13):1317–29.

19. del Zoppo GJ, Higashida RT, Furlan AJ, et al. PROACT: a phase II randomized trial of recombinant pro-urokinase by direct arterial delivery in acute middle cerebral artery stroke. PROACT Investigators. Prolyse in acute cerebral thromboembolism. Stroke 1998;29(1):4–11.

20. Hacke W, Kaste M, Fieschi C, et al. Randomised double-blind placebo-controlled trial of thrombolytic therapy with intravenous alteplase in acute ischaemic stroke (ECASS II). Lancet 1998; 352(9136):1245–51.

21. Wahlgren N, Ahmed N, Eriksson N, et al. Multivariable analysis of outcome predictors and adjustment of main outcome results to baseline data profile in randomized controlled trials: Safe Implementation of Thrombolysis in Stroke-MOnitoring STudy (SITS-MOST). Stroke 2008;39(12):3316–22.

22. Menon BK, Saver JL, Prabhakaran S, et al. Risk score for intracranial hemorrhage in patients with acute ischemic stroke treated with intravenous tissue-type plasminogen activator. Stroke 2012; 43(9):2293–9.

23. Sandercock P, Lindley R, Wardlaw J, et al. The Third International Stroke Trial (IST-3) of thrombolysis for acute ischaemic stroke. Trials 2008;9(1):37.

24. Yaghi S, Willey JZ, Cucchiara B, et al. Treatment and outcome of hemorrhagic transformation after intravenous alteplase in acute ischemic stroke: a scientific statement for healthcare professionals from the American Heart Association/American Stroke Association. Stroke 2017;48(12):e343–61.

25. Eissa A, Krass I, Bajorek B. Optimizing the management of acute ischaemic stroke: a review of the utilization of intravenous recombinant tissue plasminogen activator (tPA). J Clin Pharm Ther 2012;37(6):620–9.

26. Jickling GC, Liu D, Stamova B, et al. Hemorrhagic transformation after ischemic stroke in animals and humans. J Cereb Blood Flow Metab 2014;34(2): 185–99.

27. Paciaroni M, Agnelli G, Corea F, et al. Early hemorrhagic transformation of brain infarction: rate, predictive factors, and influence on clinical outcome: results of a prospective multicenter study. Stroke 2008;39(8):2249–56.

28. Batchelor C, Pordeli P, d'Esterre CD, et al. Use of noncontrast computed tomography and computed

tomographic perfusion in predicting intracerebral hemorrhage after intravenous alteplase therapy. Stroke 2017;48(6):1548–53.

29. Horsch AD, Bennink E, van Seeters T, et al. Computed tomography perfusion derived blood-brain barrier permeability does not yet improve prediction of hemorrhagic transformation. Cerebrovasc Dis 2018;45(1–2):26–32.

30. Puig J, Blasco G, Daunis IEP, et al. High-permeability region size on perfusion CT predicts hemorrhagic transformation after intravenous thrombolysis in stroke. PLoS One 2017;12(11): e0188238.

31. Bonatti M, Lombardo F, Zamboni GA, et al. Iodine extravasation quantification on dual-energy CT of the brain performed after mechanical thrombectomy for acute ischemic stroke can predict hemorrhagic complications. AJNR Am J Neuroradiol 2018;39(3):441–7.

32. Charidimou A, Shoamanesh A, Wilson D, et al. Cerebral microbleeds and postthrombolysis intracerebral hemorrhage risk: updated meta-analysis. Neurology 2015;85(11):927–34.

33. Yu Y, Guo D, Lou M, et al. Prediction of hemorrhagic transformation severity in acute stroke from source perfusion MRI. IEEE Trans Biomed Eng 2017;PP(99):1.

34. Nael K, Knitter JR, Jahan R, et al. Multiparametric magnetic resonance imaging for prediction of parenchymal hemorrhage in acute ischemic stroke after reperfusion therapy. Stroke 2017; 48(3):664–70.

35. Gupta R, Sun C-HJ, Rochestie D, et al. Presence of the hyperintense acute reperfusion marker on MRI after mechanical thrombectomy for large vessel occlusion is associated with worse early neurological recovery. J Neurointerv Surg 2017;9(7):641–3.

36. Warach S, Latour LL. Evidence of reperfusion injury, exacerbated by thrombolytic therapy, in human focal brain ischemia using a novel imaging marker of early blood-brain barrier disruption. Stroke 2004;35(11 Suppl 1):2659–61.

37. Huisman TA. Intracranial hemorrhage: ultrasound, CT and MRI findings. Eur Radiol 2005;15(3):434–40.

38. Parizel P, Makkat S, Van Miert E, et al. Intracranial hemorrhage: principles of CT and MRI interpretation. Eur Radiol 2001;11(9):1770–83.

39. Reimer P, Parizel PM, Meaney JF, et al. Clinical MR imaging. Springer-Verlag Berlin Heidelberg; 2010.

40. Powers WJ, Rabinstein AA, Ackerson T, et al. 2018 guidelines for the early management of patients with acute ischemic stroke: a guideline for healthcare professionals from the American Heart Association/American Stroke Association. Stroke 2018; 49(3):e46–110.

41. Hemphill JC, Greenberg SM, Anderson CS, et al. Guidelines for the management of spontaneous intracerebral hemorrhage: a guideline for healthcare professionals from the American Heart Association/American Stroke Association. Stroke 2015; 46(7):2032–60.

42. Wada R, Aviv RI, Fox AJ, et al. CT angiography "spot sign" predicts hematoma expansion in acute intracerebral hemorrhage. Stroke 2007;38(4):1257–62.

43. Demchuk AM, Dowlatshahi D, Rodriguez-Luna D, et al. Prediction of haematoma growth and outcome in patients with intracerebral haemorrhage using the CT-angiography spot sign (PREDICT): a prospective observational study. Lancet Neurol 2012;11(4):307–14.

44. Orito K, Hirohata M, Nakamura Y, et al. Leakage sign for primary intracerebral hemorrhage: a novel predictor of hematoma growth. Stroke 2016;47(4): 958–63.

45. Li Q, Zhang G, Xiong X, et al. Black hole sign: novel imaging marker that predicts hematoma growth in patients with intracerebral hemorrhage. Stroke 2016;47(7):1777–81.

46. Li Q, Liu Q-J, Yang W-S, et al. Island sign: an imaging predictor for early hematoma expansion and poor outcome in patients with intracerebral hemorrhage. Stroke 2017;48(11):3019–25.

47. Shimoda Y, Ohtomo S, Arai H, et al. Satellite sign: a poor outcome predictor in intracerebral hemorrhage. Cerebrovasc Dis 2017;44(3–4):105–12.

48. Li Q, Zhang G, Huang YJ, et al. Blend sign on computed tomography: novel and reliable predictor for early hematoma growth in patients with intracerebral hemorrhage. Stroke 2015;46(8):2119–23.

49. Selariu E, Zia E, Brizzi M, et al. Swirl sign in intracerebral haemorrhage: definition, prevalence, reliability and prognostic value. BMC Neurol 2012; 12(1):109.

50. Morotti A, Brouwers HB, Romero JM, et al. Intensive blood pressure reduction and spot sign in intracerebral hemorrhage: a secondary analysis of a randomized clinical trial. JAMA Neurol 2017; 74(8):950–60.

51. Arboix A, Comes E, Massons J, et al. Relevance of early seizures for in-hospital mortality in acute cerebrovascular disease. Neurology 1996;47(6): 1429–35.

52. Burn J, Dennis M, Bamford J, et al. Epileptic seizures after a first stroke: the Oxfordshire Community Stroke Project. BMJ 1997;315(7122):1582–7.

53. Camilo O, Goldstein LB. Seizures and epilepsy after ischemic stroke. Stroke 2004;35(7):1769–75.

54. Huang CW, Saposnik G, Fang J, et al. Influence of seizures on stroke outcomes: a large multicenter study. Neurology 2014;82(9):768–76.

55. Reith J, Jorgensen HS, Nakayama H, et al. Seizures in acute stroke: predictors and prognostic significance. The Copenhagen Stroke Study. Stroke 1997;28(8):1585–9.

56. Berges S, Moulin T, Berger E, et al. Seizures and epilepsy following strokes: recurrence factors. Eur Neurol 2000;43(1):3–8.

57. Lamy C, Domigo V, Semah F, et al. Early and late seizures after cryptogenic ischemic stroke in young adults. Neurology 2003;60(3):400–4.

58. Paolucci S, Silvestri G, Lubich S, et al. Poststroke late seizures and their role in rehabilitation of inpatients. Epilepsia 1997;38(3):266–70.

59. Gupta SR, Naheedy MH, Elias D, et al. Postinfarction seizures. A clinical study. Stroke 1988;19(12): 1477–81.

60. Labovitz DL, Hauser WA, Sacco RL. Prevalence and predictors of early seizure and status epilepticus after first stroke. Neurology 2001;57(2):200–6.

61. Krakow K, Sitzer M, Rosenow F, et al. Predictors of acute poststroke seizures. Cerebrovasc Dis 2010; 30(6):584–9.

62. Szaflarski JP, Rackley AY, Kleindorfer DO, et al. Incidence of seizures in the acute phase of stroke: a population-based study. Epilepsia 2008;49(6): 974–81.

63. Denier C, Masnou P, Mapoure Y, et al. Watershed infarctions are more prone than other cortical infarcts to cause early-onset seizures. Arch Neurol 2010;67(10):1219–23.

64. Alberti A, Paciaroni M, Caso V, et al. Early seizures in patients with acute stroke: frequency, predictive factors, and effect on clinical outcome. Vasc Health Risk Manag 2008;4(3):715–20.

65. Thevathasan A, Naylor J, Churilov L, et al. Association between hemorrhagic transformation after endovascular therapy and poststroke seizures. Epilepsia 2018;59(2):403–9.

66. Vilela P. Acute stroke differential diagnosis: stroke mimics. Eur J Radiol 2017;96:133–44.

67. Rolak LA, Rutecki P, Ashizawa T, et al. Clinical features of Todd's post-epileptic paralysis. J Neurol Neurosurg Psychiatry 1992;55(1):63–4.

68. Hassan AE, Cu SR, Rodriguez GJ, et al. Regional cerebral hyperperfusion associated with postictal paresis. J Vasc Interv Neurol 2012;5(1):40–2.

69. Kubiak-Balcerewicz K, Fiszer U, Naganska E, et al. Differentiating stroke and seizure in acute setting-perfusion computed tomography? J Stroke Cerebrovasc Dis 2017;26(6):1321–7.

70. Rennebaum F, Kassubek J, Pinkhardt E, et al. Status epilepticus: clinical characteristics and EEG patterns associated with and without MRI diffusion restriction in 69 patients. Epilepsy Res 2016;120: 55–64.

71. Lansberg MG, O'Brien MW, Norbash AM, et al. MRI abnormalities associated with partial status epilepticus. Neurology 1999;52(5):1021–7.

72. Chu K, Kang DW, Kim JY, et al. Diffusion-weighted magnetic resonance imaging in nonconvulsive status epilepticus. Arch Neurol 2001;58(6):993–8.

73. Senn P, Lovblad KO, Zutter D, et al. Changes on diffusion-weighted MRI with focal motor status epilepticus: case report. Neuroradiology 2003;45(4): 246–9.

74. Szabo K, Poepel A, Pohlmann-Eden B, et al. Diffusion-weighted and perfusion MRI demonstrates parenchymal changes in complex partial status epilepticus. Brain 2005;128(Pt 6):1369–76.

75. Briellmann RS, Wellard RM, Jackson GD. Seizure-associated abnormalities in epilepsy: evidence from MR imaging. Epilepsia 2005;46(5):760–6.

76. Nguyen D, Kapina V, Seeck M, et al. Ictal hyperperfusion demonstrated by arterial spin-labeling MRI in status epilepticus. J Neuroradiol 2010;37(4):250–1.

77. Warach S, Levin JM, Schomer DL, et al. Hyperperfusion of ictal seizure focus demonstrated by MR perfusion imaging. AJNR Am J Neuroradiol 1994; 15(5):965–8.

78. Kanazawa Y, Morioka T, Arakawa S, et al. Nonconvulsive partial status epilepticus mimicking recurrent infarction revealed by diffusion-weighted and arterial spin labeling perfusion magnetic resonance images. J Stroke Cerebrovasc Dis 2015; 24(4):731–8.

79. Yacoub HA, Fenstermacher N, Castaldo J. Postictal Todd's paralysis associated with focal cerebral hypoperfusion on magnetic resonance perfusion studies. J Vasc Interv Neurol 2015;8(2):32–4.

80. Leonhardt G, de Greiff A, Weber J, et al. Brain perfusion following single seizures. Epilepsia 2005;46(12):1943–9.

81. Donaire A, Carreno M, Gomez B, et al. Cortical laminar necrosis related to prolonged focal status epilepticus. J Neurol Neurosurg Psychiatry 2006; 77(1):104–6.

82. Cianfoni A, Caulo M, Cerase A, et al. Seizure-induced brain lesions: a wide spectrum of variably reversible MRI abnormalities. Eur J Radiol 2013; 82(11):1964–72.

83. Glauser T, Shinnar S, Gloss D, et al. Evidence-based guideline: treatment of convulsive status epilepticus in children and adults: report of the guideline committee of the American Epilepsy Society. Epilepsy Curr 2016;16(1):48–61.

84. Hacke W, Schwab S, Horn M, et al. 'Malignant' middle cerebral artery territory infarction: clinical course and prognostic signs. Arch Neurol 1996; 53(4):309–15.

85. von Kummer R, Meyding-Lamade U, Forsting M, et al. Sensitivity and prognostic value of early CT in occlusion of the middle cerebral artery trunk. AJNR Am J Neuroradiol 1994;15(1):9–15 [discussion: 16–8].

86. Krieger DW, Demchuk AM, Kasner SE, et al. Early clinical and radiological predictors of fatal brain swelling in ischemic stroke. Stroke 1999;30(2): 287–92.

87. Kucinski T, Koch C, Grzyska U, et al. The predictive value of early CT and angiography for fatal hemispheric swelling in acute stroke. AJNR Am J Neuroradiol 1998;19(5):839–46.

88. Kasner SE, Demchuk AM, Berrouschot J, et al. Predictors of fatal brain edema in massive hemispheric ischemic stroke. Stroke 2001;32(9):2117–23.

89. Mori K, Aoki A, Yamamoto T, et al. Aggressive decompressive surgery in patients with massive hemispheric embolic cerebral infarction associated with severe brain swelling. Acta Neurochir (Wien) 2001;143(5):483–91 [discussion: 491–2].

90. Manno EM, Nichols DA, Fulgham JR, et al. Computed tomographic determinants of neurologic deterioration in patients with large middle cerebral artery infarctions. Mayo Clin Proc 2003; 78(2):156–60.

91. Barber PA, Demchuk AM, Zhang J, et al. Computed tomographic parameters predicting fatal outcome in large middle cerebral artery infarction. Cerebrovasc Dis 2003;16(3):230–5.

92. Maramattom BV, Bahn MM, Wijdicks EF. Which patient fares worse after early deterioration due to swelling from hemispheric stroke? Neurology 2004;63(11):2142–5.

93. Lee SJ, Lee KH, Na DG, et al. Multiphasic helical computed tomography predicts subsequent development of severe brain edema in acute ischemic stroke. Arch Neurol 2004;61(4):505–9.

94. Ryoo JW, Na DG, Kim SS, et al. Malignant middle cerebral artery infarction in hyperacute ischemic stroke: evaluation with multiphasic perfusion computed tomography maps. J Comput Assist Tomogr 2004;28(1):55–62.

95. Park J, Goh DH, Sung JK, et al. Timely assessment of infarct volume and brain atrophy in acute hemispheric infarction for early surgical decompression: strict cutoff criteria with high specificity. Acta Neurochir (Wien) 2012;154(1):79–85.

96. Thomalla G, Hartmann F, Juettler E, et al. Prediction of malignant middle cerebral artery infarction by magnetic resonance imaging within 6 hours of symptom onset: a prospective multicenter observational study. Ann Neurol 2010;68(4):435–45.

97. Kruetzelmann A, Hartmann F, Beck C, et al. Combining magnetic resonance imaging within six-hours of symptom onset with clinical follow-up at 24 h improves prediction of 'malignant' middle cerebral artery infarction. Int J stroke 2014;9(2):210–4.

98. Thomalla GJ, Kucinski T, Schoder V, et al. Prediction of malignant middle cerebral artery infarction by early perfusion- and diffusion-weighted magnetic resonance imaging. Stroke 2003;34(8): 1892–9.

99. Oppenheim C, Samson Y, Manai R, et al. Prediction of malignant middle cerebral artery infarction by diffusion-weighted imaging. Stroke 2000;31(9): 2175–81.

100. Foerch C, Otto B, Singer OC, et al. Serum S100B predicts a malignant course of infarction in patients with acute middle cerebral artery occlusion. Stroke 2004;35(9):2160–4.

101. Bektas H, Wu TC, Kasam M, et al. Increased blood-brain barrier permeability on perfusion CT might predict malignant middle cerebral artery infarction. Stroke 2010;41(11):2539–44.

102. Torbey MT, Bosel J, Rhoney DH, et al. Evidence-based guidelines for the management of large hemispheric infarction: a statement for health care professionals from the Neurocritical Care Society and the German Society for Neuro-intensive Care and Emergency Medicine. Neurocrit Care 2015;22(1):146–64.

103. Videen TO, Zazulia AR, Manno EM, et al. Mannitol bolus preferentially shrinks non-infarcted brain in patients with ischemic stroke. Neurology 2001; 57(11):2120–2.

104. Koenig MA, Bryan M, Lewin JL 3rd, et al. Reversal of transtentorial herniation with hypertonic saline. Neurology 2008;70(13):1023–9.

105. Bereczki D, Liu M, Prado GF, et al. Cochrane report: a systematic review of mannitol therapy for acute ischemic stroke and cerebral parenchymal hemorrhage. Stroke 2000;31(11):2719–22.

106. Diringer MN, Scalfani MT, Zazulia AR, et al. Cerebral hemodynamic and metabolic effects of equiosmolar doses mannitol and 23.4% saline in patients with edema following large ischemic stroke. Neurocrit Care 2011;14(1):11–7.

107. Vahedi K, Hofmeijer J, Juettler E, et al. Early decompressive surgery in malignant infarction of the middle cerebral artery: a pooled analysis of three randomised controlled trials. Lancet Neurol 2007; 6(3):215–22.

108. Boyd LA, Hayward KS, Ward NS, et al. Biomarkers of stroke recovery: consensus-based core recommendations from the stroke recovery and rehabilitation roundtable. Neurorehabil Neural Repair 2017;31(10–11):864–76.

109. Puig J, Blasco G, Schlaug G, et al. Diffusion tensor imaging as a prognostic biomarker for motor recovery and rehabilitation after stroke. Neuroradiology 2017;59(4):343–51.

110. Klingbeil J, Wawrzyniak M, Stockert A, et al. Resting-state functional connectivity: an emerging method for the study of language networks in post-stroke aphasia. Brain Cogn, in press.

111. Emeriau S, Soize S, Riffaud L, et al. Parenchymal FLAIR hyperintensity before thrombolysis is a prognostic factor of ischemic stroke outcome at 3 Tesla. J Neuroradiol 2015;42(5):269–77.

Reperfusion Changes After Stroke and Practical Approaches for Neuroprotection

Jae H. Choi, MD, MS[a,b,c,*], John Pile-Spellman, MD[a,c]

KEYWORDS

- Acute ischemic stroke • Ischemia/reperfusion • Reperfusion injury • Hemorrhagic transformation
- Neuroprotection • Ischemic conditioning • Therapeutic hypothermia • Selective brain cooling

KEY POINTS

- Early reperfusion therapy with systemic thrombolysis and endovascular mechanical devices improves outcome in patients with acute ischemic stroke.
- Reperfusion is not without risk and may paradoxically exacerbate ischemia-induced damages and result in reperfusion injury.
- Reperfusion injury is caused by ischemia-induced structural and functional changes that are sustained or amplified by reperfusion and includes hyperperfusion, impairment of vasomotor regulation, and disruption of the blood-brain barrier.
- The underlying mechanisms that promote the occurrence of such changes include excitotoxicity, ion disturbance, free radical production, inflammation, and apoptosis.
- Pleiotropic mechanism of action, endogenous properties, targeted delivery to the organ of interest, and improved speed and depth of cooling make selective brain hypothermia a promising adjunct neuroprotective strategy to counter ischemic and reperfusion injury.

INTRODUCTION

The principle concept of treatment of acute ischemic stroke aims at reperfusion of the ischemic region.[1] Reperfusion is the most intuitive countermeasure when blood has stopped, which is the direct translation of *ischemia*, a term of Greek origin. Dependent on a constant instream of oxygen and glucose, the glucose content of the affected brain tissue is quickly depleted, albeit compensation is possible with sufficient collateral perfusion, when a blood supplying artery acutely occludes and ischemia ensues.[2] Current reperfusion strategies involve pharmacologic therapy (recombinant

tissue plasminogen activator [rtPA]), mechanical (stent-retriever devices) and physical methods (suction devices), and any combinations thereof.[1,3] With the latest endovascular devices, reperfusion is successfully achieved in 70% to 80% of cases.[4–8] Clinical trials have shown that early reopening of the vessel and reperfusing the affected tissue with blood from the circulation reduce infarct size and improves clinical outcome.

If performed early and guided by clinical and imaging-based selection criteria, ischemic tissue may be salvaged with reperfusion therapy.[1] Reperfusion is also associated, however, with several molecular pathways that lead to local functional

a Center for Unruptured Brain Aneurysms, Neurological Surgery PC, 1991 Marcus Avenue, Suite 108, Lake Success, NY 11042, USA; b Department of Neurology, State University of New York Downstate Medical Center, 450 Clarkson Avenue, Brooklyn, NY 11203, USA; c Hybernia Medical LLC, 626 RexCorp Plaza, Uniondale, NY 11556, USA
* Corresponding author. Center for Unruptured Brain Aneurysms, Neurological Surgery PC, 1991 Marcus Avenue, Suite 108, Lake Success, NY 11042.
E-mail address: jae.h.choi.0524@gmail.com

Neuroimag Clin N Am 28 (2018) 663–682
https://doi.org/10.1016/j.nic.2018.06.008
1052-5149/18/© 2018 Elsevier Inc. All rights reserved.

and structural changes and may ultimately lead to cell death despite full restoration of cerebral blood flow (CBF) (Figs. 1–6A–D).[9,10] Clinically, these pathways may manifest as intracerebral hemorrhage, brain edema, failure of ischemia regression, and neurologic worsening. These unwanted effects arising from recanalizing an occluded vessel, also known as reperfusion injury, were described first in a canine coronary model where early reperfusion after coronary ligation produced ischemic myocardial damages much more pronounced than the damages found during long-term occlusion.[11] Reperfusion injury, thus, is not unique to the brain but also occurs after reperfusion therapy after myocardial and limb ischemia.[11,12] In addition, reperfusion injury after pharmacolytic therapy, for example, with rtPA, may be an aggregate result of reperfusion-related mechanisms, on one hand, and thrombolytic and other molecular activities of rtPA, on the other.[13]

Complications of reperfusion therapy are not uncommon and among the most feared is hemorrhagic transformation (Tables 1–4). Hemorrhagic transformation is divided into the clinically relevant symptomatic type and less critical asymptomatic types. Hemorrhagic transformation is also part of the natural history of ischemic stroke and ischemic injury itself, however, thus occurring in patients without early recanalization (see Table 1).[4,5,14–18] Hemorrhagic transformation is only 1 of multiple clinical manifestations of reperfusion injury and there are several functional and structural changes that constitute the basis of this phenomenon. Underlying those functional and structural changes are molecular mechanisms that are promoted by reperfusion and trigger cascades that may prevent the recovery of ischemic brain tissue despite successful reperfusion.

This article reviews the mechanisms involved in the occurrence of reperfusion injury after stroke. Neuroprotective strategies are discussed that are unrelated to the concept of reperfusion but use endogenous properties, including selective brain hypothermia.

CLINICAL FACTORS OF REPERFUSION INJURY

Reperfusion therapy is associated with improved outcome after acute ischemic stroke (see Tables 1 and 2). This is true for intravenous (IV) rtPA with and without endovascular mechanical intervention (vs placebo or rtPA alone, respectively). Application of either treatment modality or combined modalities results in more successful recanalization (vs spontaneous recanalization) and better outcome (modified Rankin scale [mRS] 0–2 and mortality).[19] In large artery occlusion, it has been shown that endovascular intervention with preceding IV rtPA is superior to IV rtPA alone in terms of successful recanalization and clinical outcome without significantly increasing the risk of intracranial hemorrhage (ICH).[20] The odds of good outcome (mRS score 0–2 at 90 days) are significantly increased (vs placebo) when rtPA is given within 3 hours (odds ratio [OR] 1.75; 95% CI, 1.35–2.27) and 4.5 hours (OR 1.26; 95% CI, 1.05–1.51) from symptom onset.[21] Likewise, the odds of good outcome are significantly improved with endovascular intervention (vs tissue plasminogen activator [tPA] alone) when performed within 3 hours (OR 2.83; 95% CI, 2.07–3.86), 6 hours (OR 2.32; 95% CI, 1.56–3.44), and 8 hours (OR 2.03; 95% CI, 1.03–3.99) from symptom onset.[22] Hereby, a higher degree of recanalization is associated with improved outcome. In a study of 100 patients undergoing endovascular therapy,[23] recanalization to Thrombolysis in Cerebral Infarction (TICI) Grade 0 to 2a versus TICI 2b to 3 resulted in good outcome (mRS 0–2 at day 90) in 24% and 57% of the patients, respectively (P = .001) (see Tables 3 and 4). Also, the overall positive correlation between outcome and improving Thrombolysis in Myocardial Infarction (TIMI) and TICI scores was significant (P = .023 and P = .008).

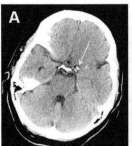 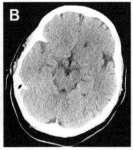 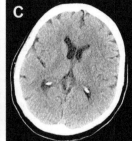 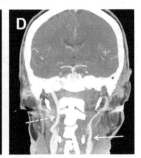

Fig. 1. Acute occlusion of the left internal carotid artery (ICA) in a 68 year-old woman. Baseline noncontrast CT approximately 1.5 hours from symptom onset with clot in the distal ICA/M1 (*solid yellow arrow*) (*A–C*). CT angiogram (coronal cut) shows no flow in the left ICA (*solid white arrow*); the right ICA is present (*dashed white arrow*) (*D*).

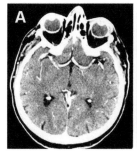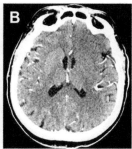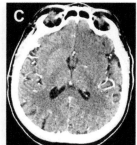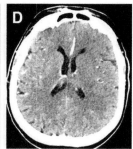

Fig. 2. On same CT angiogram as in Fig. 1 (transverse cuts), symmetric flow in contrast-enhanced cerebral arteries suggesting sufficient collateralization; in bilateral comparison, asymmetry in density between territories of the anterior circulations (A–D).

Reperfusion therapy is not without risk, however, especially with the administration of rtPA. A meta-analysis, including 3391 patients treated with rtPA and 3365 patients in the control group, found increased odds for fatal ICH with rtPA therapy (OR 7.14; 95% CI, 3.98–12.79) that was significant across the investigated ranges of treatment time-window (<3 h to >4.5 h), age (≤80 and >80 y), and baseline National Institutes of Health Stroke Scale (NIHSS) scores (0 to >22).[21] In the European Cooperative Acute Stroke Study (ECASS) II trial, 11.8% of patients treated with rtPA had parenchymal hemorrhage (PH) (Table 5).[24] The multivariate logistic model revealed increased odds for PH with rtPA therapy (OR 3.61; 95% CI, 1.78–7.31,) age (OR 1.04; 95% CI, 1.00–1.08), attenuation of density on baseline CT (OR 2.64; 95% CI, 1.59–4.39), prior congestive heart failure (OR 2.57; 95% CI, 1.16–5.71), and baseline systolic blood pressure (OR 1.02; 95% CI, 1.00–1.03 per 1–mm Hg increment).[25]

PH is associated with symptomatic ICH (SICH), which is often detrimental (mortality rates of 45%–83%).[14,16,25–28] Although the definitions of SICH vary among studies, they all include neurologic deterioration as the clinical component (Table 6).[29] Unlike PH, hemorrhagic infarction–type hemorrhagic transformation (see Table 5) has been shown to be inversely associated with early neurologic deterioration (OR 0.2; 95% CI, 0.1–0.6) and 90-day mortality (OR 0.2; 95% CI, 0.07–0.60).[30] Because rtPA administration is associated with both better recanalization and improved outcome compared with placebo, on one hand, and increased risk of SICH, on the other, it is difficult to determine, by reviewing the clinical risk factors alone, how recanalization and improved perfusion promotes reperfusion injury. It may also be a reasonable hypothesis that rtPA use and recanalization are cofactors for reperfusion injury. In addition to its fibrinolytic property, rtPA may cause systemic coagulopathy[31,32] and has been found to increase the activities of matrix metallopeptidase (MMP)-9 and N-methyl-D-aspartate (NMDA) excitotoxicity, mechanisms that are involved in the breakdown of the blood-brain barrier.[33,34] A meta-analysis involving 2066 acute ischemic stroke patients did not find any association between recanalization and SICH.[19] This analysis was performed, however, in a subset of only 678 patients. Furthermore, recanalization was quantified using the TIMI score with TIMI 2 to 3 defined as successful recanalization. Unlike the TICI scale, which is now routinely used for stroke trials, the TIMI scale does not distinguish between 2° of partial recanalization, that is, 2a and 2b

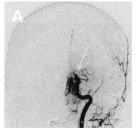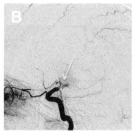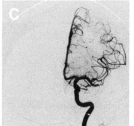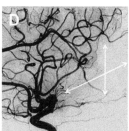

Fig. 3. Patient received IV tPA and was transferred to the angiography room for endovascular revascularization therapy. Cerebral angiogram with injection into the left ICA shows occlusion of same artery in the distal portion (solid yellow arrow) (A, B). Reperfusion into the left anterior circulation after reopening of the ICA approximately 4 hours from symptom onset with presentation of the left anterior cerebral artery and middle cerebral artery branches, except for the lower division of the MCA (space covered by solid white arrows) (C, D).

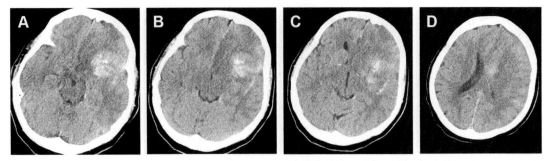

Fig. 4. Control CT shows inhomogeneous hyperdense area within the left middle cerebral artery territory suggestive of contrast extravasation and cerebral edema with beginning midline shift 8 hours postreperfusion (A–D).

(see **Tables 3** and **4**). The latest acute stroke trials define TICI 2b/3 as successful recanalization. By using the TIMI scale, the study may have lumped together successful recanalization with less successful ones, thereby reducing the true impact of recanalization on reperfusion injury.

Another meta-analysis of data from 55 studies, including 65,264 acute ischemic stroke patients treated with rtPA and with subsequent ICH in 3953 patients, found the following clinical factors associated with ICH (factors with low heterogeneity only): higher age versus lower age with cutoff at 65 years (OR 1.78; 95% CI, 1.17–2.71), renal impairment (OR 2.79; 95% CI, 1.19–6.54), congestive heart failure (OR 1.96; 95% CI, 1.30–2.94), atrial fibrillation (OR 1.86; 95% CI, 1.50–2.31); diabetes (OR 1.54; 95% CI, 1.18–2.02), prior hypertension (OR 1.50; 95% CI, 1.18–1.89), ischemic heart disease (OR 1.54; 95% CI, 1.08–2.20), prestroke statin medication (OR 1.72; 95% CI, 1.14–2.61), increasing blood glucose level (OR 1.10; 95% CI, 1.05–1.14), increasing baseline NIHSS (OR 1.08, 95%CI 1.06–1.11), lower Alberta Stroke Program Early CT Score (ASPECTS) score versus higher score with cutoff at 5 points (OR 3.46, 95%CI 1.92–6.21), and leukoaraiosis (OR 2.45; 95% CI, 1.64–3.66).[29] These results suggest that age, systemic and ischemic premorbid conditions, conditions associated with cardioembolic source,

and increased baseline stroke severity are associated with the development of post-tPA reperfusion injury. Overall, this indicates that increased vascular vulnerability and reduced capacity for repair and compensation may be underlying mechanisms for reperfusion injury. Why prior statin use is associated with SICH is undetermined. One plausible explanation is that patients with higher baseline stroke risk and more premorbid conditions were more likely to be prescribed statin medication.

A Chinese study sought to determine factors associated with SICH in 632 acute ischemic stroke patients treated with endovascular mechanical devices.[35] SICH occurred in 16% of treated patients. IV and intra-arterial (IA) thrombolytics use was similar between the SICH and non-SICH groups, with 32% (IV) and 16% (IA). Large-artery atherosclerosis was the cause of stroke in greater than 30% of cases, with the remainder having a cardioembolic source as the cause. Identified predictors of SICH after endovascular treatment included the following: cardioembolic cause (OR 1.91; 95% CI, 1.13–3.25), baseline ASPECTS score less than 6 (OR 2.27; 95% CI, 1.24–4.14), time from symptom onset to groin puncture greater than 270 min (OR 1.70; 95% CI, 1.03–2.80), poor collaterals (OR 1.97; 95% CI, 1.16–3.36), passes of retriever greater than 3 (OR 2.55;

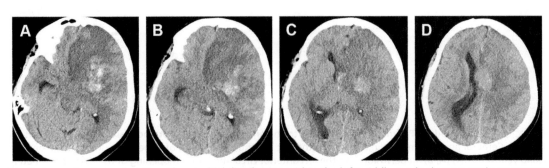

Fig. 5. Increasing hyperdensity with petechial distribution within the left middle cerebral artery territory suggestive of hemorrhagic transformation and progressive midline shift 14 hours postreperfusion (A–D).

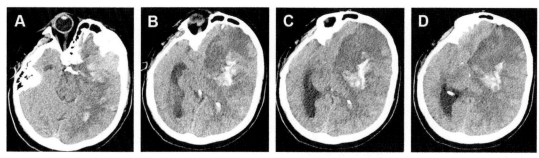

Fig. 6. Infarcted left anterior circulation territory with hyperdense demarcation in the anterior cerebral artery and upper division of the middle cerebral artery territory. Progressive hemorrhagic transformation with confluent hyperdense areas within the left middle cerebral artery territory and further demarcation with midline shift 21 hours postreperfusion (A–D).

95% CI, 1.40–4.65), and baseline neutrophil/lymphocyte ratio (OR 2.07; 95% CI, 1.24–3.46). The results of this study again suggest that cardioembolic cause and increased baseline stroke severity promote the development of reperfusion injury. This study is interesting, because all patients were treated with mechanical devices with only one-third receiving thrombolytics. Angiographic assessment of the degree of recanalization was determined in all patients. Patients with successful recanalization (TICI 2b/3) experienced hemorrhage less frequently (75.2% vs 86.3%), confirming the favorable benefit-to-risk ratio of early reperfusion therapy. In the multivariate analysis, however, it was not associated with a reduction in SICH risk. Furthermore, administration of thrombolytics was not significant in the univariate analysis and thus was not included in the final multivariate model for predictors of SICH. Given absent relationship between thrombolytic drug and ICHs in this study and lack of association between degree of recanalization and reduction in risk of hemorrhage, this may introduce the possibility that some factors related with reperfusion are involved in the occurrence of reperfusion injury. In addition, the results suggest that reduced collateral perfusion and neutrophil-mediated inflammation may play an important role.

FUNCTIONAL AND STRUCTURAL FACTORS OF REPERFUSION INJURY AND UNDERLYING MOLECULAR MECHANISMS

After cerebral ischemia and reperfusion, there is a marked increase in CBF in the previously ischemic region. This hyperperfusion phase may last several hours to more than a day postreperfusion.[36–39] In a study involving 10 acute ischemic stroke patients with spontaneous recanalization between 5 hours and 18 hours post–symptom onset, the changes in cerebral hemodynamic and metabolic parameters were assessed with PET with oxygen 15.[40]

During the acute phase of reperfusion, there was a significant increase in CBF, cerebral blood volume (CBV), cerebral metabolic rate of oxygen ($CMRO_2$), and a reduced oxygen extraction fraction (OEF) in the peri-infarct region, with average changes of +74%, +20%, +34%, and −22%, respectively, compared with the respective contralateral region. The ratio CBF/CBV was also elevated in the ipsilateral region by an average +48%. On repeat imaging 26 days later, all parameters significantly decreased in the previously ischemic region compared with the values of the acute phase, and the absolute values were similar to the contralateral values, except for the ipsilateral CBV, which was slightly lower. In the infarcted region, which was significantly smaller than the hyperperfused peri-infarct region (mean ±SD, 2.2 cm^2 ± 3.2 cm^2 vs 9.9 cm^2 ± 7.5 cm^2; $P = .005$), the parameters were similar to the ones of the contralateral side during the acute phase. From the acute phase to the chronic phase, CBF, $CMRO_2$, and OEF were significantly reduced. Neither CBV nor CBF/CBV values differed between sides or between the 2 measurements. The results of the study suggest that after ischemia-reperfusion there is a prolonged phase of hyperperfusion (CBF increase) that may be related to increased metabolic rate in the peri-infarct region, for example, due to increased protein synthesis. The increase in CBV, however, suggests a dysfunction or impairment of vasomotor regulation, so-called vasoplegia, with significantly dilated arteries within the peri-infarct area. Paradoxically, OEF is decreased during this period, which may indicate true hyperperfusion, which is beyond what is necessary for the metabolic demand (luxury perfusion). The changes in the infarcted region from acute to chronic indicate reduction of tissue metabolic rate due to cell death. Because all patients survived and no hemorrhage occurred, the investigators concluded that postreperfusion hyperperfusion may be a marker for good prognosis.

Table 1
Study characteristics and results of control groups

	National Institute of Neurological Disorders and Stroke	European Cooperative Acute Stroke Study III	Prolyse in Acute Cerebral Thromboembolism II	Interventional Management of Stroke III	Multicentre Randomised Controlled Trial of Endovascular Treatment for Acute Ischaemic Stroke in the Netherlands	Endovascular Treatment for Small Core and Anterior Circulation Proximal Occlusion with Emphasis on Minimizing CT to Recanalization Times	Endovascular Therapy Following Imaging Evaluation for Ischemic Stroke 3
Patients (N)	312	403	59	222	267	150	90
Median NIHSS	15	10	17	16	18	17	16
Treatment window	3 h	4.5 h	6 h	3 h	6 h	12 h	16 h
Sympt. ICH	0.6%	0.2%	2%	5.9%	6.4%	2.7%	4%
Asympt. ICH	2.9%	17.4%	11%	18.9%			
Timing of ICH	24 h	7 d	24 h	30 h	7 d	7 d	36 h
Sympt. ICH criteria	Suspicion or neurologic decline	NIHSS increase	NIHSS increase	Neurologic decline	NIHSS increase	NIHSS increase	NIHSS increase
Sympt. edema	9% of sympt. ICH; 4% of all ICH	7.2%					
Hemicraniectomy or malignant stroke					4.9%	10.7%	

Abbreviations: Asympt, asymptomatic; Sympt, symptomatic.

Table 2
Study characteristics and results of interventional groups

	National Institute of Neurological Disorders and Stroke	European Cooperative Acute Stroke Study III	Prolyse in Acute Cerebral Thromboembolism II	Interventional Management of Stroke III	Multicentre Randomised Controlled Trial of Endovascular Treatment for Acute Ischaemic Stroke in the Netherlands	Endovascular Treatment for Small Core and Anterior Circulation Proximal Occlusion with Emphasis on Minimizing CT to Recanalization Times	Endovascular Therapy Following Imaging Evaluation for Ischemic Stroke 3
n	312	418	121	434	233	165	92
Median NIHSS	15	9	17	17	17	16	16
Sympt. ICH	6.40%	2.40%	10%	6.20%	7.70%	3.60%	7%
Asympt. ICH	4.50%	24.60%	25%	27.40%			
Sympt. edema	9% of sympt. ICH 4% of all ICH	6.90%					
Hemicraniectomy or malignant stroke					6%	4.80%	

Abbreviations: Asympt., asymptomatic; Sympt., symptomatic.

Table 3
Thrombolysis in myocardial infarction scale

Thrombolysis in Myocardial Infarction Grade	Definition
0	Absence of any antegrade flow beyond the target occlusion (no perfusion)
1	Antegrade flow beyond the target occlusion, without distal branch filling (penetration without perfusion).
2	Delayed antegrade flow with some filling of the distal branches (partial perfusion).
3	Normal flow, which fills all distal branches (complete perfusion).

In contrast, another study in 221 acute ischemic stroke patients found that hyperperfusion (advanced MR imaging and arterial spin-labeling technique) was a predictor of hemorrhagic transformation, which occurred in 37% of the patients (OR 3.5; 95% CI, 2.0–6.3), as were IV rtPA treatment (OR 3.1; 95% CI, 1.8–5.6), endovascular mechanical thrombectomy (OR 4.1; 95% CI, 2.0–8.5), and atrial fibrillation (OR 2.0; 95% CI, 1.1–3.9).[41] There was a trend for increased risk for PH with occurrence of hyperperfusion more than 12 hours after symptom onset (vs <12 h). Predictors of hyperperfusion

Table 4
Thrombolysis in cerebral infarction scale

Thrombolysis in Cerebral Infarction Grade	Definition
0	No perfusion
1	Antegrade perfusion beyond the occlusion, but limited distal branch filling with slow distal perfusion
2a	Antegrade perfusion of less than half of the occluded artery ischemic territory
2b	Antegrade perfusion of more than half of the target artery ischemic territory
3	Antegrade perfusion of the occluded target artery ischemic territory

included IV rtPA treatment (OR 2.7; 95% CI, 1.5–4.8) and endovascular mechanical thrombectomy (OR 2.9; 95% CI, 1.4–5.8). These results indicate that early reperfusion (<12 h from symptom onset) may reduce the risk for hemorrhagic transformation, especially PH, and that hyperperfusion is associated with recanalization therapy and probably also with HT. The odds for HT were not further increased with thrombolytics compared with endovascular therapy, which may suggest appropriate patient selection and adherence to standard treatment guidelines.

Another model for hyperperfusion-mediated ICH is carotid surgery, for example, carotid endarterectomy. The complications of this hyperperfusion syndrome have been well described and occur in 20% to 40% of patients after carotid endarterectomy,[10] during which the carotid is briefly clamped and then reperfused. Hyperperfusion syndrome is associated with partial seizures, focal neurologic deficits, headache, and ICH and is defined as CBF increase of greater than 100% from baseline. The assumed mechanism is that a vascular bed that is maximally dilated (due to vasomotor dysfunction) and that has undergone ischemic changes may be more susceptible to damages from higher perfusion pressures.[42–45] Thus, blood pressure control is critical in these patients. Symptoms have also been observed in patients with less elevated blood pressure, however, leading to the formulation of the hypothesis of normal perfusion pressure breakthrough.[46,47]

Cerebral energy metabolism is primarily defined by the aerobic glycolytic pathway, which ends in oxidative phosphorylation in the mitochondrion resulting in the production of ATP and heat.[48] CBF is coupled to $CMRO_2$, which remains relatively constant globally but may show patterns of focal variation or metabolic activation, a phenomenon that is exploited in functional MR imaging studies.[49] CBF is largely regulated by nitric oxide–mediated vasomotor tone of cerebral arteries and is held at approximately 50 mL/100 g/min for an average $CMRO_2$ of 150 μmol O_2/100 g/min and cerebral glucose metabolism of 25 μmol glucose/100 g/min over a wide range of cerebral perfusion pressure (cerebral autoregulation).[46,48,50–52] With a sudden and marked reduction of perfusion, glucose must be extracted from the tissue stores. Brain glucose content, however, is only 130 μmol glucose/100 g and is depleted in 5 minutes to 6 minutes. The reason brain tissue remains salvageable for hours after an occlusion is because of collaterals.[53] As such, good collateralization has been shown to be associated with lower baseline severity (NIHSS) and higher rates of reperfusion (TICI 2b/3).[54,55] In one study,

Table 5
Imaging-based classification of hemorrhagic transformation postrecanalization

National Institute of Neurological Disorders and Stroke		European Cooperative Acute Stroke Study	
HI	Punctate hypodensity or hyperdensity within the vascular territory	HI-1	Petechiae
		HI-2	More confluent petechiae
PH	Homogeneous, hyperdense area with sharp border	PH-1	Hyperdense lesion <30% of infarcted area, mild mass effect
		PH-2	Hyperdense lesion >30% of infarcted area, significant mass effect

Abbreviation: HI, hemorrhagic infarct.

outcome was similar in patients with poor (n = 31) or good (n = 29) baseline collaterals, if reperfusion was successful. In another study in 119 acute ischemic stroke patients, good collaterals were associated with perilesional hyperperfusion (OR 5.05; 95% CI, 1.62–15.7), which was defined as the penumbral CBF greater than 130% of the healthy contralateral hemisphere.[53] The presence of perilesional hyperperfusion improved reperfusion (TICI 2b/3; OR 7.5; 95% CI, 1.6–35.1) and penumbral salvage (final infarct size < penumbra; OR 6.64; 95% CI, 1.8–24.49). Hemorrhagic transformation occurred in 17% in patients with hyperperfusion, whereas only 1% of patients without hyperperfusion were affected. All hemorrhages, however, were petechial type bleeds.

Ischemia and reperfusion are often accompanied by cerebral edema. Two types of edema are distinguished from each other: (1) cytotoxic edema, which is part of the pathway leading to cell death, and (2) vasogenic edema, which is a sign for disruption of the blood-brain barrier, that is, breakdown of endothelial cell lining and extracellular matrix. Cytotoxic edema shows as a hyperintense signal on diffusion-weighted imaging, whereas the vasogenic edema-related signal is less pronounced and variable.[56,57]

The molecular mechanisms of ischemia and reperfusion help understand the functional and structural changes over time. With ischemia and consequential metabolic depression after depletion of energy stores, inhibition and failure of the Na^+/K^+ pump lead to anoxic depolarization that is characterized by reduction of extracellular Na^+, Cl^- and rise in extracellular $K+$.[58] Diminishing oxidative phosphorylation and continuing glycolytic activity with accumulation of lactate result in a reduction of pH.[59] Depolarization and NMDA-receptor activation leads to Ca^{2+} influx into the cell.[60–64] NMDA-receptor activation is amplified by continuously elevated glutamate levels.[65–67] A rise in intracellular $Ca2^+$ activates nitric oxide synthase (NOS) and cyclooxygenase-2, leading to vasodilation and endothelial dysfunction, and free radical generation, which is exacerbated by acidity.[68,69] The thrombolytic drug, rtPA, has been found to impair vascular reactivity in arteries, which is amplified during ischemia.[70] Proinflammatory cytokines, such as interleukin-1α, interleukin-1β, and tumor necrosis factor α, increase early during ischemia.[71–75] Inflammatory responses include 1. activation of nuclear factor κ light chain enhancer of activated B cells, a strong regulator of cell-mediated immunity against infections,[76–78] 2. mitogen-activated protein kinases that induce the translation of proinflammatory proteins,[79–81] and 3. up-regulation of cell adhesion molecules on endothelial cells enabling the accumulation and transmigration of neutrophils.[82–84] Increase in matrix zinc-metalloproteinases leads to degradation of extracellular matrix.[85–87] Up-regulation of the BAX and calpain genes promote apoptosis.[88–91]

With successful reperfusion, however, the molecular changes from transient focal ischemia are

Table 6
Definition of symptomatic hemorrhage from the literature

Hemorrhage Definition	N studies (N)	Hemorrhage (CI)	Heterogeneity
Any hemorrhage with any neurologic deterioration	26	5.3% (4.6%–6.0%)	High
Any hemorrhage with significant neurologic deterioration	12	6.5% (5.8%–7.2%)	Low
Any PH with or without neurologic deterioration	9	12.2% (8.6%–15.7%)	High
PH with significant neurologic deterioration	8	4.1% (2.7%–5.5%)	High

not simply reverted to baseline conditions. Experiments in animal stroke models and in vitro models found that K[+] levels fluctuated for hours after reperfusion and Ca2[+] levels remained elevated in the infarcted area.[92–94] Despite sufficient delivery of nutrients, ATP production does not recover and glucose utilization remains reduced.[95,96] Furthermore, MMP activity stays elevated.[85] Free radical levels increase during reperfusion and cause single-strand DNA breaks, whereas these DNA breaks are usually not detected even at the end of prolonged ischemia.[97–101] Cytoskeletal damages are also amplified with reperfusion.[102] These findings suggest that many functional and structural changes are induced by reperfusion after temporary ischemia.[103] The changes are most prominent in the infarcted region and to a lesser degree in the peri-infarct area or penumbra. The structural damages are mostly attributable to free radicals and to the recruitment of leukocytes that exacerbate the destructive processes, plausible mechanisms for endothelial damages and cell death.[104–106] These changes cause vessels to become leaky and promote the breakdown of the blood-brain barrier. As a consequence, brain edema, ICH, and infarct progression may manifest as clinical findings.

Clinical investigations have been performed to better identify stroke patients who are at high risk for reperfusion injury using advanced brain imaging. In a study of 144 acute ischemic stroke patients, the investigators found that hyperintense signals in the sulcal CSF space corresponding to the site of the stroke (observed in follow-up gadolinium-enhanced, magnetic resonance–fluid-attenuated inversion recovery sequence imaging in 47 patients) occurred more often in patients who later suffered hemorrhagic transformation (vs without; 73% vs 25%, $P<.001$).[107] This enhancement of the CSF space, a sign of blood-brain barrier disruption, was also associated with reperfusion (OR 4.09; 95% CI, 1.28–13.1). Similar findings were reported with blood brain permeability measurements in acute ischemic stroke patients undergoing endovascular treatment with dynamic susceptibility contrast imaging.[108] In another study in 51 stroke patients, greater ipsilateral reductions of apparent diffusion coefficient to 70 ± 13%, CBV to 31 ± 26%, and CBF to 28 ± 19% (of values from the healthy contralateral side) were associated with hemorrhagic transformation ($P<.01$).[109] Hemorrhage occurred in 19 patients and reperfusion was established in 18 of 19 patients. In a third study with CT-MRI coregistration in 146 ischemic stroke patients, a CT-perfusion threshold of ipsilateral relative CBF and relative CBV of 2.5% of the values from the contralateral side and

reperfusion greater than 6 hours from symptom onset were associated with PH.[110] These results suggest that blood-brain barrier disruption is related to reperfusion and increases the risk for hemorrhagic transformation. Furthermore, severity and duration of ischemic damage are risk factors for breakdown of the blood-brain barrier and, thus, hemorrhagic transformation.

PRACTICAL NEUROPROTECTIVE STRATEGIES WITH ENDOGENOUS PROPERTIES: SELECTIVE BRAIN HYPOTHERMIA

With the improvement in understanding of the mechanisms involved in ischemia and reperfusion-mediated damages an impressive number of drugs (more than 1000) have been investigated for their neuroprotective properties.[111] They include Ca2[+]-channel antagonists (eg, nimodipine, papaverine, nicardipine, lubeluzole, and magnesium sulfate), NMDA receptor antagonists and γ-aminobutyric acid agonists (eg, ARL 15896, selfotel, dextrorphan, and clomethiazole), antioxidants (eg, ebselen, NXY-059, tirilazad, and simvastatin), anti-inflammatory drugs (eg, corticoids, tacrolimus, acetaminophen, nonsteroidal anti-inflammatory drugs, and rovelizumab), antiapoptotic agents (eg, growth factors and erythropoietin), oxygen delivery, and various thrombolytic agents, among others. Unfortunately, the translational efforts over the past half-century have been rarely successful and, to date, systemic rtPA administration and endovascular mechanical thrombectomy are the only Food and Drug Administration–approved first-line interventions in the treatment of acute ischemic stroke. Numerous trials have been conducted and many are ongoing, with drugs selected according to their mechanisms and current scientific understanding, that counter a specific element or cascade in the complex chain of reactions that result in ischemic and reperfusion injury and, ultimately, cell death.

One unconventional method is ischemic preconditioning, which is derived from the observation that brief episodes of ischemia (several minutes) with intermittent reperfusion lead to significant protection of the myocardium or brain from subsequent long-term ischemia.[112–117] As such, the infarct size in preconditioned dogs was only 25% of that in control animals. Significant reductions in myocardial infarct size have been found with preconditioning followed by more than 3 hours of ischemia in rats compared with not preconditioned controls (infarct volume 23 mm[3] vs 69 mm[3] 4 days postischemia).[118] This ischemic tolerance is believed to be caused by tissue adapting to oxygen deprivation leading to reduced ATP depletion on ischemia,[112,119] induction of heat shock protein improving cell and tissue repair,[114,115,120] and ability of cells to buffer more $Ca2^+$,[121,122] among others. A variation of this method, called remote ischemic preconditioning, induces ischemic tolerance in the target organ by brief repeated episodes of ischemia in a remote organ.[123,124] For instance, brief episodes of limb ischemia have been shown to induce ischemic tolerance in the brain of rats with inhibition of edema formation and reduction in blood-brain barrier permeability (2 days postischemia).[125] In another experiment in rat stroke models with 120-minute occlusion of the middle cerebral artery, the effect of limb ischemia preconditioning on infarct size was compared with the effect of conditioning at the end of the occlusion period (perconditioning) and the control group.[126] After reperfusion and at 24 hours, the investigators found that perconditioning resulted in the smallest infarct size ($P<.001$), and both preconditioning and perconditioning were superior to controls ($P<.001$).

Although ischemic conditioning is effective in animal models, it may not be practical in the clinical setting of an acute ischemic event. Preconditioning is effective up to several days before the stroke incidence. The timing of the stroke, however, is rarely known in patients. Perconditioning may be relevant because this is applied at the end of the ischemic event, but with the busy and often invasive rescue protocols for acute stroke (imaging, rtPA, and endovascular interventions), this may be logistically challenging. Nonetheless, ischemic conditioning is an interesting neuroprotective concept because it exploits an inert feature of the body, the endogenous property to develop ischemic tolerance.

Another promising neuroprotective method with endogenous properties is therapeutic hypothermia. This involves the reduction of the body temperature by several degrees Celsius below normal. It is known that the metabolic rate in living systems is temperature dependent. In the brain, CBF is coupled with $CMRO_2$, meaning a reduction in $CMRO_2$ leads to a proportional reduction in CBF and vice versa. For instance, the arctic ground squirrel is capable of surviving several months of hibernation (deprived of nutrition, water, and oxygen) because of the extremely diminished metabolic rate during this phase.[127] This extreme ischemic tolerance is enabled by self-induced hypothermia when the body temperature drops even below the freezing temperature of water.[128] It may be due to this endogenous property in mammals, because animal stroke models with a body temperature reduction of as little as 2°C have conclusively shown impressive neuroprotection with an average reduction in infarct size and improvement in neurobehavioral outcome of 44% compared with the control group.[129] Hypothermia has been found to have multiple beneficial effects in ischemic conditions (pleiotropic mechanism of action), which is why this is so promising. In addition to metabolic depression via reduction of oxygen demand, hypothermia has several other effects that are beneficial in the setting of acute ischemic stroke[130–133]: hypothermia depresses excitotoxicity (neurotransmitter and ion homeostasis),[134–136] suppresses the breakdown of the blood-brain barrier (reperfusion injury and hemorrhagic transformation),[106,137–139] attenuates neutrophil infiltration (inflammation),[140,141] prevents apoptosis (cell death),[142,143] and has endogenous neuroprotective characteristics (ischemic tolerance and hibernation).

Although systemic or body hypothermia has been successfully applied in patients with out-of-hospital cardiac arrest,[144,145] neonates with ischemic encephalopathy,[146–148] and cardiac surgery,[149–151] the translation into acute stroke care has been hampered by frequent and severe complications that occur during the phases of therapeutic hypothermia.[152–156] These include shivering, pain, summit metabolism, and significant delay to target body temperature (induction phase), ion disturbance, coagulopathy, cardiac failure, arrhythmia, and infections (maintenance phase), and rebound issues with hyperthermia and elevated intracranial pressure, vasodilation, and ion disturbance (rewarming phase), among others.

Various methods and devices are used to induce systemic hypothermia, including cold fluid infusion, ice packs, surface cooling pads, esophageal closed-loop systems that circulate cold fluids within a closed tube, and intravascular (central vein) closed-loop catheters.[155] Unlike ground squirrels, however, nonhibernating mammals do not easily tolerate a reduction in body temperature, especially when they are conscious. Thus, hypothermia induction in awake stroke patients requires a strong drug regimen that includes muscle relaxants, sedatives, and analgesics.

To minimize the systemic impact of hypothermia, speed up the cooling process, and attempt to focus cooling on the tissue or organ of interest, ie, the brain, in the setting of ischemic stroke, a more targeted approach has been the object of recent development, that is, devices that induce selective brain hypothermia. The variety of technology ranges from external applications (cooling cap and head and neck wraps), endonasal devices (coolant spray and closed-loop system), and sophisticated endovascular IA catheters with embedded sensors and controllers (closed-loop type and infusion type) (Table 7). External devices are less invasive and more practical because they

Table 7
Cooling systems and their characteristics

Cooling System	Type (Manufacturer/ Company)	Setting	Speed (°C/min)	Depth (Temperature reduction from baseline (in C)	Duration
				Cooling Parameter	
Extracorporeal cooling (reintroduction of cooled blood into systemic circulation)	Systemic cooling (Medtronic, Minneapolis, MN; ThermopeutiX, San Diego, CA)	Cardiac surgery	0.5	>10	3–6 h
Systemic cooling (surface cooling pads, intravascular and esophageal closed-loop systems)	Systemic cooling (Zoll Medical Corporation, Chelmsford, MA; Cryothermic Systems; C.R. Bard, Murray Hill, NJ; Advanced Cooling Therapy, Chicago, IL)	ICU	0.05	2–3	Days
Head and neck cooling (surface pads)	Local/systemic cooling (Emcools, Traiskirchen, Austria; Natus Medical, Pleasanton, CA)	Ambulatory, emergency room, ICU	0.05–0.1	2–3	>48 h
Transnasal cooling (coolant spray and closed-loop systems)	Local cooling (BeneChill, San Diego, CA; Quickcool AB, Scheelevagen, Sweden)	Ambulatory, ER, ICU	0.05	2	1 h
Endovascular IA cooling	Local cooling	Angiography room, ICU			
Closed-loop type	(FocalCool, Mullica Hill, NJ; Acandia, Pforzheim, Germany)		0.1	2–3	2–3 h
Infusion type	(Hybernia Medical, Uniondale, NY)		0.5	3–7	2–3 h

may be used in the ambulatory or emergency care setting. Their effectiveness in cooling the brain, however, is significantly reduced because of the physiologic barriers that the cooling devices have to overcome, including scalp, fat, and muscle tissue; external circulation; bone; and dura. Internal devices, such as endovascular catheter–based systems, are more invasive and require an angiographic setting. Their cooling effectiveness is, however, high, because they directly modify the arterial input temperature (see Table 7). As such, brain cooling to moderate hypothermic temperature can be achieved within minutes.

There is an urgent need for neuroprotective therapies. With its pleiotropic mechanisms of action, therapeutic hypothermia has great potential to improve the outcome in patients with acute ischemic stroke and in settings where brain ischemia is a major or frequent complication, for example, in out-of-hospital cardiac arrest and carotid and coronary angioplasty and stenting. For therapeutic hypothermia to be applied successfully, however, in these common medical conditions and procedures, there are performance requirements that must be met by the systems that deliver brain hypothermia. The promises and challenges of selective brain hypothermia and devices are discussed.

First, brain cooling must be delivered quickly, within minutes, if possible. This is important not only in the acute setting where "time is brain" but also in the elective scenario in which significant delays to target brain temperature are impractical and not resourceful. Endovascular selective brain cooling devices have the potential to achieve brain cooling quickly because they directly modify the arterial input temperature without the need to overcome the many layers of thermal insulation. It has been shown that temperature equilibrium between modified arterial input and brain occurs within minutes.[157,158]

Second, the system should be capable of brain cooling to at least the level of moderate hypothermia (approximately 32°C–34°C), if not to the level of deep or profound hypothermia or 27°C to 31°C. There are 3 reasons that this might be beneficial. One, although the optimal depth of cooling is the subject of ongoing research, experimental results suggest that in models of cerebral ischemia the neuroprotective effect increases with the depth of brain hypothermia.[129] In addition, during circulatory arrest, the target temperature of cerebral perfusion is often as low as 18°C, which has been shown to provide excellent neuroprotection during the phases of arrest.[159,160] Furthermore, the side effects of cooling during systemic hypothermia may not necessarily apply to the scenario where the brain is cooled selectively. At least for the induction phase, there is mounting evidence for that.[157,161,162] Again, internal selective cooling devices are likely better suited to achieve the desired depths of brain hypothermia with their ability to change the arterial input temperature.

This leads to the third point, the duration of cooling, which is also the subject of continuing debate. How long should the brain be cooled—minutes, hours, or days? Categorizing cooling according to the timing and type of ischemic injury, that is, preischemic, intraischemic, postischemic with reperfusion and without reperfusion, or with edema and without edema, may help derive a meaningful practice pattern. For instance, cold brain perfusion during circulatory arrest is intraischemic, preventative cooling. Cooling is performed for the duration of the main surgery. Prevention of reperfusion injury may apply to the period immediately after revascularization procedures, such as thrombectomy, whereas cooling before ischemia onset is preischemic, for example, in procedures with risk for iatrogenic embolic events. In the case of an acute ischemic stroke from an occlusion of a major cerebral artery with beginning midline shift due to brain edema, prolonged cooling over several days may be the goal (postischemic cooling). Clinical experience with prolonged brain cooling over many hours and days (using brain-selective devices) is scarce, however, and currently exists mostly in neonates (postglobal ischemia cooling), albeit systemic hypothermia routinely ensues during this procedure. Elective carotid angioplasty and stenting is a setting where preischemic and intraischemic cooling with endovascular IA devices could be performed. Due to the fact that external selective cooling devices are less invasive than internal devices, they are better candidates for prolonged cooling. Internal devices, especially endovascular catheters that are placed in the carotid artery, are usually not indicated beyond the duration of the procedure, which may

last several hours. In addition, the brain cooling infusion system must also keep track of the overall hemodilution and ensure sufficient oxygenation of the target tissue. Nevertheless, systemic hypothermia may occur after prolonged selective brain cooling due to the venous return, regardless of the type of local cooling device.[147,163–166] Covering the patient with heating blankets during the procedure may attenuate the systemic cooling effect.[157] Also, the rewarming phase, which may take considerable time to avoid rebound issues, adds to the overall duration that the system must be capable of performing safely. Endonasal cooling devices, although less invasive than endovascular catheters, are usually not used for more than an hour due to the cold stress to the mucous membrane.

As discussed previously, invasiveness, ease of use, and resource demand are important points to consider when developing selective brain cooling devices. For instance, the use of endovascular devices for selective brain hypothermia may be justifiable in settings where catheter intervention is the main procedure, for example, thrombectomy in acute ischemic stroke or carotid angioplasty and stenting. In an intensive or emergency care-based treatment setting, however, selective brain cooling with an endovascular device poses an unnecessary risk and uses resources beyond economic meaningfulness. This issue becomes even more prominent with extracorporeal blood cooling concepts that involve handling of blood outside the body system, which is considered high risk and usually requires the support from perfusion specialists. In cases of intractable seizures or rapidly progressing inflammatory diseases of the central nervous system, however, endovascular selective brain hypothermia may be an appealing option to investigate.

The combined use of selective and systemic cooling systems offers advantages that make it a promising clinical approach. Induction of cooling and moderate to deep brain hypothermia is achieved quickly with selective cooling devices and brain cooling is maintained over several hours. This may avoid some immediate countermechanisms against cooling, such as shivering and rapid rise in body metabolism. If prolonged hypothermia is indicated, the switch to a systemic hypothermia system is possible. Furthermore, selective brain cooling over several hours may already induce some level of systemic hypothermia, which serves as a bridge to systemic cooling.

Ultimately, the assessment of the benefits and risks of selective brain hypothermia as a standalone, adjunct, or bridging procedure must be determined in clinical trials testing the available systems in various settings. The ideal cooling system that achieves brain cooling selectively and quickly, to levels of profound hypothermia and over a duration that is sufficient for the brain to repair itself and regenerate may be unrealistic. Each selective cooling system, however, comes with distinct advantages and drawbacks that not only create challenges but also offer room for potential to achieve clinical benefit. Ingenuity in engineering, materials with excellent conductive or insulating properties, embedded sensors, and feedback-regulated smart controllers are essential in developing selective brain hypothermia systems that are able to overcome the clinical barriers against cold stress. Last but not least, the systems must be practical, be usable, and come adapted to the current clinical workflow and should offer diagnostic features with capability of monitoring local temperature, blood flow, and metabolic parameters to allow dosing of hypothermia treatment and physiology-driven care.

SUMMARY

Reperfusion therapy is the most effective treatment and the standard of care in acute ischemic stroke. Numerous trials have conclusively demonstrated that early reperfusion improves clinical outcome when based on specific selection criteria. Paradoxically, reperfusion can amplify and exacerbate the molecular changes that are triggered by ischemia. Those include excitotoxicity, ion disturbance, free radical production, inflammation, and apoptosis. Sustenance and amplification of those processes promote endothelial dysfunction, hyperperfusion, and the breakdown of the blood brain barrier. Clinical manifestations include hemorrhagic transformation, brain edema, infarct progression, and neurologic worsening. Based on the understanding of the mechanisms involved in ischemic injury, more than 1000 drugs and interventions have been selected due to their specific property to modify a single reaction or aspect within the injury cascade and studied. Rarely have they been positive. More promising interventions include those with endogenous properties, specifically procedures that induce ischemic tolerance and have multiple neuroprotective properties (pleiotropic mechanism of action). Ischemic preconditioning and remote ischemic conditioning can induce ischemic tolerance in the brain. Ischemic conditioning is less practical in the setting of acute ischemic stroke, however, because the timing of stroke must be known in advance. Therapeutic hypothermia exploits the fact that metabolism (oxygen demand) is temperature dependent and hibernating animals show profound tolerance to ischemia because of deep hypothermia during hibernation. In addition, hypothermia is characterized by pleiotropic mechanism of action resulting in tremendous neuroprotection in animal stroke models. Selective brain hypothermia is a novel concept that can provide targeted cooling of the brain, which would improve speed and depth of cooling and may avoid the many complications of systemic hypothermia.

REFERENCES

1. Jauch ED, Saver JL, Adams HP, et al. Guidelines for the early management of patients with acute ischemic stroke. Stroke 2013;44:870–947.
2. Siesjo BK. Brain energy metabolism. New York: Wiley and Sons; 1978.
3. Powers WJ, Derdeyn CP, Biller J, et al. 2015 American Heart Association/American Stroke Association Focused update of the 2013 guidelines for the early management of patients with acute ischemic stroke regarding endovascular treatment. Stroke 2015;46:3020–35.
4. Berkhemer OA, Fransen PS, Beumer D, et al, MR CLEAN Investigators. A randomized trial of intra arterial treatment for acute ischemic stroke. N Engl J Med 2015;372(1):11–20.
5. Goyal M, Demchuk AM, Menon BK, et al, ESCAPE Trial Investigators.. Randomized assessment of rapid endovascular treatment of ischemic stroke. N Engl J Med 2015;372(11):1019–30.
6. Campbell BC, Mitchell PJ, Kleinig TJ, et al, EXTEND-IA Investigators. Endovascular therapy for ischemic stroke with perfusion-imaging selection. N Engl J Med 2015;372(11):1009–18.
7. Saver JL, Goyal M, Bonafe A, et al, SWIFT PRIME Investigators. Stent-retriever thrombectomy after intravenous t-PA vs.t-PA alone in stroke. N Engl J Med 2015;372(24):2285–95.
8. Jovin TG, Chamorro A, Cobo E, et al, REVASCAT Trial Investigators. Thrombectomy within 8 hours after symptom onset in ischemic stroke. N Engl J Med 2015;372(24):2296–306.
9. Pan J, Konstas AA, Bateman B, et al. Reperfusion injury following cerebral ischemia: pathophysiology, MR imaging, and potential therapies. Neuroradiology 2007;49:93–102.
10. Karapanayioitides T, Meuli R, Devuyst G, et al. Postcarotid endarterectomy hyperperfusion or reperfusion syndrome. Stroke 2005;36:21–6.
11. Jennings RB, Sommers HM, Smyth GA, et al. Myocardial necrosis induced by temporary occlusion of a coronary artery in the dog. Arch Pathol 1960;70:68–78.
12. Beyersdorf F, Matheis G, Kruger S, et al. Avoiding reperfusion injury after limb revascularization: experimental observations and recommendations for clinical application. J Vasc Surg 1989;9:757–66.

13. Yaghi S, Willey JZ, Cucchiara B, et al. Treatment and outcome of hemorrhagic transformation after intravenous alteplase in acute ischemic stroke. Stroke 2017;48:e343–61.

14. National Institute of Neurological Disorders and Stroke rt-PA Stroke Study Group. Tissue plasminogen activator for acute ischemic stroke. N Engl J Med 1995;333:1581.

15. Hacke W, Kaste M, Bluhmki E, et al. Thrombolysis with alteplase 3 to 4.5 hours after acute ischemic stroke. N Engl J Med 2008;359:1317–29.

16. Furlan A, Higashida R, Wechsler L, et al. Intra-arterial prourokinase for acute ischemic stroke. The PROACT II study: a randomized controlled trial. Prolyse in Acute Cerebral Thromboembolism. JAMA 1999;282:2003–11.

17. Broderick JP, Palesch YY, Demchuk AM, et al, Interventional Management of Stroke (IMS) III Investigators. Endovascular therapy after intravenous t-PA versus t-PA alone for stroke. N Engl J Med 2013; 368:1265.

18. Albers GW, Marks MP, Kemp S, et al. Thrombectomy for stroke at 6 to 16 hours with selection by perfusion imaging. N Engl J Med 2018;378:708–18.

19. Rha JH, Saver JL. The impact of recanalization on ischemic stroke outcome. Stroke 2007;38:967–73.

20. Badhiwala JH, Nassiri F, Alhazzani W, et al. Endovascular thrombectomy for acute ischemic stroke: a meta-analysis. JAMA 2015;314(17):1832–43.

21. Emberson J, Lees KR, Lyden P, et al. Effect of treatment delay, age, and stroke severity on the effects of intravenous thrombolysis with alteplase for acute ischaemic stroke: a meta-analysis of individual patient data from randomised trials. Lancet 2014;384:1929–35.

22. Saver JL, Goyal M, van der Lugt A, et al. Time to treatment with endovascular thrombectomy and outcomes from ischemic stroke: a meta-analysis. JAMA 2016;316(12):1279–88.

23. Marks MP, Lansberg MG, Mlynash M, et al. Correlation of AOL recanalization, TIMI reperfusion and TICI reperfusion with infarct growth and clinical outcome. J Neurointerv Surg 2014;6(10):724–8.

24. Hacke W, Kaste M, Fieschi C, et al. Randomised double-blind placebo-controlled trial of thrombolytic therapy with intravenous alteplase in acute ischaemic stroke (ECASS II). Second European-Australasian Acute Stroke Study Investigators. Lancet 1998;352(9136):1245–51.

25. Intracerebral hemorrhage after intravenous t-PA therapy for ischemic stroke. The NINDS t-PA Stroke Study Group. Stroke 1997;28:2109–18.

26. Larrue V, von Kummer R, Muller A, et al. Risk factors for severe hemorrhagic transformation in ischemic stroke patients treated with recombinant tissue plasminogen activator. A Secondary Analysis of the European-Australasian Acute Stroke Study (ECASS II). Stroke 2001;32:438–41.

27. Larrue V, von Kummer R, del Zoppo G, et al. Hemorrhagic transformation in acute ischemic stroke. Potential contributing factors in the European Cooperative Acute Stroke Study. Stroke 1997;28:957–60.

28. Trouillas P, von Kummer R. Classification and pathogenesis of cerebral hemorrhages after thrombolysis in ischemic stroke. Stroke 2006;37:556–61.

29. Whiteley WN, Bruins K, Fernandes P, et al. Risk factors for intracranial hemorrhage in acute ischemic stroke patients treated with recombinant tissue plasminogen activator. A systematic review and meta-analysis of 55 studies. Stroke 2012;43:2904–9.

30. Berger C, Fiorelli M, Steiner T, et al. Hemorrhagic transformation of ischemic brain tissue: asymptomatic or symptomatic. Stroke 2001;32:1330–5.

31. Matosevic B, Knoflach M, Werner P, et al. Fibrinogen degradation coagulopathy and bleeding complications after stroke thrombolysis. Neurology 2013;80:1216–24.

32. Yaghi S, Boehme AK, Dibu J, et al. Treatment and outcome of thrombolysis-related hemorrhage: a multicenter retrospective study. JAMA Neurol 2015;72:1451–7.

33. Wang X, Tsuji K, Lee SR, et al. Mechanisms of hemorrhagic transformation after tissue plasminogen activator reperfusion therapy for ischemic stroke. Stroke 2004;35:2726–30.

34. Ning M, Furie KL, Koroshetz WJ, et al. Association between tPA therapy and raised early matrix metalloproteinase-9 in acute stroke. Neurology 2006;66:1550–5.

35. Hao Y, Yang D, Wang H, et al. Predictors for symptomatic intracranial hemorrhage after endovascular treatment of acute ischemic stroke. Stroke 2017; 48(5):1203–9.

36. Cipolla MJ, McCall AL, Lessov N, et al. Reperfusion decreases myogenic reactivity and alters middle cerebral artery function after focal cerebral ischemia in rats. Stroke 1997;28:176–80.

37. Cipolla MJ, Curry AB. Middle cerebral artery function after stroke: the threshold duration of reperfusion for myogenic activity. Stroke 2002;33:2094–9.

38. Tamura A, Asano T, Sano K. Correlation between rCBF and histological changes following temporary middle cerebral artery occlusion. Stroke 1980;11:487–9.

39. Gourley JK, Heistad DD. Characteristics of reactive hyperemia in the cerebral circulation. Am J Physiol 1984;246:H52–8.

40. Marchal G, Furlan M, Beaudouin V, et al. Early spontaneous hyperperfusion after stroke. A marker of favourable tissue outcome? Brain 1996;119:409–19.

41. Yu S, Liebeskind DS, Dua S, et al. Postischemic hyperperfusion on arterial spin labeled perfusion MRI

is linked to hemorrhagic transformation in stroke. J Cereb Blood Flow Metab 2015;35:630–7.

42. Morgan MK, Johnston I, Besser M, et al. Cerebral arteriovenous malformations, steal, and the hypertensive breakthrough threshold. An experimental study in rats. J Neurosurg 1987;66:563–7.

43. Huang Duong D, Young WL, Vang MC, et al. Feeding artery pressure and venous drainage pattern are primary determinants of hemorrhage from cerebral arteriovenous malformation. Stroke 1998;29:1167–76.

44. Olsen TS, Larsen B, Skriver EB, et al. Focal cerebral hyperemia in acute stroke. Incidence, pathophysiology and clinical significance. Stroke 1981; 12:598–607.

45. Macfarlane R, Moskowitz MA, Sakas DE, et al. The role of neuroeffector mechanisms in cerebral hyperperfusion syndromes. J Neurosurg 1991;75:845–55.

46. Jorgensen LG, Schroeder TV. Defective cerebrovascular autoregulation after carotid endarterectomy. Eur J Vasc Surg 1993;7:370–9.

47. Spetzler RF, Wilson CB, Weinstein P, et al. Normal perfusion pressure breakthrough theory. Clin Neurosurg 1978;25:651–72.

48. Yablonskiy DA, Ackerman JJH, Raichle ME. Coupling between changes in human brain temperature and oxidative metabolism during prolonged visual stimulation. Proc Natl Acad Sci U S A 2000;97:7603–8.

49. Hyder F, Kida I, Behar KL, et al. Quantitative functional imaging of the brain: towards mapping neuronal activity by BOLD fMRI. NMR Biomed 2001;14(7–8):413–31.

50. Derdeyn CP, Videen TO, Yundt KD, et al. Variability of cerebral blood volume and oxygen extraction: stages of cerebral haemodynamic impairment revisited. Brain 2002;125:595–607.

51. Hatazawa J, Fujita H, Kanno I, et al. Regional cerebral blood flow, blood volume, oxygen extraction fraction, and oxygen utilization rate in normal volunteers measured by the autoradiographic technique and the single breath inhalation method. Ann Nucl Med 1995;9:15–21.

52. Hawkins RA, Phelps ME, Huang SC, et al. Effect of ischemia on quantification of local cerebral glucose metabolic rate in man. J Cereb Blood Flow Metab 1981;1:37–51.

53. Bhaskar S, Bivard A, Stanwell P, et al. Baseline collateral status and infarct topography in postischaemic perilesional hyperperfusion: an arterial spin labelling study. J Cereb Blood Flow Metab 2017;37:1148–62.

54. Marks MP, Lansberg MG, Miynash M, et al. Effect of collateral blood flow on patients undergoing endovascular therapy for acute ischemic stroke. Stroke 2014;45:1035–9.

55. Bang OY, Saver JL, Kim SJ, et al. Collateral flow averts hemorrhagic transformation after endovascular therapy for acute ischemic stroke. Stroke 2011;42:2235–9.

56. Schaefer PW, Gonzalez RG, Hunter G, et al. Diagnostic value of apparent diffusion coefficient hyperintensity in selected patients with acute neurologic deficits. J Neuroimaging 2001;11:369–80.

57. Ay H, Buonanno FS, Schaefer PW, et al. Posterior leukoencephalopathy without severe hypertension: utility of diffusion-weighted MRI. Neurology 1998; 51:1369–76.

58. Goldman DE. Potential, impedance and rectification in membranes. J Gen Physiol 1944;27:37–48.

59. Gevers W. Generation of protons by metabolic processes in heart cells. J Mol Cell Cardiol 1977;11: 867–74.

60. Lipton P, Raley PKM, Lobner D. Long-term inhibition of synaptic transmission and macromolecular synthesis following anoxia in the rat hippocampal slice: interaction between Ca and NMDA receptors. In: Somjen G, editor. Mechanisms of cerebral hypoxia and stroke. New York: Springer; 1998. p. 229–49.

61. Rader RK, Lanthorn TH. Experimental ischemia induces a persistent depolarization blocked by decreased calcium and NMDA antagonists. Neurosci Lett 1989;99:125–30.

62. Lauritzen M, Hansen AJ. The effect of glutamate receptor blockade on anoxic depolarization and cortical spreading depression. J Cereb Blood Flow Metab 1992;12:223–9.

63. Kral T, Luhmann THJ, Mittman T, et al. Role of NMDA receptors and voltage-activated calcium channels in an in vitro model of cerebral ischemia. Brain Res 1993;612:278–88.

64. Grigg JJ, Anderson EG. Competitive and noncompetitive N-methyl-D-aspartate antagonists modify hypoxia-induced membrane potential changes and protect rat hippocampal slices from functional failure: a quantitative comparison. J Pharmacol Exp Ther 1990;253:130–5.

65. Baker CJ, Fiore AJ, Frazzini VI, et al. Intraischemic hypothermia decreases the release of glutamate in the cores of permanent focal cerebral infarcts. Neurosurgery 1995;36:994–1001.

66. Benveniste H, Drejer J, Schousboe A, et al. Elevation of the extracellular concentrations of glutamate and aspartate in rat hippocampus during transient cerebral ischemia monitored by intracerebral microdialysis. J Neurochem 1984;43:1369–74.

67. Miyashita K, Nakajima T, Ishikawa A, et al. An adenosine uptake blocker, propentofylline, reduces glutamate release in gerbil hippocampus following transient forebrain ischemia. Neurochem Res 1992;17:147–50.

68. Iadecola C, Xu X, Zhang F, et al. Marked induction of calcium-independent nitric oxide synthase activity after focal ischemia. J Cereb Blood Flow Metab 1995;15:52–9.

69. Nogawa S, Zhang F, Ross ME, et al. Cyclooxyge-nase-2 gene expression in neurons contributes to ischemic brain damage. J Neurosci 1997;17:2746–55.

70. Cipolla MJ, Lessov N, Clark WM. Postischemic attenuation of cerebral artery reactivity is increased in the presence of tissue plasminogen activator. Stroke 2000;31:940–5.

71. Degraba TJ. The role of inflammation after acute stroke. Utility of pursuing anti-adhesion molecule therapy. Neurology 1998;51(Suppl 3):S62–8.

72. Chamorro A, Hallenbeck J. The harms and benefits of inflammatory and immune responses in vascular disease. Stroke 2006;37:291–3.

73. Zheng Z, Yenari MA. Post-ischemic inflammation: molecular mechanisms and therapeutic implications. Neurol Res 2004;26:884–92.

74. Nawashiro H, Tasaki K, Ruetzler A, et al. TNF-alpha pretreatment induces protective effects against focal cerebral ischemia in mice. J Cereb Blood Flow Metab 1997;17:483–90.

75. Allan SM, Rothwell NJ. Cytokines and acute neuro-degeneration. Nat Rev Neurosci 2001;2:734–44.

76. Baeuerle PA, Henkel T. Function and activation of NF-kappa B in the immune system. Annu Rev Immunol 1994;12:141–79.

77. Siebenlist U, Franzoso G, Brown K. Structure, regulation and function of NFk B. Annu Rev Cell Biol 1994;10:405–55.

78. Schneider A, Martin-Villalba A, Weih F, et al. NF-kappaB is activated and promotes cell death in focal cerebral ischemia. Nat Med 1999;5:554–9.

79. Irving EA, Bamford M. Role of mitogen- and stress-activated kinases in ischemic injury. J Cereb Blood Flow Metab 2002;22(6):631–47.

80. Irving EA, Barone FC, Reith AD, et al. Differential activation of MAPK/ERK and p38/SAPK in neurones and glia following focal cerebral ischaemia in the rat. Brain Res Mol Brain Res 2000;77(1):65–75.

81. Zhang QG, Wang RM, Yin XH, et al. Knock-down of POSH expression is neuroprotective through down-regulating activation of the MLK3-MKK4-JNK pathway following cerebral ischaemia in the rat hippocampal CA1 subfield. J Neurochem 2005;95(3):784–95.

82. Wang X, Feuerstein GZ. Induced expression of adhesion molecules following focal brain ischemia. J Neurotrauma 1995;12(5):825–32.

83. Zhang RL, Chopp M, Zaloga C, et al. The temporal profiles of ICAM-1 protein and mRNA expression after transient MCA occlusion in the rat. Brain Res 1995;682(1–2):182–8.

84. Garcia JH, Liu KF, Relton JK. Interleukin-1 receptor antagonist decreases the number of necrotic neurons in rats with middle cerebral artery occlusion. Am J Pathol 1995;147:1477–86.

85. Heo JH, Lucero J, Abumiya T, et al. Matrix metallo-proteinases increase very early during experimental focal cerebral ischemia. J Cereb Blood Flow Metab 1999;19:624–33.

86. Rosenberg GA. Matrix metalloproteinases in neuro-inflammation. Glia 2002;39(3):279–91.

87. Rosenberg GA, Cunningham LA, Wallace J, et al. Immunohistochemistry of matrix metalloprotei-nases in reperfusion injury to rat brain: activation of MMP-9 linked to stromelysin-1 and microglia in cell cultures. Brain Res 2001;893(1–2):104–12.

88. Chen J, Zhu RL, Nakayama M. Expression of the apoptosis-effector gene, BAX, is upregulated in vulnerable hippocampal CA1 neurons following global ischemia. J Neurochem 1996;67:64–71.

89. Hara A, Iwai T, Niwa M. Immunohistochemical detection of BAX and Bcl-2 proteins in gerbil hip-pocampus following transient forebrain ischemia. Brain Res 1996;711:249–53.

90. Nath R, Stafford D, Allen H, et al. Nonerythroid alpha-spectrin breakdown by calpain and inter-leukin 1-beta-converting-enzyme-like proteases in apoptotic cells: contributory roles of both protease families in neuronal apoptosis. Biochem J 1996;319:683–90.

91. Squier MKT, Miller ACK, Malkinson AM, et al. Calpain activation in apoptosis. J Cell Physiol 1994;159:229–37.

92. Gido G, Kristian T, Siesjo BK. Extracellular potassium in a neocortical core area after transient focal ischemia. Stroke 1997;28:206–10.

93. Ikonomidou C, Mosinger JL, Salles KS, et al. Sensitivity of the developing rat brain to hypobaric/ischemic damage parallels sensitivity to N-methyl-D-aspartate neurotoxicity. J Neurosci 1989;9:2809–16.

94. Kristian T, Gido G, Kuroda S, et al. Calcium metabolism in focal and penumbral tissues in rats subjected to transient middle cerebral artery occlusion. Exp Brain Res 1998;120:503–9.

95. Zhao W, Belayev WL, Ginsberg M. Transient middle cerebral artery occlusion by intraluminal suture. II. Neurological deficits and pixel-based correlation of histopathology with local blood flow and glucose utilization. J Cereb Blood Flow Metab 1997;17:1281–90.

96. Belayev L, Zhao W, Busto R, et al. Transient middle cerebral artery occlusion by intraluminal suture. I. Three-dimensional autoradiographic image analysis of local cerebral glucose metabolism-blood flow interrelationships during ischemia and early recircula-tion. J Cereb Blood Flow Metab 1997;17:1266–80.

97. Dirnagl U, Lindauer U, Schreiber S. Global cerebral ischemia in the rat: online monitoring of oxygen free radical production using chemiluminescence in vivo. J Cereb Blood Flow Metab 1995;15:929–40.

98. Oliver CN, Starke-Reed PE, Stadtman ER, et al. Oxidative damage to brain proteins, loss of gluta-mine synthetase activity and production of free

radicals during ischemia/reperfusion-induced injury to gerbil brain. Proc Natl Acad Sci U S A 1990;87:5144–7.

99. Phillis JW, O'Regan MHO. Mechanismsofglutamateand aspartate release in the ischemic rat cerebral cortex. Brain Res 1996;730:150–64.

100. Sakamoto A, Ohnishi ST, Ohnishi T, et al. Relationship between free radical production and lipid peroxidation during ischemia-reperfusion injury in the rat brain. Brain Res 1991;554:186–92.

101. Yoshida S, Abe K, Busto R, et al. Influence of transient ischemia in lipidsoluble antioxidants, free fatty acids and energy metabolites in rat brain. Brain Res 1982;245:307–16.

102. Harada K, Fukuda S, Kunimoto M, et al. Distribution of ankyrin isoforms and their proteolysis after ischemia and reperfusion in rat brain. J Neurochem 1997;69:371–6.

103. Kalimo H, Olsson Y, Paljarvi L, et al. Structural changes in brain tissue under hypoxic-ischemic conditions. J Cereb Blood Flow Metab 1982;1(suppl2):S19–22.

104. Kumura E, Yoshimine T, Tanaka S, et al. Generation of nitric oxide and superoxide during reperfusion after focal ischemia in rats. Am J Physiol 1996;270:C748–52.

105. Olesen S-P. Free oxygen radicals decrease electrical resistance of microvascular endothelium in brain. Acta Physiol Scand 1987;129:181–7.

106. Peters O, Back T, Lindauer U, et al. Increased formation of reactive oxygen species after permanent and reversible middle cerebral artery occlusion in the rat. J Cereb Blood Flow Metab 1998;18:196–205.

107. Warach S, Latour LL. Evidence of reperfusion injury, exacerbated by thrombolytic therapy, in human focal brain ischemia using a novel imaging marker of early blood–brain barrier disruption. Stroke 2004;35(suppl I):2659–61.

108. Leigh R, Christensen S, Campbell BCV, et al. Pretreatment blood–brain barrier disruption and post-endovascular intracranial hemorrhage. Neurology 2016;87:263–9.

109. Fiehler J, Remmele C, Kucinski T, et al. Reperfusion after severe local perfusion deficit precedes hemorrhagic transformation: an MRI study in acute stroke patient. Cerebrovasc Dis 2005;19:117–24.

110. Renu A, Laredo C, Tudela R, et al. Brain hemorrhage after endovascular reperfusion therapy of ischemic stroke: a threshold-finding whole-brain perfusion CT study. J Cereb Blood Flow Metab 2017;37(1):153–65.

111. O'Collins VE, Macleod MR, Donnan GA, et al. 1,026 experimental treatments in acute stroke. Ann Neurol 2006;59:467–77.

112. Murry CE, Jennings RB, Reimer KA. Preconditioning with ischemia: a delay of lethal cell injury in isChemic myocardium. Circulation 1986;74:1124–36.

113. Reimer KA, Murry CE, Yamasawa I, et al. Four brief periods of myocardial ischemia cause no cumulative ATP loss or necrosis. Am J Physiol 1986;251:H1306–15.

114. Kirino T, Tsujita Y, Tamura A. Induced tolerance to ischemia in gerbil hippocampal neurons. J Cereb Blood Flow Metab 1991;11:299–307.

115. Liu Y, Kato H, Nakata N, et al. Temporal profile of heat shock protein 70 synthesis in ischemic tolerance induced by preconditioning ischemia in rat hippocampus. Neuroscience 1993;56:921–7.

116. Kitagawa K, Matsumoto M, Tagaya M, et al. Ischemic tolerance phenomenon found in the brain. Brain Res 1990;528:21–4.

117. Heurteaux C, Lauritzen I, Windmann C, et al. Essential role of adenosine, adenosine A1 receptors, and ATP-sensitive K1 channels in cerebral ischemic preconditioning. Proc Natl Acad Sci U S A 1995;92:4666–70.

118. Matsushima K, Hakim AM. Transient forebrain ischemia protects against subsequent focal ischemia without changing cerebral perfusion. Stroke 1995;26:1047–52.

119. Dunn JF, Wu Y, Zhao Z, et al. Training the brain to survive stroke. PLoS One 2012;7(9):e45108.

120. Abe H, Nowak TS. Gene expression and induced ischemic tolerance following brief insults. Acta Neurobiol Exp 1996;56:3–8.

121. Ohta S, Furuta S, Matsubara I, et al. Calcium movement in ischemia-tolerant hippocampal CA1 neurons after transient forebrain ischemia in gerbils. J Cereb Blood Flow Metab 1996;16:915–22.

122. Shimazaki K, Nakamura T, Nakamura K. Reduced calcium elevation in hippocampal CA1 neurons of ischemia-tolerant gerbils. Neuroreport 1998;9:1875–8.

123. Frank A, Bonney M, Bonney S, et al. Myocardial ischemia reperfusion injury: from basic science to clinical bedside. Semin Cardiothorac Vasc Anesth 2012;16(3):123–32.

124. Tapuria N, Kumar Y, Habib MM, et al. Remote ischemic preconditioning: a novel protective method from ischemia reperfusion injury–a review. J Surg Res 2008;150:304–30.

125. Wei D, Ren C, Chen X, et al. The chronic protective effects of limb remote preconditioning and the underlying mechanisms involved in inflammatory factors in rat stroke. PLoS One 2012;7(2):e30892.

126. Hahn CD, Manlhiot C, Schmidt MR, et al. Remote ischemic per-conditioning. A novel therapy for acute stroke? Stroke 2011;42:2960–2.

127. Drew KL, Buck CL, Barnes BM, et al. Central nervous system regulation of mammalian hibernation: implications for metabolic suppression and ischemia tolerance. J Neurochem 2007;102(6):1713–26.

128. Drew KL, Harris MB, LaManna JC, et al. Hypoxia tolerance in mammalian heterotherms. J Exp Biol 2004;207:3155–62.

129. van der Worp HB, Sena ES, Donnan GA, et al. Hypothermia in animalmodels of acuteischaemic stroke: a systematic review andmeta-analysis. Brain 2007;130:3063–74.

130. Rosomoff HL, Holaday DA. Cerebral blood flow and cerebral oxygen consumption during hypothermia. Am J Physiol 1954;179(1):85–8.

131. Michenfelder JD, Milde JH, Katusic ZS. Postischemic canine cerebral blood flow is coupled to cerebral metabolic rate. J Cereb Blood Flow Metab 1991;11:611–6.

132. Mori K, Maeda M, Miyazaki M, et al. Effects of mild (33 degrees C) and moderate (29 degrees C) hypothermia on cerebral blood flow and metabolism, lactate, and extracellular glutamate in experimental head injury. Neurol Res 1998;20:719–26.

133. Walter B, Bauer R, Kuhnen G, et al. Coupling of cerebral blood flow and oxygen metabolism in infant pigs during selective brain hypothermia. J Cereb Blood Flow Metab 2000;20:1215–24.

134. Sick TJ, Xu G, Perez-Pinzon MA. Mild hypothermia improves recovery of cortical extracellular potassium ion activity and excitability after middle cerebral artery occlusion in the rat. Stroke 1999;30:2416–21.

135. Nakashima K, Todd MM. Effects of hypothermia on the rate of excitatory amino acid release after ischemic depolarization. Stroke 1996;27:913–8.

136. Busto R, Globus MY, Dietrich WD, et al. Effect of mild hypothermia on ischemia-induced release of neurotransmitters and free fatty acids in rat brain. Stroke 1989;20:904–10.

137. Kumura E, Yoshimine T, Iwatsuki KI, et al. Generation of nitric oxide and superoxide during reperfusion after focal cerebral ischemia in rats. Am J Physiol 1996;270:c748–52.

138. Huang ZG, Xue D, Preston E, et al. Biphasic opening of the blood-brain barrier following transient focal ischemia: effects of hypothermia. Can J Neurol Sci 1999;26:298–304.

139. Kidwell CS, Saver JL, Starkman S, et al. Late secondary ischemic injury in patients receiving intraarterial thrombolysis. Ann Neurol 2002;52:698–703.

140. Ishikawa M, Sekizuka E, Sato S, et al. Effects of moderate hypothermia on leukocyte- endothelium interaction in the rat pial microvasculature after transient middle cerebral artery occlusion. Stroke 1999;30:1679–86.

141. Toyoda T, Suzuki S, Kassell NF, et al. Intraischemic hypothermia attenuates neutrophil infiltration in the rat neocortex after focal ischemia-reperfusion injury. Neurosurgery 1996;39:1200–5.

142. Wang LM, Yan Y, Zou LJ, et al. Moderate hypothermia prevents neural cell apoptosis following spinal cord ischemia in rabbits. Cell Res 2005;15:387–93.

143. Xu L, Yenari MA, Steinberg GK, et al. Mild hypothermia reduces apoptosis of mouse neurons in vitro early in the cascade. J Cereb Blood Flow Metab 2002;22:21–8.

144. Hypothermia After Cardiac Arrest Study Group. Mild therapeutic hypothermia to improve the neurologic outcome after cardiac arrest. N Engl J Med 2002;346:549–56.

145. Bernard SA, Gray TW, Buist MD, et al. Treatment of comatose survivors of out-of-hospital cardiac arrest with induced hypothermia. N Engl J Med 2002;346:557–63.

146. Eicher DJ, Wagner CL, Katikaneni LP, et al. Moderate hypothermia in neonatal encephalopathy: efficacy outcomes. Pediatr Neurol 2005;32:11–7.

147. Gluckman PD, Wyatt JS, Azzopardi D, et al. Selective head cooling with mild systemic hypothermia after neonatal encephalopathy: multicentre randomised trial. Lancet 2005;365:663–70.

148. Shankaran S, Laptook AR, Ehrenkranz RA, et al. Whole-body hypothermia for neonates with hypoxiaischemic encephalopathy. N Engl J Med 2005;353:1574–84.

149. The Warm Heart Investigators. Randomised trial of normothermic versus hypothermic coronary bypass surgery. Lancet 1994;343:559–63.

150. Regragui I, Birdi I, Izzat MB, et al. The effects of cardiopulmonary bypass temperature on neuropsychologic outcome after coronary artery operations: a prospective randomized trial. J Thorac Cardiovasc Surg 1996;112:1036–45.

151. Plourde G, Leduc AS, Morin JE, et al. Temperature during cardiopulmonary bypass for coronary artery operations does not influence postoperative cognitive function: a prospective, randomized trial. J Thorac Cardiovasc Surg 1997;114:123–8.

152. De Georgia MA, Krieger DW, Abou-Chebl A, et al. Cooling for acute ischemic brain damage (COOL AID): a feasibility trial of endovascular cooling. Neurology 2004;63:312–7.

153. Lyden PD, Allgren RL, Ng K, et al. Intravascular cooling in the treatment of stroke (ICTuS): early clinical experience. J Stroke Cerebrovasc Dis 2005;14:107–14.

154. Andresen M, Gazmuri JT, Marín A, et al. Therapeutic hypothermia for acute brain injuries. Scand J Trauma Resusc Emerg Med 2015;23:42.

155. Polderman KH. Induced hypothermia and fever control for prevention and treatment of neurological injuries. Lancet 2008;371(9628):1955–69.

156. Yenari MA, Hemmen TM. Therapeutic hypothermia for brain ischemia: where have we come and where do we go? Stroke 2010;41:72–4.

157. Choi JH, Marshall RS, Neimark MA, et al. Selective brain cooling with endovascular intracarotid infusion of cold saline: a pilot feasibility study. AJNR Am J Neuroradiol 2010;31:928–34.

158. Choi JH, Mangla S, Barone FC, et al. Rapid and selective brain cooling and maintenance of selective cooling with intra-carotid cold fluid infusion is feasible and safe. Eur Stroke J 2016; 1(suppl.):391.

159. Chau KH, Ziganshin BA, Elefteriades JA. Deep hypothermic circulatory arrest: real-life suspended animation. Prog Cardiovasc Dis 2013; 56:81–91.

160. Kaneko T, Aranki SF, Neely RC, et al. Is there a need for adjunct cerebral protection in conjunction with deep hypothermic circulatory arrest during noncomplex hemiarch surgery? J Thorac Cardiovasc Surg 2014;148:2911–7.

161. Peng X, Wan Y, Liu W, et al. Protective roles of intra-arterial mild hypothermia and arterial thrombolysis in acute cerebral infarction. Springerplus 2016;5: 1988.

162. Chen J, Liu L, Zhang H, et al. Endovascular hypothermia in acute ischemic stroke. Pilot Study of selective intra-arterial cold saline infusion. Stroke 2016;47:1933–5.

163. Neimark MA, Konstas AA, Choi JH, et al.The role of intracarotid cold saline infusion on a theoretical brain model incorporating the Circle of Willis and cerebral venous return. Proceedings of the 29th Annual International Conference of the IEEE EMBS, Lyon, France, August 23–26, 2007.

164. Abou-Chebl A, Sung G, Barbut D, et al. Local brain temperature reduction through intranasal cooling with the RhinoChill device. Preliminary safety data in brain-injured patients. Stroke 2011;42:2164–9.

165. Mattingly TK, Denning LM, Siroen KL, et al. Catheter based selective hypothermia reduces stroke volume during focal cerebral ischemia in swine. J Neurointerv Surg 2016;8:418–22.

166. Cattaneo G, Schumacher M, Maurer C, et al. Endovascular cooling catheter for selective brain hypothermia: an animal feasibility study of cooling performance. AJNR Am J Neuroradiol 2016;37(5): 885–91.

Economic and Societal Aspects of Stroke Management

Govind Mukundan, MD*, David J. Seidenwurm, MD

KEYWORDS

- Stroke • Health care • Cost • Economics • CMS • Payer

KEY POINTS

- Efforts like performance measures help measure quality objectively and benchmark care to evolving standards to reward those who deliver superior care while sometimes relatively penalizing those who fail.
- On a more basic level, although appearing daunting, these constructs actually help shed light and improve transparency in an often-opaque health care delivery system and ultimately help cement the trust of the consumer and payers.
- Other payment models like bundled payments hope to squeeze out inefficiency and increase quality by reducing care fragmentation and aligning the interests of the health care providers with payers and patients by sharing risk and the attendant rewards.

STROKE AND PUBLIC POLICY

Time is brain[1]

It is the purpose of this order to ensure that health care programs administered or sponsored by the Federal Government promote quality and efficient delivery of health care through the use of health information technology, transparency regarding health care quality and price, and better incentives for program beneficiaries, enrollees, and providers.

—*Executive Order of the President, August 26, 2006.[2]*

Stroke is a major health burden worldwide with attendant mortality, morbidity, and cost. In 2010, there were approximately 16.9 million strokes and an estimated 33 million stroke survivors worldwide.[3]

In the United States, approximately 780,000 people present with new or recurrent strokes every year.[4] Also, in the United States, stroke is the third leading cause of death, with ischemic stroke resulting in 8% 30-day mortality (20% for hemorrhagic stroke). Stroke is the leading cause of disability as well.[5] Lastly, the mortality rate for ischemic stroke increases with age, especially older than 65 years. Currently, the numbers of stroke survivors, disability adjusted life years, as well as mortality are increasing, despite a stable incidence over the last 20 years.[5] This finding highlights the paradoxic relationships between quality of care, quality of life, and technological progress. This paradox is significant, in that the patient experience of stroke is not well captured in these aggregate statistics and patient preferences are difficult to ascertain in stroke populations.

In addition to morbidity, mortality, and human suffering is the staggering financial and economic cost of the disease, driven in large part by

Disclosures: Nothing to disclose.
Department of Medical Imaging, Sutter Health, 1500 Expo Parkway, Sacramento, CA 95815, USA
* Corresponding author.
E-mail address: soyuz123@gmail.com

Neuroimag Clin N Am 28 (2018) 683–689
https://doi.org/10.1016/j.nic.2018.06.009
1052-5149/18/© 2018 Elsevier Inc. All rights reserved.

disability and long-term associated care. A 2010 study by Guilhaume and colleagues[4] cited the direct health care cost alone at $65.5 billion for this disease in the United States. This figure does not capture the losses to the economy from lost labor or opportunity costs for stroke survivors and their caregivers.

In economics, value is defined as perceived benefit per unit of cost. Today, value and cost are overarching concerns in the delivery of health care services in the United States. This concern is driven by the awareness of stakeholders, including health care consumers, payers, and indeed the public at large, that health care costs have dramatically outpaced the cost of most other goods and services, increasing from around 3% of the gross domestic product (GDP) in the 1940s to 17.3% in 2009 in the United States.[6] In aggregate, however, the results of the US health care system are often worse than those of other countries that often deliver superior results with lower cost systems.[7] This finding suggests that the benefits from the price paid by health care consumers is not optimal for the cost incurred. Many factors contribute to this phenomenon, including Baumol cost disease, payment policies, and political preferences. The impact on stroke incidence and stroke-related disability is just another example of a more generalized pattern in the American health care system.

For example, consider resource availability. Resource availability is a critical factor in the social determinants of the burden of stroke care among nations. However, once a sufficient level is reached, it is not clear whether the presence or application of additional resources, contribute significantly to meaningful stroke outcomes. It seems that the countries with the greatest density of advanced imaging tools are not necessarily those with the best stroke outcomes. The United States is currently second worldwide in the number of MR imaging examinations per 1000 inhabitants and leads the world by far in the number of computed tomography (CT) examinations per 1000 inhabitants.[8] In addition, the United States leads the world in MR imaging units per million inhabitants; we are a distant second to Australia in the number of CT units per million inhabitants, perhaps owing to the sparsely distributed population of that continental nation.[9,10]

This prevalence of technical resources in the United States compared with other nations does not correlate well with utilization in stroke-specific diagnoses. Data from the Organization for Economic Co-operation and Development (OECD) on a small number of relatively comparable countries suggest that the United States' advantage in the number of MR imaging and CT imaging instruments and the number of examinations performed do not correlate with higher utilization in stroke populations, especially in the younger age groups.[11] This finding may reflect access to health insurance, distortions related to disincentives to serve less affluent populations, or other sources of health care disparities. The United States is evidently in the middle of the pack or a bit better than average in stroke mortality.[12] However, it is important to point out that mortality at 7 days, 30 days, or even at 1 year may not be the best indicator of quality stroke care because some individuals and cultural groups may value some impaired health states as worse than death.

It is, therefore, necessary to consider a variety of demand-side and supply-side factors in evaluating international differences in stroke care and the societal preferences that produce these results. The percent of the GDP that a nation spends on stroke care seems closely related to the proportion of the GDP that a country spends on health care in general, though there are important differences. For example, Australia spends 2.0% of its GDP on health care and 0.16% on stroke, whereas the United States spends just less than 3.0% of health care expenditures on stroke, amounting to approximately 0.4% of the GDP.[11] The differences among nations in the distribution of care within these various-sized buckets are also striking. For example, the Netherlands spends a strikingly low proportion of its cerebrovascular disease budget on hospitals and nursing home care and correspondingly more on home health care than the United States, Australia, and Canada.[11] It is challenging to reconcile these differences with much shorter lengths of stay for stroke patients in US hospitals, until one realizes that the costs of comparable services in the United States are quite a bit higher than in the rest of the world.[13]

Factors that affect the demand for health care services related to stroke include the availability of health care coverage and out-of-pocket cost sharing by patients. These impacts are stronger in countries like Mexico, South Korea, and the United States than they are in other OECD nations.[14] Additionally, out-of-pocket spending as a proportion of health care expenditures seems comparable between the United States and other industrialized nations; however, because the proportion of GDP spent on health care is higher in the United States, the patient-borne burden may be higher, especially in groups with less than the median income. Recent changes in health care insurance product design in the United States have likely altered this trend in an unfavorable direction at upper-middle-income levels and favorably in lower-income groups, though aggregate national level data collected comparably internationally are not available since this trend has been fully realized in the United States. It must also be noted that the theory behind patient contribution to cost control is not fully applicable to stroke care, because the emergent care required to ensure the most favorable possible outcomes are not accessible to comparison shopping or reference price strategies. Thus, provider-level incentives are thought to be more efficacious.

Value-based health care reform is grounded on the assumption that health care is a rational enterprise with rational actors making rational decisions to accept the highest quality at the optimal cost. Mirroring management techniques that have been shown to increase productivity and reduce cost in other enterprises,[15] this has been translated to the health care enterprise with pay-for-performance measures in which even small incentives have been shown to increase the quality of care in controlled studies.[16,17]

This shift to value-based systems for health care services payment, including stroke, is executed in the pay-for-performance programs that are administered by payer entities, including the Centers for Medicare and Medicaid Services (CMS). Pay for performance is defined as any payment scheme that aligns the incentives of the provider with the patients, with the process, it is hoped, resulting in increasing quality and decreasing cost. To make this happen, performance measures have to be developed that can demonstrate the quality of a health care product at a delivery site. A performance measure is defined as a quantifiable indicator of a specific health care product, expressed as a proportion or percentage of patients treated according to a specified standard or achieving a relative or absolute final or intermediate clinical or patient-reported outcome. Performance measures usually focus on structures, processes, or outcomes.[18] A performance measure is developed in a multistage process that starts with the clinical area of interest. This measure is something that can be developed by any organization or individual and is not limited to large, well-established programs. Then follows evidence research, including a search for gaps in guideline-recommended care, followed by specification of the measure in terms of readily available administrative or clinical data elements, and, crucially, testing of feasibility, validity, and utility in actual practice. A public comment period is frequently a part of the process, as measure developers understand that input from engaged stakeholders in diverse practice settings or patients with varying perspectives can improve metrics with their unique and valuable suggestions. Often, the most challenging aspect of validation is demonstrating the ability of the metric to discriminate among providers along meaningful dimensions of quality. The final step is submission for National Quality Forum (NQF) endorsement and then availability for value-based compensation in private or public programs.

Table 1 illustrates an example of a stroke measure (hemorrhage or infarction), the Merit-Based Incentive Payment System (MIPS).

The intracranial hemorrhage or cerebral infarction cost measure evaluates the cost to Medicare for services provided by an attributed clinician and other clinicians and providers during an episode of care. A cost/resource use–type measure type, it falls under the rubric of the Human and Health Services National Quality Strategy priority of making health care affordable. This measure can be feasibly reported using claims based data and the steward, the CMS.

Table 1	
Example of a stroke measure: Merit-Based Incentive Payment System	
Cost Measure:	It applies to inpatient care of Medicare beneficiaries hospitalized for an intracranial hemorrhage or cerebral infarction.
Calculated by:	It is calculated by determining the risk-adjusted episode cost, averaged across all of a clinician's episodes during the measurement period. The cost of each episode is the sum of the cost to Medicare for services performed by the attributed clinician and other health care providers during the episode window (from the trigger date to 90 d after the trigger date).
Formula:	([observed/expected payment − standardized Medicare cost for all episodes for specific clinician] × national average episode)/total number of episodes from intracranial hemorrhage or cerebral infarction episode group attributed to specific clinician

Measure under consideration (MUC) ID: MUC17-363: intracranial hemorrhage or cerebral infarction cost measure.

Analysis by the CMS Innovation Center of the measure shows that it has conditional support for rulemaking, if submitted, with full development and testing for reliability and face validity completed at both the clinician and group level. This measure evaluates a critical quality objective of the MIPS domain of cost efficiency and reduction, not fully addressed by other measures in the program set. This cost/resource measure is evidence based and linked to outcomes. In addition, this measure evaluates a performance gap, that of variability in spending per risk-adjusted episode of care for providers and clinician groups ending from June 1, 2016 through May 31, 2017. The recommendation by the CMS Innovation Center is for this measure to be submitted to the NQF for review and endorsement, although this has not yet been done. Therefore, the measure is not yet in use.

Medicine rapidly evolves for the better. As a result, there is a life cycle for clinical interventions, and a performance measure is no exception. A NQF fully endorsed measure is evaluated every 3 years for maintenance and enhancement to update the measure to current evidence and best practices. For example, a NQF measure that included stroke pathology, Physician Quality Reporting System measure 10 measuring the rate of documentation of infarct, hemorrhage, or mass on head CT and MR imaging reports was deemed to lack evidence to support whether this documentation rate had any impact on clinical outcomes and was retired.[19] However, updates to the specifications may be done at any time as well as harmonization with other measures, if applicable. The measure steward performs the maintenance of the measure, and a lapse in this will lead to loss of NQF endorsement. For example, the same parameters for the National Institute of Neurological Disorders and Stroke's exclusion criteria to be reported at emergent head CT were included in a subsequent metric promulgated by the American Academy of Neurology (AAN[20]) that included time parameters and other evidence-based components in a more stringent performance measure for stroke imaging.

Another pillar of the drive toward the redesign of medical care delivery in the United States is the bundled or episode payments scheme championed by the CMS.[21,22] This scheme bases payments on a bundle of services for an entire episode of care with a defined initiation event and termination. This scheme rolls in the services provided across a range of specialties, including radiology, to a defined episode of care, with the aim of avoiding care fragmentation and sharing the financial risk and performance accountability with the participating organization and clinicians,

thus, leading to higher quality and lower cost for care. The CMS Innovation Center, set up under the Affordable Care Act, calls its initiative the Bundled Payments for Care Improvement (BPCI) and is targeted at hospital delivered care, one of which is of course stroke, under the stroke diagnosis-related group (DRG). This initiative trials 4 models of bundled payments for acute care, including the first model whereby Medicare pays the hospital a discounted rate based on the inpatient prospective payment system rate and the providers separately under the fee-for-service schedule. This model participation concluded in December 2016. The second and third models involve reconciling Medicare fee-for-service payments for an episode of care against target payment benchmarks retrospectively with adjustment. The fourth evolved model is whereby the hospital receives the entire payment for a care bundle and the providers then make the appropriate no-pay claims to Medicare to receive payment from the hospital for their component of care delivered.[22]

The BPCI as of October 2017 has 1191 participants in phase 2 made up of 252 awardees and 939 episode initiators. Participants include acute care hospitals (396 total), physician group practices, home health agencies, and inpatient rehabilitation facilities.

Stroke DRGs included in this project include[22]

61	Acute ischemic stroke with use of thrombolytic agent with major complication or comorbidity
62	Acute ischemic stroke with use of thrombolytic agent with complication or comorbidity
63	Acute ischemic stroke with use of thrombolytic agent without complication or comorbidity or major complication or comorbidity
64	Intracranial hemorrhage or cerebral infarction with major complication or comorbidity
65	Intracranial hemorrhage or cerebral infarction with complication or comorbidity or tissue plasminogen activator in 24 hours
66	Intracranial hemorrhage or cerebral infarction without complication or comorbidity or major complication or comorbidity

Recent updates to this program indicate a trend toward emphasis on voluntary participation and primacy of clinician control of the care processes. The results of these innovations on clinical- and patient-reported outcomes will inform on the shape of stroke care in future payment models, as CMS innovations often spread to the private sector when favorable results are demonstrated in the Medicare population.

The lack of correlation between the resources applied to stroke prevention, treatment, and poststroke management both at the macro level and at the level of the individual care unit suggests that there is substantial room for improvement in the quality of stroke care while simultaneously improving the value received for the costs expended. For this reason, bundled payments and costs-of-care metrics have been proposed as refinements to existing payment methodologies.

Value-based payment methodologies have unique challenges in stroke care. Principal among these challenges is that, at the current time, systems and methods of acute stroke care in the United States are undergoing substantial, not to say spectacular, changes. Before the now validated and convincing value of intra-arterial mechanical thrombectomy in acute stroke, the argument that less was more may have had some currency.[23,24] Now, that point of view is no longer tenable for acute strokes that present within the first 24 hours (and are eligible for interventional therapy). Therefore, the modeling for a bundled payment plan is substantially more complex and must be priced to include, and even encourage, the performance of appropriate expensive and technologically demanding interventions when clinically indicated. It must also be stated, as has been shown repeatedly, that because patients value the health states produced by stroke more negatively than physicians do, it is incumbent on us to provide appropriate incentives to ensure that we treat patients according to their desires rather than ours. That means that any payment scheme must incentivize aggressive stroke treatment whenever a net benefit is achievable in a patient who is a member of a favorable cohort.

In order to properly price a radiology stroke care bundle, it is necessary to determine the relative distribution of various types of strokes; one must also estimate the frequency with which certain events will take place within a model of optimal care for each of those categories.[21] Initially, one would begin with a population assessment of the relative, mix of ischemic stroke and transient ischemic attack, parenchymal hemorrhage, and subarachnoid hemorrhage. Within each category,

payment would certainly be granted for a noncontrast CT scan for each patient. Beyond that, things may become substantially more complicated. In the ischemic category, one must estimate the relative distribution of patients who will arrive within 3.0, 4.5, 6.0, 16.0, and 24.0 hours of the event and then allocate to those categories increasingly complex imaging triage procedures in the appropriate proportion to reflect the expected frequencies of clinical severity. Further, one must define from the somewhat heterogeneous literature the appropriateness and delivery of vascular intervention. These estimates must be high enough to reflect patient preferences for stroke-related health states that account for substantial acceptance of therapeutic complications, if the absolute number of favorable outcomes can be increased in a population of patients who have had a stroke. Another area of controversy that must be resolved in the pricing of a radiology stroke care bundle is the frequency of advanced imaging and of additional imaging follow-up after the initial event. There is not only great heterogeneity in this area but also scientific controversy.

Another layer of complexity in creating any radiology stroke care payment bundle is the requirement of a quality outcome measure that properly reflects patient preferences. Fortunately, this aspect of stroke care payment modeling is far less complex and more highly developed through consensus-driven processes. There are substantial consensus and empirical data regarding the use of the modified Rankin score (mRS) of 2 or less as the definition of a favorable outcome. However, a pay-for-value scheme that would only reward the frequency with which this level of favorable outcome is achieved would not meet the goals of a patient-centric payment model because it might paradoxically influence patient selection to achieve a higher percentage of favorable outcomes among those treated, while resulting simultaneously in a net decrease in the absolute number of favorable outcomes among a population of patients who have had a stroke by excluding from treatment those patients whose proportion of favorable outcomes, while greater than untreated patients, might be lower than those selected in a different manner, for example, by anatomic rather than functional cerebral imaging.

Because the ideal radiological payment model for stroke is probably unachievable at present, because of the scientific uncertainty and technical complexity, intermediate steps are more likely to drive progress in realizing value-based payment for the near future. The AAN's recent stroke and stroke rehabilitation quality measures update provides a road map for guidance in this process.[25] It is easy to imagine, and to hope for, payment models that reward successful completion of the National Institutes of Health's stroke scale, assessment of fibrinolytic and intravascular treatment eligibility, initiation of appropriate fibrinolytic treatment, and interpretation of brain and vascular imaging within specified time frames. In patients who were judged eligible for endovascular treatment, it would seem appropriate to reward systems of care that achieve rapid brain and vascular imaging reported in a manner that explicitly addresses the intravascular therapy triage features, achieves rapid door-to-puncture times, rapid door-to-vascular reperfusion times, and report outcomes in a reproducible incomparable manner both with respect to the angiographic result using TICI and the clinical result, perhaps using a mRs.

Certainly, some humility is required here. Although it is certainly desirable to improve the quality of care once a stroke has occurred, the greatest potential for the reduction in the societal burden of stroke is likely to be achieved through primary and secondary prevention, poststroke complication prevention, and appropriate rehabilitation. Aggressive management of hypertension, dyslipidemia, and diabetes has the greatest potential within the medical system for reducing the global stroke burden. However, these measures are not likely to achieve the greatest benefit without accompanying approaches that facilitate healthier behaviors outside the medical system. Agricultural and farm subsidy policies that encourage healthier diets, urban planning, transportation, and housing policies that facilitate pedestrian mobility and safety will also contribute. Architectural designs that encourage reasonable use of stairs to facilitate exercise in the course of everyday life will help prevent stroke, and built environment designs that mitigate the effects of disability will encourage the integration of stroke survivors into everyday life. Thus, the radiological, medical, and payer communities must play their role in a stroke prevention, care, and rehabilitation project that encompass the larger community as well.

What does all of this mean in the context of physicians treating patients who have had a stroke from the neuroradiologist reading the acute stroke head CT or the neurointerventionalist performing an emergent large vessel thrombectomy? Clearly the health care landscape has radically changed. Today the consumer, payers, and providers of the health care product largely realize that we have finite resources, uneven quality, waste, and increasing costs for treating expanding pools of disease like stroke. There is near universal understanding that this requires payment models that optimize quality while minimizing waste.

Less apparent effects on cost in medicine are practice variations like heterogeneous imaging protocols and practices without a clear effect on outcome. For example, a retrospective analysis of Medicare fee-for-service claims for elderly patients who were admitted for hemorrhagic stroke with 1-year follow-up demonstrated no significant difference in mortality when correlated with intensity of CT imaging utilization per episode of care, adjusting for risk.[26] In addition, a higher rate of physician consults correlated with higher utilization of CT imaging for these patients; between institutions, there was variability in intensity of CT imaging use by up to 6-fold. Although morbidity was not a study variable, this variability in imaging utilization and physician consults between institutions without significant mortality difference raises serious concerns as to the benefit obtained from these medical interventions, not to mention the additional radiation dose and cost from CT imaging that these patients received.

Efforts like performance measures help measure quality objectively and benchmark care to evolving standards to reward those who deliver superior care while sometimes relatively penalizing those who fail. On a more basic level, although seemingly daunting, these constructs actually help shed light and improve transparency in an often-opaque health care delivery system and ultimately help cement the trust of the consumer and payers.

Other payment models like bundled payments hope to squeeze out inefficiency and increase quality by reducing care fragmentation and aligning the interests of the health care providers with payers and patients by sharing the risk and the attendant rewards. However, on a more granular level, the valuation of services of the various providers and their specialties and the mechanics of bundled care payments will be important questions to be answered as these models are applied in pilot programs.

REFERENCES

1. Gomez C. Time is brain. J Stroke Cerebrovasc Dis 1993;3:1–2.
2. Available at: https://georgewbushwhitehouse. archives.gov/news/releases/2006/08/20060822-2. html. Accessed September 7, 2018.
3. Feigin VL, Forouzanfar MH, Krishnamurthi R, et al. Global and regional burden of stroke during 1990–2010: findings from the Global Burden of Disease Study 2010. Lancet 2014;383:245–54.

4. Guilhaume C, Saragoussi D, Cochran J, et al. Modeling stroke management: a qualitative review of cost-effectiveness analyses. Eur J Health Econ 2010;11(4):419–26.

5. Collins TC, Petersen NJ, Menke TJ, et al. Short-term, intermediate-term, and long-term mortality in patients hospitalized for stroke. J Clin Epidemiol 2003;56(1):81–7.

6. National Health Expenditure Projections 2009-2019, The Centers for Medicare and Medicaid Services. Available at: https://www.cms.gov/NationalHealth ExpendData/downloads/proj2009.pdf. Accessed September 7, 2018.

7. D. Squires, Explaining High Health Care Spending in the United States: An International Comparison of Supply, Utilization, Prices, and Quality, The Commonwealth Fund, May 2012. Available at: https://www.commonwealthfund.org/publications/ issue-briefs/2012/may/explaining-high-health-care-spending-united-states-international.

8. OECD. 2018. Computed tomography (CT) exams (indicator). https://doi.org/10.1787/3c994537-en. Accessed February 11, 2018.

9. OECD. 2018. Magnetic resonance imaging (MRI) units (indicator). https://doi.org/10.1787/1a72e7d1-en. Accessed February 10, 2018.

10. OECD. 2018. Computed tomography (CT) scanners (indicator). https://doi.org/10.1787/bedece12-en. Accessed February 10, 2018.

11. Moon L, Moïse P, Jacobzone St, et al. "Stroke Care in OECD Countries: A Comparison of Treatment, Costs and Outcomes in 17 Countries," OECD Health Working Papers 5, OECD Publishing; 2003.

12. OECD Health Data: Health expenditure and financing: Health expenditure indicators." OECD Health Statistics (database). Available at: https://www.oecd-ilibrary.org/social-issues-migration-health/data/oecd-health-statistics_health-data-en.

13. Austin B, Frakt AB, Michael E, et al. The importance of relative prices in health care spending. JAMA 2018;319(5):441–2.

14. Institute of Medicine. Coverage matters: insurance and health care. Washington, DC: Institute of Medicine; 2001.

15. Bloom N, Eifert B, Mahajan A, et al. Does management matter? Evidence from India. National Bureau of Economic Research 2011. Available at: http://www.nber.org/papers/w16658.

16. Campbell SM, Reeves D, Kontopantelis E, et al. Effects of pay for performance on the quality of primary care in England. N Engl J Med 2009;361(4):368–78.

17. Peterson LA, Woodard LD, Urech T, et al. Does pay-for-performance improve the quality of health care? Ann Intern Med 2006;145(4):265–72.

18. Donabedian A. The quality of care. How can it be assessed? JAMA 1988;260(12):1743–8.

19. National Quality Forum. Neurology endorsement maintenance—phase I technical report. Available at: http://www.qualityforum.org/Publications/2012/12/Neurology_Endorsement_Maintenance_-_Phase_I_Technical_Report.aspx. Accessed September 7, 2018.

20. Available at: https://www.aan.com/siteassets/home-page/policy-and-guidelines/quality/quality-measures/15strokeandrehabmeasureset_pg.pdf. Accessed September 7, 2018.

21. Seidenwurm D, Lexa FJ. A radiologist's primer on bundles and care episodes. J Am Coll Radiol 2016;13(9):1029–31.

22. Available at: https://innovation.cms.gov/initiatives/bundled-payments/. Accessed September 7, 2018.

23. Albers GW, Marks MP, Kemp S. Thrombectomy for stroke at 6 to 16 hours with selection by perfusion imaging. N Engl J Med 2018. https://doi.org/10.1056/NEJMoa1713973.

24. Nogueira RG, Jadhav AP, Haussen DC, et al. Thrombectomy 6 to 24 hours after stroke with a mismatch between deficit and infarct. N Engl J Med 2018;378(1):11–21.

25. Latorre JGS, Flanagan S, Phipps MS, et al. Quality improvement in neurology: stroke and stroke rehabilitation quality measurement set update. Neurology 2017;89(15):1619–26.

26. Bekelis K, Fisher ES, Labropoulos N, et al. Variations in the intensive use of head CT for elderly patients with hemorrhagic stroke. Radiology 2015;275(1):188–95.

Health Care Organization for the Management of Stroke: The French Perspective

Jean-Pierre Pruvo, MD, PhD[a],*, Jerome Berge, MD[b],
Gregory Kuchcinski, MD[c], Martin Bretzner, MD[c],
Xavier Leclerc, MD, PhD[a], Lotfi Hacein-Bey, MD[d,e]

KEYWORDS

- Acute stroke • Mechanical thrombectomy • Neurointerventional units • Imaging-based triaging
- Telestroke • Simulation-based training • Interventionalist

KEY POINTS

- In Western Europe, the incidence of stroke is on the rise, expected to reach 3 million in the year 2035.
- The cost to society from the burden of disease and health care expenditures was €45 billion euros ($54 billion) in 2015 and growing.
- Effective treatments now exist, including thrombolysis and mechanical thrombectomy.
- Resulting challenges are on medical practice, including reliable triaging of patients; logistics, including fast patient transfer; and quality specialty training of interventionalists.
- Solutions considered by French medical and government leadership and comparisons to logistical solutions implemented in Germany are discussed.

INTRODUCTION

Stroke is a major pandemic, with an estimated annual worldwide 13 million events, most (9.5 million) consistent with ischemic strokes, resulting in more than 5 million fatalities.[1] Also worldwide, an estimated 18 million stroke survivors pose all kinds of major daily challenges to individuals, families, societies, and national health care systems.[2] Although humans are affected in similar ways throughout the world, differences in disease prevalence, culture, and health care systems account for significant variations in societal responses to the major challenges presented by stroke management. This article, after a brief review of the current status of stroke in Western Europe, discusses issues encountered by the medical—more specifically the neuroradiological—community in France in managing stroke and specific solutions, such as MR imaging–based triaging of patients, using a nationwide telestroke network, simulation-based training methods, and discussions on best possible interventionalist profiles.

Disclosure Statement: The authors have no disclosures to declare in relation with this article.
[a] Neuroradiology Department, Lille University Medical Center, Lille University, INSERM U1171, CHU Lille, Lille F-59000, France; [b] Interventional Neuroradiology, Radiology Department, Bordeaux University Medical Center, Bordeaux 33000, France; [c] Neuroradiology Department, Lille University Medical Center, CHU Lille, Lille F-59000, France; [d] Interventional Neuroradiology and Neuroradiology, Department of Medical Imaging, Sutter Health, Sacramento, CA 95815, USA; [e] Radiology Department, University of California Davis Medical School of Medicine, 4860 Y Street, Sacramento, CA 95817, USA
* Corresponding author. Neuroradiology, Radiology Department, Lille University Medical Center, Lille F-59000, France.
E-mail address: jppruvo@gmail.com

neuroimaging.theclinics.com

THE BURDEN OF DISEASE IN EUROPE

In developed countries, stroke constitutes one of the greatest health care problems, because it remains the third cause of death—the first cause of death in women—and, more importantly, the first cause of acquired disability.[3] Worse, the World Health Organization predicts an increase in the incidence of stroke in developed countries over the next 5 years.[4] Furthermore, more strokes are currently reported to occur in developed countries compared with developing countries, with lower mortality rates, resulting in comparatively more stroke survivors.[5]

A useful measure of the impact of stroke—or any large-scale disease—is the burden of disease, which can be thought of as the gap between actual and ideal health status of a society, the ideal situation being defined by the World Health Organization as the entire population living to an advanced age and free of disease or disability. The burden of disease is defined as the sum of disability-adjusted life-years (DALYs) across a population.[5,6] DALYs represent the sum of years lost from early death added to the sum of years lived with a disability and can be thought of as 1 lost year of healthy life.

In Western Europe, the number of years lived with disability due to ischemic stroke is steadily increasing.[5] Also in Western Europe, owing to the aging population, current estimates for 2035 suggest an annual incidence of stroke of 3 million and 4.6 million stroke survivors, significant increases in comparison to the 1.8 million strokes and 3.7 million survivors in 2015. The Global Burden of Disease Study 2016 report also predicts for future years a higher incidence of strokes in women and the highest growth in prevalence in Germany, Ukraine, Italy, and France.[2]

The economic burden of stroke for Europe was estimated in 2015 at approximately 45 billion euros ($54 Billion),[6,7] of which 44%, that is, €20 billion ($24 billion) were represented by direct health care costs.

CURRENT STATE OF STROKE TREATMENT IN EUROPE

Dreadful as it is, stroke no longer equates with certainty of death or major permanent disability previously meant for mankind. Effective treatments now exist, in the form of intravenous (IV) thrombolysis, mechanical thrombectomy, and—hopefully soon—various neuroprotective measures.

The European Cooperative Acute Stroke Study III (ECASS III) demonstrated the effectiveness of IV thrombolysis within 4.5 hours of stroke onset, and, for a decade now, IV tissue plasminogen activator (t-PA) has been established as standard of care.[8] More recently, several trials have also established the effectiveness of mechanical thrombectomy in acute ischemic stroke from large vessel occlusion (LVO), also now standard of care.[9–16] The average proportion of stroke patients that are eligible for mechanical thrombectomy (with LVO) is 10.4% (ranging between 4% and 17% in various studies).[13,17,18] The statistical probability of a good outcome is far superior for those patients compared with IV thrombolysis, with a number needed to treat as low as 2.6 for mechanical thrombectomy versus a number needed to treat ranging from 8 to 14 for IV t-PA alone (respectively, within the 0–3 hour and 0–4.5 hour time windows), meaning that for 2.6 treated patients, 1 will return to functional independency (defined as modified Rankin scale ≤2) within 3 months.[19]

Furthermore, in patients with LVO, the benefit of mechanical thrombectomy was shown to extend beyond the traditional 6-hour time window,[20,21] although within specific limitations of small infarct core size and large salvageable tissue volume (penumbra), requiring rigorous selection with advanced imaging—preferably MR imaging based—to establish eligibility for treatment.

For all patients, reperfusion must be achieved as quickly as possible. Factors consistently shown to have a significant impact time to reperfusion are (1) treatment in large-volume, specialized centers; (2) close control of workflow; and (3) aggressive time goals.[22] When patients must be transferred to a high-level (comprehensive) stroke center, which can provide mechanical thrombectomy, treatment is delayed by 100 minutes on average (275 minutes to reperfusion vs 179 minutes) with a resultant significantly lesser chance of a good outcome.[22]

In Europe and for the year 2016, of an estimated 192,614 strokes eligible for mechanical thrombectomy, only 25,576 patients (13%) were treated. Within Europe, Western European countries perform by far the largest numbers of mechanical thrombectomy procedures. Although this can be partly explained by the presence of a tight, long-established stroke network, effective reimbursement schedules to medical facilities for devices due to modern, up-to-date national health care systems are an important factor as well. Again, in 2016, of the 25,576 patients treated in Europe (28 countries in the European Union) with mechanical thrombectomy, a vast majority (41.5%) were treated in 2 countries, Germany (n = 6000) and France (n = 4589).

A comparison between France (population, 68 million) and Germany (population, 83 million) reveals similar percentages of stroke interventions for LVO in both countries, 3.8% in France versus 3.5% in Germany (**Table 1**). Germany, however, possesses many more stroke units globally (n = 279 vs 172), and 3 times as many comprehensive, thrombectomy-capable stroke centers compared with France (n = 114 vs 37) (see **Table 1**). France has 135 primary stroke centers (thrombolysis-capable only) and 37 comprehensive stroke centers, primarily large academic medical centers, in which thrombectomy procedures can be performed. In Germany, there are 162 primary stroke centers, which may drip and ship eligible patients with LVO to 107 comprehensive stroke centers; in addition, 10 telestroke units are present throughout Germany (see Table 1).[23]

A STRONG NATIONAL COMMITMENT TO STROKE TREATMENT

As in all countries, the medical community and the French government are strongly committed to "ensure equal access to health care for all patients throughout the nation."

It has been estimated that for each additional point in the National Institutes of Health Stroke Scale of patients, the total cost of health care increases by 15% over 5 years.[24] Consequently, even modest improvements in patient outcomes are cost effective at the scale of society. Studies in the United States have demonstrated cost effectiveness of mechanical thrombectomy for each quality-adjusted life year (QALY) gained, ranging between $9386 to $16,001. QALYs are

considered the current economic standard in health care assessment; in Europe, treatment is considered cost effective if its cost compared with standard or no therapy (QALY1-QALY0) is less than $50,000.[25-27] A study performed in the United Kingdom found the cost of a mechanical thrombectomy procedure of €3000 to €5000 ($3600–$6000) to be largely compensated for by gains in neurologic function; savings in hospital time, rehabilitation, and home care; and return to work, and estimated that for each treated patient, there was an average $11,651 in savings compared with untreated patients, indicating high cost-effectiveness.[28]

CHOICE OF MR IMAGING–BASED TRIAGING OF STROKE

There is a strong impetus in France in favor of MR imaging for the triaging of stroke patients. Most academic medical centers in France, and many community centers have 24/7 MR imaging coverage. New echo planar–based MR imaging protocols allow the reliable evaluation of acute ischemic stroke patients under 10 minutes. Recent improvements in MR imaging technique allow scan time shortening, including (1) reduction of phase field of view without aliasing, (2) partial k-space sampling allowing data acquisition shortening, and (3) multislice acquisition with signal-to-noise preservation (multiband technique). By combining these techniques in stroke evaluation, high-quality studies may be obtained with scan times under 6 minutes. An example of such protocols uses the following sequences: diffusion-weighted imaging (DWI) (40 s), T2* (1 min), fluid-attenuated inversion recovery (FLAIR) (2 min), and time-of-flight magnetic resonance angiography (MRA) (2 min). An optional 50-second gadolinium-based perfusion may be added in stroke patients seen within the 6-hour to 24-hour time window.[29-31]

DWI, the current gold standard for the detection of acute infarction, in particular small infarcts, multiple bilateral cardioembolic lesions, small cortical infarcts, posterior fossa ischemic lesions, and lacunar infarcts, maintains significant superiority over CT. CT also currently lacks accurate, validated threshold values to sort out infarction from penumbra.

- A major advantage of MR imaging compared with CT is superior accuracy in diagnosing stroke mimics, which have been reported to occur in as many as 38% of patients presenting to the emergency department with a presumptive diagnosis of stroke.[32] Common

Table 1
Comparative stroke management in France and Germany in 2016

	France	Germany
Population (millions)	68	83
Ischemic strokes/y	130,000	200,000
Mechanical thrombectomy procedures	4589 (3.8%)	6000 (3.5%)
Comprehensive stroke centers	37 (20%)	114 (40%)
Regional stroke units (drip and ship)	135	162
Telestroke units	—	10
Total number of stroke units	172	279

stroke mimics include seizures, demyelinating diseases, headaches, psychogenic disorders, brain tumors, and vertigo.[32]

- Major previous concern for missing or underdiagnosing cerebral hemorrhage is addressed by a 1-minute T2* sequence, which has high specificity in demonstrating hematomas.[33,34]
- In addition, T2* is superior to CT in showing microbleeds, the clinical significance of which remains debated. Charidimou and colleagues[35] found microbleeds in 17% of 790 acute stroke patients before IV t-PA. The presence of a small number of microbleeds should not constitute a contraindication to IV t-PA. Symptomatic hemorrhagic transformation was reported in 7.4% with microbleeds versus 4.4% without microbleeds.[35] If 10 or more microbleeds are present, however, the risk of hemorrhagic transformation increases steeply.[36]
- Also, the T2* sequence has demonstrated high specificity in showing offending intraarterial thrombi.[37–39] Furthermore, clot length may be accurately measured on T2* sequences.[40] Clot length is a predictive marker for success (if $\leq$8 mm) or failure of IV thrombolysis.[41]
- DWI-measured infarct core volume measurement is a major determinant of treatment decision making and the current gold standard. A core infarct target volume less than or equal to 70 mL highly correlates with positive outcomes with successful recanalization. Infarct volume greater than or equal to 100 mL suggests a high risk of hemorrhagic transformation, and volume greater than or equal to 145 mL may herald malignant edema.[42–44]
- Particularly important in the 6-hour to 24-hour window, the penumbra may be evaluated by the time-to-maximum (Tmax) function on perfusion imaging, which requires the use of gadolinium contrast. Arterial spin labeling may allow soon to evaluate tissue at risk without the use of contrast; however, current techniques are lengthy, especially on 1.5T scanners.[45]
- Several surrogate markers for penumbra volume have been described, some useful and practical. A patient's clinical status, that is, National Institutes of Health Stroke Scale greater than or equal to 8, correlates with a large penumbra.[46] The apparent diffusion coefficient volume has been suggested as a penumbral marker.[47] The MRA/DWI mismatch has been described as a predictor of response to recanalization.[48] Perhaps the most practical of those surrogate techniques is the FLAIR vascular hypersignal,[49] which merely represents stagnant flow in cortical vessels. The observation that patients with a mismatch DWI/FLAIR vascular hypersignal may have better outcomes[49] has led to the suggestion that FLAIR imaging may be an alternative to perfusion imaging.

Compared with MR imaging, CT is more readily available and more technically practical (Table 2). The only clinical parameter, however, for which CT may have superiority over MR imaging, is the evaluation of intracranial arteries, as summarized in Table 3.

The combination of an effective patient triaging system, a strong tradition in neurointerventional medicine, and the positive results of recent mechanical thrombectomy trials have resulted in an approximately 5-fold increase in the numbers of patients treated in France between 2014 and 2017, whereas the neurointerventional workforce has grown little during the same period (Table 4).

Although current official previsions in France are for 10,000 annual thrombectomy procedures in 2020, and 13,600 in 2025, if considering that 10% to 15% of 130,000 stroke patients per year in France are eligible for intervention, the number may soon amount to 15,000 patients/y, a 3-fold increase in procedural volume in comparison to 2017. Furthermore, actual numbers may be even higher, considering the extension of interventional time windows and a strong trend toward treating increasingly older patients.

Consequently, major additional challenges will soon be facing interventional neuroradiologists, the stroke community, and health care systems not only in France but also worldwide. The issue is compounded by the fact that almost half of stroke therapeutic interventions take place during nights and weekends, resulting in significant strain and even burnout on treating teams.

Table 2
Comparison of technical parameters of CT and MR imaging for stroke evaluation

Technical Parameter	CT	MR Imaging
Availability	Yes	Variable
Scan time	Fast	10 min
Imaging coverage	Limited	Whole brain
Artefacts	Rare	Frequent
Radiation exposure	12 mSv	No
Contraindications	Rare	Frequent

Table 3
Comparison of clinical parameters of CT and
MR imaging for stroke evaluation

Clinical Parameter	CT	MR Imaging
Hemorrhage	+	+
Stroke mimics	+	++
Infarct core	+	++
Posterior fossa	−	++
Lacunar infarct	−	++
Salvageable tissue	+	+
Intracranial vessels	++	+
Practical considerations	++	+

LOGISTICAL CHALLENGES AND SOLUTIONS

On a national level, the goal of the French government is to develop a stroke center–ready proximity network. Access to care for patients who live in rural areas remains a major issue. Major discussions are constantly taking place between medical societies and government officials to weigh the benefits of centralization as opposed to the opening of new centers in some parts of the country to extend coverage, with current plans to add 10 thrombectomy capable centers throughout France.

Prehospital triaging of patients has been steadily improving over the past few years in a consistent manner throughout the country.

Telestroke units are being actively developed. Telestroke allows to overcome the scarcity of resources in rural areas and community hospitals by the delivery of high-level expertise. In France, several regional telestroke systems have been developed in ways that have demonstrated safety and effectiveness.[50,51]

For example, in Northern France (Hauts-de-France), the authors developed in 2012 a rotational MR imaging–based telestroke network, which resulted in a significant and measurable increase in the rate of IV thrombolysis in emergency departments.[52] Furthermore, access to MR imaging for general neurologists combined to 24/7 availability

Table 4
Recent growth in mechanical thrombectomy
procedures in France

Year	Number of Mechanical Thrombecomies	Number of Neurointerventionalists
2014	1222	104
2015	2918	110
2016	4589	113
2017	5591	115

of specialized neuroradiologists led to an extremely low rate (<1%) of stroke mimics receiving IV t-PA.

Transport systems for fast patient transfer are constantly being improved, not only on the ground but also with the increasing use of helicopters in rural and underserved areas. Discussions are under way to decide whether to transfer patients by helicopter only to large-volume (≥500 patients/y) centers or to geographically closer, midlevel, thrombectomy-capable centers.

Currently, approximately 60% of stroke patients are admitted and managed in dedicated stroke units. Communication between physicians and hospital administrators are taking place at national and regional levels to improve subspecialty care of stroke patients.

Currently available evidence of cost effectiveness comes in support of obtaining the government's help on various levels. Coding schedules for procedures are constantly re-evaluated to help subsidize this effort. In addition, cost-benefit analyses are regularly undertaken by the medical leadership.

MANPOWER AND TRAINING CHALLENGES AND SOLUTIONS

Perhaps the most difficult challenge is to find ways to rapidly increase the workforce without sacrificing quality of care. Table 4 shows a modest increase in the number of trained neurointerventionalists in France between 2014 and 2017, whereas the number of stroke interventions increased 5-fold during the same time period. In 2017, each French neurointerventionalist performed on average 50 thrombectomy procedures (many more in centers that perform ≥500 annual procedures), twice the average number of procedures performed by their German colleagues. Although large numbers may yield higher levels of expertise to the benefit of patients, this constitutes a significant strain on physicians in an already thin-spread system, with resultant limited room left for growth.

Therefore, solutions are being considered by specialized societies involving various disciplines within radiology and neurology working with government officials.

- The obvious initial measure decided at a national level is to significantly increase the number of training positions in interventional neuroradiology over the next few years. Although this will definitely provide some breathing room for currently overburdened teams and will guarantee long-term quality manpower, particularly in major centers, the effect is expected to be neither immediate nor massive.

Table 5
Training pathway for stroke interventional management in Germany: De GIR/DGNR certification criteria with minimum required number of procedures

Curriculum	Indication Area	Number of Procedures for Level 2
DeGIR/DGNR	Vascular recanalization and reconstruction (non-neurovascular) (aorta, peripheral, hemodialysis shunts) (module A)	150
	Vascular embolization procedures (module B)	100
	Miscellaneous procedures including vascular foreign body removal, TIPSS, venous access (module C)	100
	Minimally invasive tumor therapy including tumor embolization, chemoembolization and SIRT (module D)	100
	Neurovascular revascularization including carotid and stroke (module E)	**100 (including at least 30 extracranial and at least 30 intracranial procedures)**
	Neurovascular embolization (aneurysms, malformations, AV fistula) (module F)	100 (including at least 50 intracranial procedures)

Abbreviations: SIRT, selective internal radiation therapy; TIPSS, transjugular intrahepatic portosystemic shunt.
From Landwehr P, Reimer P, Bücker A, et al. DeGIR-/DGNR training programme in interventional radiology and neuroradiology. Vasa 2017;46(6):494–5.

- Therefore, a novel interventionalist profile is also being evaluated by specialized societies: in hospitals with lower volumes of stroke patients and in rural/semirural areas, peripheral vascular interventional radiologists may be trained by selected experts to perform mechanical thrombectomy procedures in addition to their daily mission of treating peripheral vascular conditions. Such solution may show immediate positive effect, particularly in large geographic rural areas that benefit from the resources of affiliated, regional, major academic centers.
- Also, the German model of training is currently being evaluated by governing bodies. The German Society of Interventional Radiology and Minimally Invasive Therapy (DeGIR) and the German Society of Neuroradiology (DGNR)[53] organize the training as follows as:
  - Level 1: basic level general interventional radiology
  - Level 2: specialized training in interventional neuroradiology, with submodules A–F representing various specialties
  - Level 3: specialists who are credentialed to train levels 1 and 2 trainees

Modules E and F levels apply to neuroradiological procedures. Module E, which concerns certification in stroke and carotid intervention, requires the independent and successful performance of 100 procedures, to include at least 30 intracranial interventions (Table 5).

Innovative training methods, such as simulation-based programs, are popular throughout Europe[54–57] and currently widely implemented in France.[57] Simulation-based training relies on predefined simulated clinical scenarios presented to participants from various multidisciplinary backgrounds in a realistic environment. Communication and behavioral issues are then reviewed at debriefing, provided by facilitators, toward addressing clinical issues in the most effective manner possible.[56] Those training methods have been shown to impact positively physicians and staff knowledge, technical skills, motivation, and self-confidence levels.[54–57] When applied to emergency departments as part of a telestroke network in Northeastern France (Lorraine), simulation training models have shown measurable additional improvements in the process of IV thrombolysis delivery.[57]

SUMMARY

Although the burden of stroke on society is expected to grow, the good news is that in increasing numbers of patients, the damage from stroke can either be reversed or significantly reduced. Therefore, organized, expert, adapted, and thoughtful responses are necessary to effectively address the challenges posed on physicians, health care systems, and societies. In France, specific solutions have included a nationwide MR imaging–based telestroke network, simulation-based learning, and novel models of interventionalist profiles.

ACKNOWLEDGMENTS

The authors gratefully acknowledge the help of Pascale Dhôte-Burger, MD, Director, Office of Stroke and Neurologic disorders, French Ministry of Health, for providing statistical data and significant support.

REFERENCES

1. Available at: https://www.scopus.com/record/display. uri?eid=2-s2.0 84994158650&doi=10.1016%2fS014 0-6736%2816%2931012 1&origin=inward&txGid=ca 61fbe3130215718dc0858d423703ef.
2. Feigin VL, Roth GA, Naghavi M, et al. Global burden of stroke and risk factors in 188 countries, during 1990-2013: a systematic analysis for the Global Burden of Disease Study 2013. Lancet Neurol 2016;15(9):913–24.
3. Roger VL, Go AS, Lloyd-Jones DM, et al. Heart disease and stroke statistics—2012 update. Circulation 2012;125(1):e2–220.
4. Truelsen T, Piechowski-Jóźwiak B, Bonita R, et al. Stroke incidence and prevalence in Europe: a review of available data. Eur J Neurol 2006;13:581–98.
5. Feigin VL, Krishnamurthi RV, Parmar P, et al. Update on the global burden of ischemic and hemorrhagic stroke in 1990-2013: the GBD 2013 study. Neuroepidemiology 2015;45(3):161–76.
6. Available at: http://www.safestroke.eu/burden-of-stroke/.
7. Atlas Writing Group, Timmis A, Townsend N, Gale C, et al. European Society of Cardiology: cardiovascular disease statistics 2017. Eur Heart J 2018;39(7): 508–79.
8. Hacke W, Kaste M, Bluhmki E, et al. Thrombolysis with alteplase 3 to 4.5 hours after acute ischemic stroke. N Engl J Med 2008;359(13):1317–29.
9. Berkhemer OA, Fransen PS, Beumer D, et al. A randomized trial of intraarterial treatment for acute ischemic stroke. N Engl J Med 2015;372:11–20.
10. Goyal M, Demchuk AM, Menon BK, et al. Randomized assessment of rapid endovascular treatment of ischemic stroke. N Engl J Med 2015;372:1019–30.
11. Saver JL, Goyal M, Bonafe A, et al. Stent-retriever thrombectomy after intravenous t-PA vs. t-PA alone in stroke. N Engl J Med 2015;372:2285–95.
12. Campbell BC, Mitchell PJ, Kleinig TJ, et al. Endovascular therapy for ischemic stroke with perfusion-imaging selection. N Engl J Med 2015; 372:1009–18.
13. Jovin TG, Chamorro A, Cobo E, et al. Thrombectomy within 8 hours after symptom onset in ischemic stroke. N Engl J Med 2015;372:2296–306.
14. Mocco J, Zaidat OO, von Kummer R, et al. Aspiration thrombectomy after intravenous alteplase versus intravenous alteplase alone. Stroke 2016; 47(9):2331–8.
15. Bracard S, Ducrocq X, Mas JL, et al. Mechanical thrombectomy after intravenous alteplase versus alteplase alone after stroke (THRACE): a randomised controlled trial. Lancet Neurol 2016;15(11):1138–47.

16. Lapergue B, Blanc R, Gory B, et al. Effect of endovascular contact aspiration vs stent retriever on revascularization in patients with acute ischemic stroke and large vessel occlusion: the ASTER randomized clinical trial. JAMA 2017;318(5):443–52.
17. Campbell BCV, Donnan GA, Lees KR, et al. Endovascular stent thrombectomy: the new standard of care for large vessel ischaemic stroke. Lancet Neurol 2015;14(8):846–54.
18. Vanacker P, Lambrou D, Eskandari A, et al. Eligibility and predictors for acute revascularization procedures in a stroke center. Stroke 2016;47(7):1844–9.
19. Wahlgren N, Moreira T, Michel P, et al. Mechanical thrombectomy in acute ischemic stroke: consensus statement by ESO-karolinska stroke update 2014/ 2015, supported by ESO, ESMINT, ESNR and EAN. Int J Stroke 2016;11(1):134–47.
20. Nogueira RG, Jadhav AP, Haussen DC, et al. Thrombectomy 6 to 24 hours after stroke with a mismatch between deficit and infarct. N Engl J Med 2018; 378(1):11–21.
21. Albers GW, Marks MP, Kemp S, et al. Thrombectomy for stroke at 6 to 16 hours with selection by perfusion imaging. N Engl J Med 2018;378(8):708–18.
22. Goyal M, Jadhav AP, Bonafe A, et al. Analysis of workflow and time to treatment and the effects on outcome in endovascular treatment of acute ischemic stroke: results from the SWIFT PRIME randomized controlled trial. Radiology 2016;279(3): 888–97.
23. Available at: http://www.dsg-info.de/stroke-units/ stroke-units-uebersicht.html.
24. Luengo-Fernandez R, Yiin GS, Gray AM, et al. Population-based study of acute- and long-term care costs after stroke in patients with AF. Int J Stroke 2013;8:308–14.
25. Kim AS, Nguyen-Huynh M, Johnston SC. A cost-utility analysis of mechanical thrombectomy as an adjunct to intravenous tissue-type plasminogen activator for acute large-vessel ischemic stroke. Stroke 2011;42:2013–8.
26. Nguyen-Huynh MN, Johnston SC. Is mechanical clot removal or disruption a cost-effective treatment for acute stroke? AJNR Am J Neuroradiol 2011;32: 244–9.
27. Patil CG, Long EF, Lansberg MG. Cost-effectiveness analysis of mechanical thrombectomy in acute ischemic stroke. J Neurosurg 2009;110:508–13.
28. Ganesalingam J, Pizzo E, Morris S, et al. Cost-utility analysis of mechanical thrombectomy using stent retrievers in acute ischemic stroke. Stroke 2015; 46(9):2591–8.
29. Tisserand M, Naggara O, Legrand L, et al. Patient "candidate" for thrombolysis: MRI is essential. Diagn Interv Imaging 2014;95(12):1135–44.
30. Nael K, Khan R, Choudhary G, et al. Six-minute magnetic resonance imaging protocol for evaluation

of acute ischemic stroke: pushing the boundaries. Stroke 2014;45(7):1985–91.

31. Benzakoun J, Maïer B, Calvet D, et al. Can a 15-sec FLAIR replace conventional FLAIR sequence in stroke MR protocols? J Neuroradiol 2017;44(3): 192–7.

32. Quenardelle V, Lauer-Ober V, Zinchenko I, et al. Stroke mimics in a stroke care pathway based on MRI screening. Cerebrovasc Dis 2016;42(3–4): 205–12.

33. Brazzelli M, Sandercock PA, Chappell FM, et al. Magnetic resonance imaging versus computed tomography for detection of acute vascular lesions in patients presenting with stroke symptoms. Cochrane Database Syst Rev 2009;(4):CD007424.

34. Oppenheim C, Touzé E, Hernalsteen D, et al. Comparison of five MR sequences for the detection of acute intracranial hemorrhage. Cerebrovasc Dis 2005;20(5):388–94.

35. Charidimou A, Gang Q, Werring DJ. Sporadic cerebral amyloid angiopathy revisited: recent insights into pathophysiology and clinical spectrum. J Neurol Neurosurg Psychiatry 2012;83(2):124–37.

36. Shoamanesh A, Kwok CS, Lim PA, et al. Postthrombolysis intracranial hemorrhage risk of cerebral microbleeds in acute stroke patients: a systematic review and meta-analysis. Int J Stroke 2013;8(5): 348–56.

37. Rovira A, Orellana P, Alvarez-Sabín J, et al. Hyperacute ischemic stroke: middle cerebral artery susceptibility sign at echo-planar gradient-echo MR imaging. Radiology 2004;232(2):466–73.

38. Liebeskind DS, Sanossian N, Yong WH, et al. CT and MRI early vessel signs reflect clot composition in acute stroke. Stroke 2011;42(5):1237–43.

39. Kimura K, Iguchi Y, Shibazaki K, et al. The presence of a right-to-left shunt is associated with dramatic improvement after thrombolytic therapy in patients with acute ischemic stroke. Stroke 2009;40(1):303–5.

40. Naggara O, Raymond J, Domingo Ayllon M, et al. T2* "susceptibility vessel sign" demonstrates clot location and length in acute ischemic stroke. PLoS One 2013;8(10):e76727.

41. Riedel CH, Zimmermann P, Jensen-Kondering U, et al. The importance of size: successful recanalization by intravenous thrombolysis in acute anterior stroke depends on thrombus length. Stroke 2011; 42(6):1775–7.

42. Davis SM, Donnan GA, Parsons MW, et al. Effects of alteplase beyond 3 h after stroke in the Echoplanar Imaging Thrombolytic Evaluation Trial (EPITHET): a placebo-controlled randomised trial. Lancet Neurol 2008;7(4):299–309.

43. Oppenheim C, Samson Y, Manaï R, et al. Prediction of malignant middle cerebral artery infarction by diffusion-weighted imaging. Stroke 2000;31(9): 2175–81.

44. Lansberg MG, Straka M, Kemp S, et al. MRI profile and response to endovascular reperfusion after stroke (DEFUSE 2): a prospective cohort study. Lancet Neurol 2012;11(10):860–7.

45. Bivard A, Krishnamurthy V, Stanwell P, et al. Arterial spin labeling versus bolus-tracking perfusion in hyperacute stroke. Stroke 2014;45(1):127–33.

46. Dávalos A, Blanco M, Pedraza S, et al. The clinical-DWI mismatch: a new diagnostic approach to the brain tissue at risk of infarction. Neurology 2004; 62(12):2187–92.

47. Drier A, Tourdias T, Attal Y, et al. Prediction of subacute infarct size in acute middle cerebral artery stroke: comparison of perfusion-weighted imaging and apparent diffusion coefficient maps. Radiology 2012;265(2):511–7.

48. Lansberg MG, Thijs VN, Bammer R, et al. The MRA-DWI mismatch identifies patients with stroke who are likely to benefit from reperfusion. Stroke 2008;39(9): 2491–6.

49. Legrand L, Tisserand M, Turc G, et al. Do FLAIR vascular hyperintensities beyond the DWI lesion represent the ischemic penumbra? AJNR Am J Neuroradiol 2015;36(2):269–74.

50. Legris N, Hervieu-Bègue M, Daubail B, et al. Telemedicine for the acute management of stroke in Burgundy, France: an evaluation of effectiveness and safety. Eur J Neurol 2016;23(9):1433–40.

51. Richard S, Lavandier K, Zioueche Y, et al. Use of telemedicine to manage severe ischaemic strokes in a rural area with an elderly population. Neurol Sci 2014;35(5):683–5.

52. Dequatre-Ponchelle N, Touzani H, Banh A, et al. Rate of intravenous thrombolysis for acute ischaemic stroke in the North-of-France region and evolution over time. J Neurol 2014;261(7):1320–8.

53. Landwehr P, Reimer P, Bücker A, et al. DeGIR-/DGNR training programme in interventional radiology and neuroradiology. Vasa 2017;46(6): 494–5.

54. Ross AJ, Reedy GB, Roots A, et al. Evaluating multi-site multiprofessional simulation training for a hyperacute stroke service using the Behaviour Change Wheel. BMC Med Educ 2015;15:143.

55. Tahtali D, Bohmann F, Kurka N, et al. Implementation of stroke teams and simulation training shortened process times in a regional stroke network-A network-wide prospective trial. PLoS One 2017; 12(12):e0188231.

56. Rudolph JW, Simon R, Rivard P, et al. Debriefing with good judgment: combining rigorous feedback with genuine inquiry. Anesthesiol Clin 2007;25(2): 361–76.

57. Richard S, Mione G, Varoqui C, et al. Simulation training for emergency teams to manage acute ischemic stroke by telemedicine. Medicine (Baltimore) 2016;95(24):e3924.

Statement of Ownership, Management, and Circulation
UNITED STATES POSTAL SERVICE® (All Periodicals Publications Except Requester Publications)

1. Publication Title	2. Publication Number	3. Filing Date
NEUROIMAGING CLINICS OF NORTH AMERICA	010 – 548	9/18/2018

4. Issue Frequency	5. Number of Issues Published Annually	6. Annual Subscription Price
FEB, MAY, AUG, NOV	4	$387.00

7. Complete Mailing Address of Known Office of Publication (Not printer) (Street, city, county, state, and ZIP+4®)

ELSEVIER INC.
230 Park Avenue, Suite 800
New York, NY 10169

Contact Person
STEPHEN R. BUSHING

Telephone (Include area code)
215-239-3688

8. Complete Mailing Address of Headquarters or General Business Office of Publisher (Not printer)

ELSEVIER INC.
230 Park Avenue, Suite 800
New York, NY 10169

9. Full Names and Complete Mailing Addresses of Publisher, Editor, and Managing Editor (Do not leave blank)

Publisher (Name and complete mailing address)

TAYLOR E BALL, ELSEVIER INC.
1600 JOHN F KENNEDY BLVD. SUITE 1800
PHILADELPHIA, PA 19103-2899

Editor (Name and complete mailing address)

JOHN VASSALLO, ELSEVIER INC.
1600 JOHN F KENNEDY BLVD. SUITE 1800
PHILADELPHIA, PA 19103-2899

Managing Editor (Name and complete mailing address)

PATRICK MANLEY ELSEVIER INC.
1600 JOHN F KENNEDY BLVD. SUITE 1800
PHILADELPHIA, PA 19103-2899

10. Owner (Do not leave blank. If the publication is owned by a corporation, give the name and address of the corporation immediately followed by the names and addresses of all stockholders owning or holding 1 percent or more of the total amount of stock. If not owned by a corporation, give the names and addresses of the individual owners. If owned by a partnership or other unincorporated firm, give its name and address as well as those of each individual owner. If the publication is published by a nonprofit organization, give its name and address.)

Full Name	Complete Mailing Address
WHOLLY OWNED SUBSIDIARY OF REED/ELSEVIER, US HOLDINGS	1600 JOHN F KENNEDY BLVD. SUITE 1800 PHILADELPHIA, PA 19103-2899

11. Known Bondholders, Mortgagees, and Other Security Holders Owning or Holding 1 Percent or More of Total Amount of Bonds, Mortgages, or Other Securities. If none, check box ▶ ☐ None

Full Name	Complete Mailing Address
N/A	

12. Tax Status (For completion by nonprofit organizations authorized to mail at nonprofit rates) (Check one)
The purpose, function, and nonprofit status of this organization and the exempt status for federal income tax purposes:
☒ Has Not Changed During Preceding 12 Months
☐ Has Changed During Preceding 12 Months (Publisher must submit explanation of change with this statement)

PS Form **3526**, July 2014 [Page 1 of 4 (see instructions page 4)] PSN 7530-01-000-9631   PRIVACY NOTICE: See our privacy policy on www.usps.com.

---

13. Publication Title	14. Issue Date for Circulation Data Below
NEUROIMAGING CLINICS OF NORTH AMERICA	MAY 2018

15. Extent and Nature of Circulation			Average No. Copies Each Issue During Preceding 12 Months	No. Copies of Single Issue Published Nearest to Filing Date
a. Total Number of Copies (Net press run)			328	483
b. Paid Circulation (By Mail and Outside the Mail)	(1)	Mailed Outside-County Paid Subscriptions Stated on PS Form 3541 (Include paid distribution above nominal rate, advertiser's proof copies, and exchange copies)	236	330
	(2)	Mailed In-County Paid Subscriptions Stated on PS Form 3541 (Include paid distribution above nominal rate, advertiser's proof copies, and exchange copies)	0	0
	(3)	Paid Distribution Outside the Mails Including Sales Through Dealers and Carriers, Street Vendors, Counter Sales, and Other Paid Distribution Outside USPS®	45	73
	(4)	Paid Distribution by Other Classes of Mail Through the USPS (e.g., First-Class Mail®)	0	0
c. Total Paid Distribution (Sum of 15b (1), (2), (3), and (4))		▶	281	403
d. Free or Nominal Rate Distribution (By Mail and Outside the Mail)	(1)	Free or Nominal Rate Outside-County Copies included on PS Form 3541	37	64
	(2)	Free or Nominal Rate In-County Copies Included on PS Form 3541	0	0
	(3)	Free or Nominal Rate Copies Mailed at Other Classes Through the USPS (e.g., First-Class Mail)	0	0
	(4)	Free or Nominal Rate Distribution Outside the Mail (Carriers or other means)	0	0
e. Total Free or Nominal Rate Distribution (Sum of 15d (1), (2), (3) and (4))		▶	37	64
f. Total Distribution (Sum of 15c and 15e)		▶	318	467
g. Copies not Distributed (See instructions to Publishers #4 (page #3))		▶	10	16
h. Total (Sum of 15f and g)		▶	328	483
i. Percent Paid (15c divided by 15f times 100)		▶	88.36%	86.30%

* If you are claiming electronic copies, go to line 16 on page 3. If you are not claiming electronic copies, skip to line 17 on page 3.

16. Electronic Copy Circulation		Average No. Copies Each Issue During Preceding 12 Months	No. Copies of Single Issue Published Nearest to Filing Date
a. Paid Electronic Copies	▶	0	0
b. Total Paid Print Copies (Line 15c) + Paid Electronic Copies (Line 16a)	▶	281	403
c. Total Print Distribution (Line 15f) + Paid Electronic Copies (Line 16a)	▶	318	467
d. Percent Paid (Both Print & Electronic Copies) (16b divided by 16c × 100)	▶	88.36%	86.3%

☒ I certify that 50% of all my distributed copies (electronic and print) are paid above a nominal price.

17. Publication of Statement of Ownership

☒ If the publication is a general publication, publication of this statement is required. Will be printed
in the NOVEMBER 2018 issue of this publication.   ☐ Publication not required

18. Signature and Title of Editor, Publisher, Business Manager, or Owner

STEPHEN R. BUSHING - INVENTORY DISTRIBUTION CONTROL MANAGER   *Stephen R. Bushing*   Date 9/18/2018

I certify that all information furnished on this form is true and complete. I understand that anyone who furnishes false or misleading information on this form or who omits material or information requested on the form may be subject to criminal sanctions (including fines and imprisonment) and/or civil sanctions (including civil penalties).

PS Form **3526**, July 2014 (Page 3 of 4)   PRIVACY NOTICE: See our privacy policy on www.usps.com

Moving?

Make sure your subscription moves with you!

To notify us of your new address, find your **Clinics Account Number** (located on your mailing label above your name), and contact customer service at:

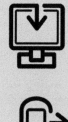

Email: journalscustomerservice-usa@elsevier.com

800-654-2452 (subscribers in the U.S. & Canada)
314-447-8871 (subscribers outside of the U.S. & Canada)

Fax number: 314-447-8029

Elsevier Health Sciences Division
Subscription Customer Service
3251 Riverport Lane
Maryland Heights, MO 63043

*To ensure uninterrupted delivery of your subscription, please notify us at least 4 weeks in advance of move.

Printed and bound by CPI Group (UK) Ltd, Croydon, CR0 4YY

03/10/2024

01040385-0011